Biodegradable Polymeric Nanocomposites

Advances in Biomedical Applications

Biodegradable Polymeric Nanocomposites

Advances in Biomedical Applications

Edited by Dilip Depan

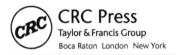

CRC Press
Taylor & Francis Group
Boca Raton London New York

CRC Press is an imprint of the
Taylor & Francis Group, an **informa** business

CRC Press
Taylor & Francis Group
6000 Broken Sound Parkway NW, Suite 300
Boca Raton, FL 33487-2742

First issued in paperback 2021

© 2016 by Taylor & Francis Group, LLC
CRC Press is an imprint of Taylor & Francis Group, an Informa business

No claim to original U.S. Government works

ISBN 13: 978-0-367-78338-9 (pbk)
ISBN 13: 978-1-4822-6051-9 (hbk)

Visit the Taylor & Francis Web site at
http://www.taylorandfrancis.com

and the CRC Press Web site at
http://www.crcpress.com

Contents

Chapter 8   Curcumin-Loaded Polymeric Nanoparticle: A Promising Route

*Chinmayee Saikia, Mandip Sarmah, Monoj K. Das,
Anand Ramteke, and Tarun K. Maji*

Chapter 9   Plastics of the Future: Innovations for Improvement and

Vinod Pravin Sharma

Nazire Deniz Yılmaz

Preface

Biomaterials based on polymers are of prime importance and are a cornerstone for biomedical applications. Biomaterials are primarily supposed to perform a time-limited architectural or a related function but, being foreign, should disappear from the body once that function has been fulfilled. A wide range of materials have been considered for biomedical applications such as drug delivery, biosensors, and tissue engineering.

Biodegradable polymers are a unique category of materials that opened up an entirely novel concept in the biomedical industry, with research more focused on the development of more sophisticated biomedical applications to solve patients' problems. The involvement of nanotechnology has further helped in making some significant advancements in this field. An overview of degradation properties and mechanism of biodegradable polymers, focusing on relevant aspects of biomedical applications, is provided in this book.

Efforts have been made to not only focus on biomaterials but also give priority to the general topics on successful designing and applications of biomaterials. So, the book presents the unique advantages and limitations of various biomaterials, such as biopolymers, ceramics, biodegradable nanocomposites, and natural products–based biomaterials. The book also deals with the state-of-the-art recent advancements in drug delivery devices.

I thank all contributors for their efforts on writing comprehensive chapters. I extend my sincere thanks to all the readers of the book and look forward to receiving comments and feedback.

Dilip Depan, PhD
Chemical Engineering Department
University of Louisiana at Lafayette
Lafayette, Louisiana

Editor

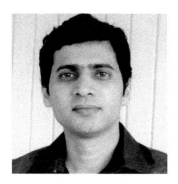

Dr. Dilip Depan is a research scientist in the Chemical Engineering Department at the University of Louisiana at Lafayette, Louisiana. He earned his PhD from the National Chemical Laboratory, Pune, India, in 2009. He has taught undergraduate courses in materials and biomaterials, and in laboratories, from 2010 at the University of Louisiana at Lafayette. Dr. Depan has an extensive research background in the modification and characterization of biomaterial surface for various biomedical applications. His recent research is focused on bone–biomaterial interaction, tissue engineering 3-D scaffolds, dental materials, nanomedicine, and engineering education.

Contributors

Diego Arce
Department of Mechanical
   Engineering
Pontifical Catholic University
   of Peru
Lima, Peru

Andreea Irina Barzic
Department of Physical Chemistry of
   Polymers
"Petru Poni" Institute of
   Macromolecular Chemistry
Iasi, Romania

Monoj K. Das
Department of Molecular Biology and
   Biotechnology
Tezpur University
Assam, India

Kishore Debnath
Department of Mechanical and
   Industrial Engineering
Indian Institute of Technology,
   Roorkee
Uttarakhand, India

Sergey V. Dorozhkin
Moscow, Russia

Silvia Ioan
Department of Physical Chemistry of
   Polymers
"Petru Poni" Institute of
   Macromolecular Chemistry
Iasi, Romania

Tarun K. Maji
Department of Chemical Sciences
Tezpur University
Assam, India

Bogdănel S. Munteanu
Faculty of Physics
"Al. I. Cuza" University
Iasi, Romania

Elena Pâslaru (Stoleru)
Department of Physical Chemistry of
   Polymers
"P. Poni" Institute of Macromolecular
   Chemistry
Iasi, Romania

Anand Ramteke
Department of Molecular Biology and
   Biotechnology
Tezpur University
Assam, India

Mehdi Sadat-Shojai
Department of Chemistry
College of Sciences
Shiraz University
Shiraz, Iran

Chinmayee Saikia
Department of Chemical Sciences
Tezpur University
Assam, India

Mandip Sarmah
Department of Chemical Sciences
Tezpur University
Assam, India

Vinod Pravin Sharma
CSIR-Indian Institute of Toxicology
   Research
Uttar Pradesh, India

Inderdeep Singh
Department of Mechanical and
   Industrial Engineering
Indian Institute of Technology, Roorkee
Uttarakhand, India

Fernando G. Torres
Department of Mechanical Engineering
Pontifical Catholic University of Peru
Lima, Peru

Cornelia Vasile
Department of Physical Chemistry of
    Polymers
"P. Poni" Institute of Macromolecular
    Chemistry
Iasi, Romania

Congming Xiao
College of Materials Science and
    Engineering
Huaqiao University
Quanzhou, Fujian, People's Republic of
    China

Nazire Deniz Yilmaz
Department of Textile Engineering
Pamukkale University
Denizli, Turkey

1 Calcium Phosphate–Reinforced Polyester Nanocomposites for Bone Regeneration Applications

Mehdi Sadat-Shojai

CONTENTS

1.1 INTRODUCTION

Defects that result in the need for bone tissue replacement pose a major clinical problem in orthopedic surgery. To restore the function of damaged or diseased bone tissue, bone replacement grafts have conventionally been used. These bone grafts are usually derived from tissues harvested from a second anatomic location of the same patient (autografts) or from other patients (allografts) [1–4]. The use of donor tissue, however, suffers from several limitations, including donor site morbidity, occurrence of immune-related problems in the recipient's body, difficulties in shaping explanted bone, limited supplies of suitable bone grafts, risk of disease transmission, and lessening or even complete loss of bone inductive factors. Additionally, both autografting and allografting require a second surgery site, which is expensive and sometimes associated with hematoma formation [2,3,5].

In the past two decades, various man-made biomaterials have offered a promising alternative approach to bone treatment. These biomaterials must be biocompatible and meet certain minimum mechanical requirements to be functional. On the other hand, techniques for bone regeneration based on tissue engineering have also been proven to be very effective [4–7]. By taking advantage of the body's natural regenerative capacity to form new bone, tissue engineering has progressed in the last two decades to become a powerful alternative for treatment of damaged bone tissues. The basic concept of tissue engineering techniques is schematically illustrated in Figure 1.1.

According to Figure 1.1, tissue engineering applies principles and methods from engineering, biology, and medicine to create constructs for regeneration of new tissues. Tissue engineering is now frequently used in conjunction with the more encompassing descriptor of regenerative medicine [3,8–10]. The aim of regenerative medicine is to recreate tissues and organs typically using a combination of cells, scaffolds, and bioactive molecules. One common approach in regenerative medicine is to isolate specific cells through a small biopsy from a patient to grow them on a 3D scaffold under controlled culture conditions. The construct is subsequently delivered to the desired site in the patient's body with the aim to direct new tissue formation into the scaffold. The scaffold must have the ability to undergo a progressive degradation as the new tissue regenerates. An alternative approach is to implant scaffolds for tissue ingrowth directly in vivo with the purpose to stimulate and direct tissue formation in situ [8].

In many cases of bone tissue engineering, development of biodegradable materials with appropriate mechanical properties, suitable degradation rate, and high osteoconductivity is desirable. Indeed, biodegradable materials, which can be resorbed in the human body fluids, are always excellent candidates to serve as scaffolding materials [11,12]. Today, these materials are usually biodegradable polymers, both natural and synthetic, such as polysaccharides, polyesters, and hydrogels [7,8].

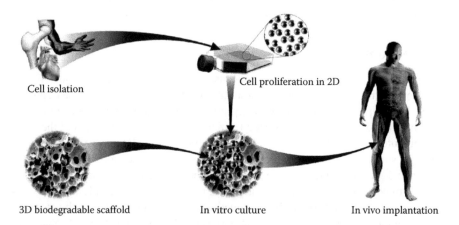

Cell isolation

Cell proliferation in 2D

3D biodegradable scaffold   In vitro culture   In vivo implantation

FIGURE 1.1 Basic principles of tissue engineering approach. Cells are first isolated and then expanded in a tissue-culture flask. Once 2D cell proliferation sufficiently occurs, they can be placed in a 3D scaffold and cultured in vitro in a bioreactor or incubator. When the engineered scaffold is matured enough, then it can be implanted in the area of defect.

Other important categories of systems are bioactive materials, mainly calcium phosphate (CaP) ceramics and bioactive glasses or glass–ceramic combinations [12–15]. However, as demonstrated by the increasing research efforts, polymer/ceramic composite systems combining the advantages of polymers and ceramics seem to be a more promising choice to fulfill many requirements of an ideal scaffold, in particular, for bone tissue engineering. Currently, various polymers and bioactive ceramics are being combined in a variety of composite systems with the aim to increase the mechanical stability of scaffold and to improve tissue–scaffold interaction [6–9].

It is obvious that the requirements of composite materials for bone tissue engineering are manifold and challenging: biocompatibility of the composite is definitely necessary; that is, the material must not elicit an unresolved inflammatory response nor demonstrate immunogenicity or cytotoxicity. The composite material should also have a suitable biodegradability at a rate commensurate with the rate of bone tissue formation. In addition, its mechanical properties must be sufficient so that the scaffold does not collapse or break during the patient's normal activities. The composite materials should also have the ability to support cell adhesion, migration, proliferation, and differentiated function [6–8,11]. As soon as a suitable composite material is selected, the next step is to fabricate a 3D scaffold. A certain minimum requirement for a 3D scaffold construct, particularly in bone tissue engineering, is a controllable interconnected porosity with a multiple pore size distribution to direct the cells to grow into the desired physical form, to facilitate diffusion of nutrients and gases, and finally to support vascularization of the ingrown tissue [8,11]. Moreover, it is desirable if the fabricated scaffold truly mimics the natural extracellular matrix (ECM) in terms of physiological functions [10,12]. Another highly desirable feature concerning the processing of bone scaffold is scalability for cost-effective industrial production [8].

Although diverse bone scaffold constructs have been developed, most of them differ substantially from natural bone either compositionally or structurally. At the lowest structural level, human bones are a natural nanocomposite consisting nano-sized CaP crystals embedded in a collagen-rich organic matrix [12,16]. Therefore, considering the bone as the biological template, nanocomposite systems comprising CaP bioceramics, especially hydroxyapatite (HAp) and tricalcium phosphate (TCP), and synthetic biodegradable polymers, especially polyesters, have attracted great attention worldwide from both academic and industrial points of view [7–9]. These nanocomposite systems can effectively combine the ductility and processability of polyester matrices and bioactivity and the osteoconductivity of CaP nanoparticles. The most widely used polyester matrices include poly(lactic acid) (PLA), poly(lactic-co-glycolic acid) (PLGA), poly(ε-caprolactone) (PCL), polyhydroxyalkanoates (PHAs), and their blends. Up to now, various combinations of synthetic polyesters and CaP nanoparticles have been developed and proved to be bioresorbable with excellent processability, bioactivity, and mechanical properties [8,9]. Accordingly, this chapter focuses on the state of the art of CaP-reinforced polyester nanocomposites for regenerative medicine and tissue engineering applications. In this chapter, we will try to provide an outline of current research on the CaP nanoparticles in the direction of nanocomposite preparation and to discuss the variety of biodegradable polyesters that have been used as orthopedic materials. Moreover, biological and mechanical characteristics of different CaP/polyester combinations, along with their degradation features with focus on bone regeneration, will be discussed and compared. This chapter is expected to be a useful reference for specialists and advanced students to gain an insight on CaP-reinforced nanocomposites with application to bone tissue engineering.

1.2   BONE AS A NANOCOMPOSITE

The design strategy of an ideal composite bone scaffold may not be straightforward without understanding the fundamentals of bone composition and architecture. As shown in Figure 1.2, humane bone can be considered a true anisotropic nanocomposite at the nanoscale level, consisting of biominerals embedded in a protein matrix, other organic materials, and water.

The biomineral phase, which is one or more types of CaPs, comprises 65%–70% of bone, water accounts for 5%–8%, and the organic phase, which is mainly in the form of collagen fibers along with a low amount of non-collagenous proteins and lipids, accounts for the remaining portion [16,17]. The collagen matrix as a structural framework gives the bone its elastic resistance and acts as a template for deposition and growth of tiny plate-like CaP minerals. Among several possibilities of CaPs, HAp has been demonstrated to possess the most similarity to these tiny biominerals [17,18]. In fact, naturally occurring CaP is usually carbonated and calcium-deficient HAp with a Ca/P ratio of less than 1.67. The bone HAp is also enriched with some trace elements (e.g., sodium, potassium, magnesium, chloride, and fluoride) for various metabolic functions [19]. Therefore, bone not only supports and protects the organs of the body but also serves as a reservoir of diverse minerals. Bone is also a good example of a renewable tissue since it has the capability of self-repairing to a certain extent [19]. Considering the natural bone as an archetype, various 3D biomaterials have been developed up to now. While less complex, the structure of these systems is usually similar to that of natural bone. Such composite materials in combination with cells and bioactive agents have also been shown to be a promising candidate as scaffolding material in bone tissue engineering.

1.3   WHY BIOACTIVE CALCIUM PHOSPHATES?

For decades, CaP ceramics have been of interest owing to their excellent biocompatibility, affinity to biopolymers, ability to replace toxic ions, and high osteogenic potential [16]. It has been well documented that CaP ceramics can promote new bone ingrowth through osteoconduction mechanism without causing any local or systemic toxicity, inflammation, or foreign body response [16,20,21]. When a CaP-based ceramic is implanted, a fibrous tissue-free layer containing biological carbonated apatite forms on its surfaces and contributes to the chemical bonding of the implant to the host bone, resulting in earlier implant stabilization and superior fixation of the implant to the surrounding tissues. This carbonated apatite that forms on the implant is chemically and structurally similar to the minerals found in human bone [8,16]. The in vivo bone-bonding behavior of CaP ceramics, which is referred to as bioactivity, can also be reproduced in contact with biological fluids, especially

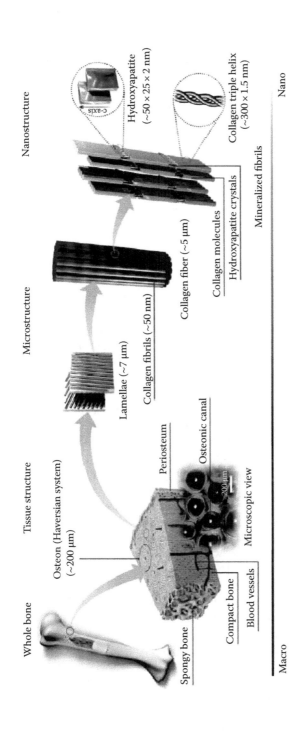

FIGURE 1.2 The hierarchical structure of typical bone at various length scales. The microstructure of cortical or compact bone consists of Haversian systems (circles in cross section and microscopic view) with osteonic canals and lamellae, and at the nanoscale, the structural framework is collagen fibers composed of bundles of mineralized collagen fibrils. (Reprinted from Sadat-Shojai, M. et al., *Acta Biomater.*, 9, 7591, 2013. With permission.)

TABLE 1.1

Ion Concentrations in a Typical Supersaturated SBF Solution and in the Human Blood Plasma

Ion	Ion Concentrations (mM)	
	Blood Plasma	SBF
Na^+	142.0	142.0
K^+	5.0	5.0
Mg^{2+}	1.5	1.5
Ca^{2+}	2.5	2.5
Cl^-	103.0	147.8
HCO_3^-	27.0	4.2
HPO_4^{2-}	1.0	1.0
SO_4^{2-}	0.5	0.5
pH	7.40	7.40

Source: Reprinted from Sadat-Shojai, M. et al., *J. Cryst. Growth.*, 361, 73, 2012. With permission.

simulated body fluid (SBF) with an ion concentration nearly equal to that of human blood plasma [8,22]. Table 1.1 represents the ionic composition of a typical SBF solution and compares it with that of human plasma. Currently, CaP is commonly the material of choice for various biomedical applications, for example, as a replacement for bony and periodontal defects, alveolar ridge, middle ear implants, tissue engineering systems, drug-delivery agent, dental materials, and bioactive coating on metallic osseous implants [16]. The general importance of CaP ceramics has also led to numerous nonmedical industrial applications, for example, as a catalyst for chemical reactions, host materials for lasers, ion conductors, and gas sensors [16].

As a result of the bone-like apatite-forming ability, addition of CaP particles into a polymeric phase should potentially have the dual effect of improving the bioactivity and mechanical properties of the resulting system. The significant increase in bioactivity of polymeric matrix with the addition of CaP particles has been demonstrated in a vast number of studies both in vitro and in vivo (see Section 1.5.1). Table 1.2 shows the most important CaP phases, which usually appear as trace impurities during the synthesis of a specific phase [16]. Among the various CaP structures, nanosized HAp, also known as HAp nanoparticles, with appropriate stoichiometry, morphology, and purity, has stimulated the most interest in various biomedical applications. Nanosized HAp, which has a grain size less than 100 nm in at least one direction, has high surface activity and an ultrafine structure similar to the mineral found in hard tissues [16]. Therefore, incorporation of nanosized HAp into the polymer matrix is assumed to mimic the structure of natural bone. It is well-known that bioceramics that mimic the bone mineral in composition and structure can more readily promote osteointegration and subsequent bone tissue formation. In other words, as the biological HAps found in physiological hard tissues are nanoscopic plate-like crystals that are a few nanometers in thickness and tens of nanometers in length, it is believed

TABLE 1.2
Main Calcium Phosphate (CaP) Salts

Name	Symbol(s)	Formula	Ca/P
Monocalcium phosphate monohydrate	MCPM and MCPH	$Ca(H_2PO_4)_2 \cdot H_2O$	0.5
Monocalcium phosphate anhydrous	MCPA and MCP	$Ca(H_2PO_4)_2$	0.5
Dicalcium phosphate dihydrate (Brushite)	DCPD	$CaHPO_4 \cdot 2H_2O$	1.0
Dicalcium phosphate anhydrous (Monetite)	DCPA and DCP	$CaHPO_4$	1.0
Octacalcium phosphate	OCP	$Ca_8(HPO_4)_2(PO_4)_4 \cdot 5H_2O$	1.33
α-Tricalcium phosphate	α-TCP	$Ca_3(PO_4)_2$	1.5
β-Tricalcium phosphate	β-TCP	$Ca_3(PO_4)_2$	1.5
Amorphous calcium phosphate	ACP	$Ca_x(PO_4)_y \cdot nH_2O$	1.2–2.2
Hydroxyapatite	HA and HAp	$Ca_{10}(PO_4)_6(OH)_2$	1.67

Source: Reprinted from Sadat-Shojai, M. et al., *Acta Biomater.*, 9, 7591, 2013. With permission.

that nanosized HAp paralleling natural bone minerals is the best choice to be used in combination with polymeric systems [16]. Studies have shown that biomaterials based on nanosized HAp exhibit enhanced resorbability and much higher bioactivity than micron-sized ceramics [23–25]. Release of calcium ions from nanosized HAp is also similar to that from biological apatite and significantly faster than that from coarser crystals. In addition, new models for nanoscale enamel and bone demineralization suggest that demineralization reactions may be inhibited when particle sizes fall into certain critical nanoscale levels [26]. Some studies have also reported that nanosized HAp possesses a significant capability of decreasing apoptotic cell death and hence improving cell proliferation and cellular activity related to bone growth [23,27]. The improved cell proliferation and differentiation may be due to superior surface functional properties of nanosized HAp compared to its microphase counterpart; indeed, nanosized HAp has higher surface area and surface roughness, resulting in better cell adhesion and cell–matrix interactions [16,23,24]. Therefore, in recent years, bioceramics and biocomposites based on nanosized HAp have been the most promising materials for a variety of biomedical applications.

Considering these points regarding nanosized HAp, one may conclude that this type of CaP is the exclusive structure adapted for application in orthopedic application. However, one key reason that makes CaP ceramics a promising scaffolding material is the possibility of controlling its phase composition and thus its critical characteristics such as the rate of bioresorption. It is well known that in vitro and in vivo biological and mechanical properties of CaP particles, such as strength, toxicity to cells, osseointegrativity, and bioresorbability, are strongly affected by their structural characteristics [16]. For example, octacalcium phosphate (OCP) (Table 1.2) has been demonstrated to be more resorbable than HAp or β-TCP [28] and hence may be considered for those bone treatments needing a shorter recovery time; similarly, amorphous CaP (Table 1.2), which usually appears as an intermediate during the formation of other CaP phases, has been proven to have high biodegradability and excellent biocompatibility, and it can be used as filler in polymeric composites to provide sustained release of calcium and phosphate ions [29–31]. The chemistry and microstructure of CaPs can be simply tailored by varying either synthesis method or processing parameters involved in a specific procedure [12,16]. Accordingly, it is now possible to engineer CaP particles with, for example, a degradation rate or a particle size specific to a particular application of bone tissue engineering. Preparation of an engineered CaP powder is, however, still connected with a number of problems, including difficulties in controlling phase composition, size and size distribution, crystallinity, and degree of particle agglomeration; hence, extensive efforts have been made to develop new routes possessing precise control over the crystallographic and chemical structure of powder. In Ref. [16], we have classified the preparation methods of CaP powders, especially nanosized HAp, into five groups as follows:

1. *Dry methods*: These methods, which can be identified in contrast to wet methods where a solvent is always used, can be performed in two main ways: solid-state synthesis and mechanochemical process. These methods have the convenience of producing highly crystalline HAp from relatively inexpensive raw materials. The main disadvantage is the large size of particles in the case of solid-state synthesis and the low-phase purity of powder in the case of mechanochemical process. In recent years, progress in preparing CaP powder using dry methods, especially solid-state method, has been very slow.

2. *Wet methods*: CaP powder generated from a typical dry method is usually large in size and irregular in shape. Therefore, wet methods have conventionally been applied to the preparation of CaP particles having a regular morphology. For this, aqueous solutions of various sources for phosphate and calcium ions are employed and CaP crystals are normally produced by precipitation. Wet processes can be performed by a number of technical routes classified into six groups: conventional chemical precipitation, hydrolysis method, sol–gel method, hydrothermal method, emulsion method, and sonochemical method. Wet chemical reactions have the advantages in precise control over the morphology and the mean size of powder; however, difficulties in controlling the crystallinity and phase purity of nanoparticles and some technically intricate and time-consuming details make some wet procedures unsuitable for scaling up to produce large quantities of powder.

3. *High-temperature processes*: These methods, which have the convenience of avoiding undesirable CaP phases, are used to produce HAp with high crystallinity and good chemical homogeneity. Two possible routes for high-temperature synthesis are combustion method and pyrolysis process, of which the former has received more attention. Poor control over the processing variables and generation of secondary aggregates, especially during pyrolysis, are the main disadvantages.

4. *Synthesis from biogenic sources*: To produce CaP ceramics, various natural materials, mainly bone waste, eggshells, exoskeleton of marine organisms, naturally derived biomolecules, and biomembranes, have been employed over the past decade. This field is expected to attract more attention in the

near future due to the better physicochemical properties of the powder generated from biogenic sources.

5. *Combination procedures*: These methods, as relatively new strategies, employ two or more distinct procedures to synthesize CaP nanoparticles. In general, combination procedures open exciting possibilities to improve the characteristics of powder.

As reviewed in Refs. [12,16], wet processes are the most promising approaches for preparation of CaP powder. Solution-based reactions, which are accomplished in an organic solvent or, more usually, in water, can be conducted at ambient temperature or elevated temperatures. Moreover, reactions can be performed by a number of technical routes involving diverse chemicals and auxiliary additives and apparatus. Figure 1.3 shows a schematic diagram of the steps involved in a simple chemical precipitation of CaP particles, along with the parameters proposed to affect the characteristics of the powder.

According to Figure 1.3, a typical procedure involves the drop-wise addition of one reagent to another under continuous and gentle stirring, while the molar ratio of elements (Ca/P) is kept at stoichiometry according to its ratio in CaP powder (e.g., 1.67 for HAp). As the last step, the resultant suspension may be either aged under atmospheric pressure or treated at elevated temperatures and pressures (i.e., hydrothermal conditions). It is well known that pH value and heat treatment employed during the precipitation reaction and/or the aging step are the most important factors affecting the structural and morphological characteristics of CaP particles [32,33]. For example, as we indicated in Ref. [22], the aspect ratio of fibrous nanoparticles steeply decreases with increasing pH value. In addition, different morphologies ranging from rod-like to spherical nanoparticles with various characteristics can be simply obtained by controlling the driving force of the chemical reaction.

In Figure 1.4, we summarized our recent results on the preparation of CaP powder under different hydrothermal conditions. According to Figure 1.4, the high pH value results in an isotropic or weak-anisotropic growth; that is, the crystallites can grow to form spherical nanoparticles or at most very short nanorods. However, with a decrease in pH value of suspension, an anisotropic growth occurs; that is, crystallites will grow into 1D nanorods or 2D nanoplates. Additionally, more complicated shapes, including 3D feathery structures, 3D microcubes, and 3D microfibers, are only obtained if the pH value decreases to 4, a pH at which dicalcium phosphate anhydrous (DCPA), dicalcium phosphate dehydrate (DCPD), and OCP become dominant (Figure 1.4 and Table 1.2). Indeed, the lower the synthetic pH, the more complicated the shapes of the CaP crystals formed. More recent approaches propose synthesis routes based on various additives to control the characteristic of powder. A well-known example is based on the biomimetic templating systems in which morphology and crystallinity can be controlled at significantly lower temperatures and pHs. In this strategy, various macromolecules act as a soft temporary template or nucleation centers to modulate the morphology and to increase crystallinity. Indeed, macromolecules adsorb on the crystal surface and influence the crystal growth. Besides macromolecules, attempts have also been made to control the characteristics of CaP powder using small organic compounds [16].

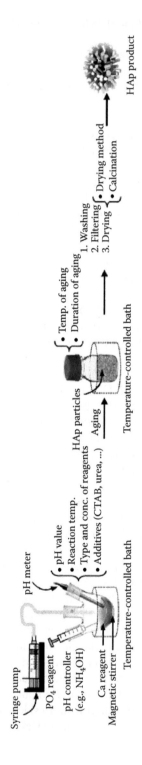

FIGURE 1.3 Preparation of CaP nanoparticles via chemical precipitation. (Reprinted from Sadat-Shojai, M. et al., *Acta Biomater.*, 9, 7591, 2013. With permission.)

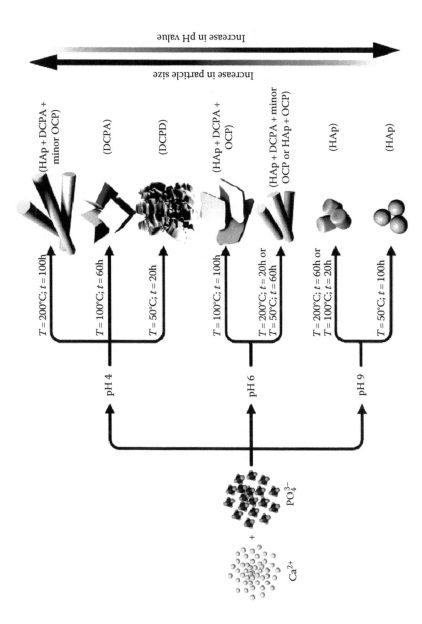

FIGURE 1.4 Effect of different hydrothermal conditions on phase, morphology, and particle size of CaP powder. (Reprinted from Sadat-Shojai, M. et al., *J. Cryst. Growth*, 361, 73, 2012. With permission.)

1.4   WHY POLYESTERS?

Biodegradable polymers that can be resorbed at the body pH are widely used in tissue engineering due to their biocompatibility, design flexibility, light weight, ductile nature, and sometimes due to their possible functional groups availability [7,8,19]. These polymers usually have chemical bonds that can undergo hydrolysis upon exposure to human body fluids [19]. Collagen, gelatin, starch, chitosan, and saturated aliphatic polyesters are the most attractive examples of biodegradable polymers, of which, in this chapter, we will focus on the FDA-approved biodegradable polyester family. Indeed, contrary to the natural polymers (e.g., collagen and chitosan), polyesters have the potential to be produced under controlled conditions and, therefore, they exhibit in general more predictable and reproducible mechanical and physical characteristics. A further advantage is the control of their impurities. Several possible risks such as toxicity, immunogenicity, and favoring of infections are lower for pure synthetic polyesters with a well-known and simple composition [8]. In Figure 1.5, we have shown the chemical structure of the most common biodegradable polyesters being investigated for tissue engineering applications.

Biocompatible and biodegradable polyesters have been demonstrated to have the ability to support cell attachment, cell growth, and cell differentiation in vitro [6,8,9]. In addition, these polymeric materials have been shown to support tissue formation in vivo with minimal inflammation [34,35]; accordingly, a number of studies have also examined their effectiveness for bone tissue repair, on the basis of their ability to support osteoblast cell development. For example, pure polyhidroxybutyrate (PHB) or PHB composites containing HAp particles have been shown to effectively support cellular processes without any significant toxicity [6,36]. Similar results have also been demonstrated for PLA, poly(glycolic acid) (PGA), and their copolymers [8,29,37,38]. On the other hand, in vitro growth of osteoblasts on porous PHA scaffolds with a significant increase in osteocalcin expression and alkaline phosphatase (ALP) activity has been reported over a 60-day growth period [39]. Recently, Kumarasuriyar et al. [40] examined the attachment characteristics, self-renewal capacity, and osteogenic potential of preosteoblast-like MC3T3-E1 S14 when cultured on solvent-cast PHA films for over 2 weeks. They found that time-dependent cell attachment was accelerated on polyester compared with collagen, but delayed compared with tissue-culture polystyrene (TCP). Moreover, cell number, expression of ALP, and osteopontin were comparable for cells grown on polyester and TCP and also increased over time, demonstrating the ability of the PHA to support osteoblast cell functions. Several other studies have demonstrated that bone cells can effectively make cell–cell and cell–substrate contacts on pure polyesters or polyesters integrated with bioactive inorganic minerals [36–38]. In conclusion, although some further in vitro and in vivo assays are still required, biocompatible polyesters having a predictable biodegradation kinetic are currently known as one of the suitable candidates for treating patients suffering from damaged or lost bone tissue.

Among the several biodegradable polyesters, saturated poly(α-hydroxy esters), especially PLA, PGA, and their copolymers (i.e., PLGA), are the most often utilized polymers for bone tissue engineering applications, partly because of their well-known structure, as well as their excellent processability, biocompatibility,

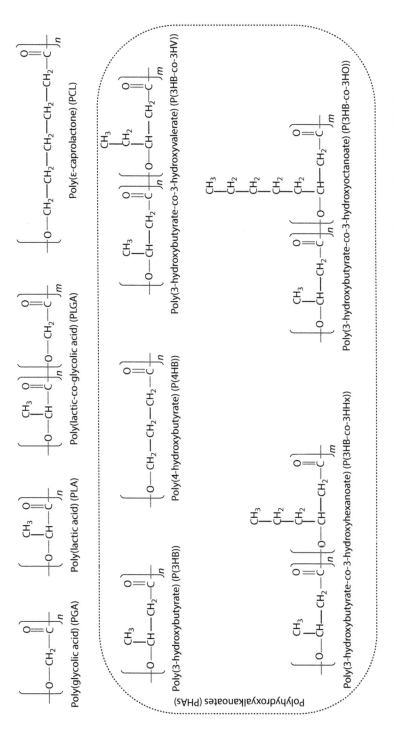

FIGURE 1.5 Chemical structure of the most common biodegradable polyesters being investigated for tissue engineering applications.

and biodegradability [8,24,29]. Depending on the property requirement by different applications, poly(α-hydroxy esters) can be either blended or composed with other polymers and bioactive fillers to further adjust their mechanical and physical characteristics. PLA exists in three forms: L-PLA (PLLA), D-PLA (PDLA), and racemic mixture of D,L-PLA (PDLLA) [8]. Depending on its stereochemistry, PLA requires around 12–24 months to finish the degradation, while the PGA is completely degraded only after around 6–12 months [41,42]. Therefore, copolymers of PLA and PGA, i.e., PLGA (Figure 1.5), may be more flexible for clinical applications, since its degradation rate can be simply adjusted by controlling the ratio of lactide (LA) to glycolide (GA). The chemical properties of various polyesters, including poly(α-hydroxy esters), allow their hydrolytic degradation through de-esterification [8]. Once degraded, the monomeric components of polymer should be removed by natural pathways. It is known that body already contains highly regulated mechanisms for completely removing monomeric components of lactic and glycolic acids. Indeed, PGA is converted to metabolites or eliminated by other mechanisms, and PLA can be broken down into nontoxic metabolites by bio-organisms. On the other hand, PLA, PGA, and PLGA can be easily processed and their mechanical properties, especially their strength and stiffness, are adjustable over a wide range, in particular, by manipulating their molecular weight. In addition, PLA of low molecular weight can be combined with active agents such as growth factors and antibiotics to establish locally acting drug-delivery systems [8]. Despite the excellent features of PLA and PLGA with respect to the scaffold performance, these polymers undergo a bulk erosion process such that they can cause scaffolds to fail prematurely [8]. Moreover, their toughness, hydrophilicity, and heat distortion temperature are not satisfactory [43,44]. Blending these polyesters with other biodegradable polymers can solve some of these problems. For example, PLA/PCL blends have been shown to have improved mechanical properties compared to the bare PLA [45–47]. PCL-based constructs have also been used as drug-delivery systems to entrap antibiotic drugs, increasing bone ingrowth and regeneration [48].

As shown in Figure 1.5, other aliphatic polyesters used in tissue engineering are polyhydroxyalkanoates (PHAs), which represent a range of polymers obtained by bacterial fermentation. A wide range of microorganisms have shown the capability to generate these polyesters under unbalanced growth conditions [49,50]. PHA polymers are generally biodegradable and thermoprocessable, making them attractive for application as degradable tissue engineering scaffolds. So far, more than 100 different types of PHA with diverse structures have been produced; however, only a few of them, particularly poly(3-hydroxybutyrate) (P(3HB)), poly(3-hydroxybutyrate-co-3-hydroxyvalerate) (P(3HB-co-3HV)), poly(4-hydroxybutyrate) (P(4HB)), poly(3-hydroxybutyrate-co-3-hydroxyhexanoate) (P(3HB-co-3HHx)), and poly(3-hydroxybutyrate-co-3-hydroxyoctanoate) (P(3HB-co-3HO)) (Figure 1.5), have been demonstrated to be suitable for tissue engineering applications. Due to the variable structures of PHAs, a wide range of mechanical properties and degradation rates can be achieved. P(3HB) or simply PHB, as the simplest and the most common member of the PHA family, has been demonstrated to have piezoelectric properties, which can stimulate bone growth and aid in bone healing [51,52]. The fact that PHB of low molecular weight occurs naturally in human body and that its molecules decompose into 3-hydroxybutyric acid, a normal constituent of human blood, provides further evidence of the biocompatibility and nontoxicity of this polymer [53,54]. Doyle et al. [55] have demonstrated that implanted PHB can produce a consistent favorable bone tissue adaptation response with no evidence of an undesirable chronic inflammatory response after implantation periods of up to 12 months. Although the PHB implants show no evidence of extensive structural breakdown in vivo, but their usefulness can be limited by their brittleness. The incorporation of hydroxyvalerate units into the PHB chains has been shown to improve both the ductility and processability of the polyester, allowing for the appropriate shape, form, and porosity of the scaffold to be created [11,56,57]. Similar to PHB, the bacterially derived P(3HB-co-3HV), or simply PHBV, has been demonstrated to be biodegradable and piezoelectric and thus might promote bone growth in vivo [51,56]. This copolyester can be composed of hydroxybutyrate (HB) with between 0% and 24% of hydroxyvalerate (HV) appearing randomly throughout the polymer chain [57]. Together with high biocompatibility, PHBV usually has a longer degradation time than PLA or PLGA, which will allow the scaffolds to maintain its mechanical integrity until the sufficient bone growth occurs in vivo. In addition, its rate of degradation can be tuned by altering its molecular weight and hydroxyvalerate content [36,52,56,58]. Accordingly, PHBV-based scaffolds may be a suitable candidate to support the long-term bone regeneration. Currently, PHB- and PHBV-based scaffolds containing CaP nanoparticles have been developed for bone tissue repair. However, a drawback of PHAs is their time-consuming extraction process from bacterial cultures, which is the main challenge for industrial production of PHA polyesters.

1.5 CaP/POLYESTER NANOCOMPOSITES

Some basic requirements have been accepted for designing bone scaffolds. First, biocompatibility and bioactivity of the scaffolding material are imperative. Indeed, the biological response should be optimized with respect to both encouraging bone regeneration and inhibiting pro-inflammation. In other words, an ideal bone scaffold should support osteoblast-mediated bone deposition along with differentiation of undifferentiated stem cells into osteogenic cells (osteoinductive) and, at the same time, support the ingrowth of vasculature and regeneration of new bone tissue within its structural framework (osteoconductive) [8,20,21,40]. In addition, degradation products must be nontoxic and easily removed by normal metabolic pathways. As with all materials in contact with the human body, bone scaffolds should be sterilizable to prevent infection. Another key requirement is that the scaffolding material should be easy to process into the desired 3D architecture with an appropriate interconnected porosity for facilitating cell infiltration and vascularization of the ingrown tissue. Other highly important feature, particularly for bone tissue engineering, is its mechanical characteristics, for example, its stiffness and shear and compressive modulus [8,56,59].

As mentioned in Section 1.3, CaP bioceramics can be used as the scaffold matrix to support bone regeneration without any significant inflammatory response. Bonding of these bioactive ceramics to living bones has been achieved through the formation of biologically active bone-like apatite layer at the bone–implant interface.

In practice, bioactive CaP ceramics have, however, been reported to be extremely brittle and have low flexibility, fracture toughness, and formability, especially in the porous forms [8,12,60–62]. Consequently, their range of applications has usually been limited to low or non-load-bearing sites. In addition, their biodegradability is also relatively slow [19]. On the other hand, CaP ceramics can be applicable to bulk defects after only being heat treated and sintered at elevated temperatures, a process that does not allow the appropriate incorporation of active agents, like growth factors and antibiotics, in the resulting construct [12,21,61–63]. Alternatively, polyester scaffolds are more flexible and moldable but are often inert in terms of bioactivity, resulting in delay in bone healing and sometimes loosening of scaffolds in clinical applications. The scaffolds made from solely polyesters also can generate an acidic environment around the bone tissue during their degradation, thereby inducing inflammatory response and osteolytic reactions [64,65]. In addition, it can be seen that porous polymeric scaffolds usually suffer from low compressive strength and stiffness compared to the cortical and cancellous bone. Accordingly, development of CaP/polyester composite systems may be attractive as advantageous intrinsic properties of each component can be simply combined to suit better the physicochemical and biological demands of hard tissues. Indeed, the most important driving force behind the development of polymer/ceramic hybrids is probably the need for conferring bioactive behavior to the polymer matrix. In this manner, by taking advantage of the moldability of polyesters and including an optimum concentration of a bioactive CaP phase, a level of flexibility can be achieved for the fabricated composite (Figure 1.6), and at the same time, the bioactivity of polyesters can be counteracted [8]. To date, various polyesters, mainly PLA, PLGA, PCL, PHB, and PHBV, have been combined with different CaP phases, mainly HAp and TCP, via simple physical mixing or in situ preparation to produce a composite with improved bioactivity, hydrophilicity, mechanical properties, protein adsorption, and osteoconductivity.

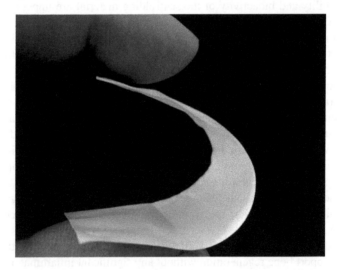

FIGURE 1.6 Photograph of a typical PHB/HAp nanocomposite film showing the relative flexibility.

The bioactivity degree of the CaP/polyester nanocomposites can be adjusted by volume fraction, size, and phase of CaP inclusions. In general, polymer nanocomposites in which the reinforcing filler has the nanoscale dimensions exhibit an outstanding improvement in their critical properties compared to either pure polymers or conventional polymer composites [66–69]. A new trend in bone tissue engineering is, therefore, to engineer organic–inorganic nanocomposites using nanosized CaP (i.e., CaP nanoparticles). Here, the reinforcing particles are comparable in size to those in natural bone, which consists of around 65%–70% CaP inclusion embedded in a collagen matrix (see Section 1.2). As reviewed in Section 1.3, CaP nanomaterials usually possess superior biological and mechanical properties over their microscale counterpart. Studies have found that, for instance, nanocrystalline HAp shows enhanced osteoblast cell adhesion, differentiation, and proliferation, and a better surface deposition of bone-like apatite, thus enhancing the formation of new bone tissue within a shorter period of time [19,23–27,70]. In particular, ceramic/polymer nanocomposites are considered one of the most promising groups of bioactive composites and have a great potential for application in bone regeneration. For example, it is suggested that polyester/nano-HAp scaffolds fabricated by thermally induced phase separation technique have an increased compressive strength and stiffness and an improved in vitro bioactivity [71]. Many studies also demonstrated that nano-CaP exposure on the surface of the composite systems resulted in an increasing bioactivity due to the presence of hydroxyl groups detected on their surface and thus an improved interaction with the osteoblast cells [6,72–74].

As other nanocomposite systems, the critical properties of a typical CaP-reinforced polyester nanocomposite are determined by four main factors, including component properties, composition, structure, and interfacial interactions between the components [75]. In addition to the kind of CaP phase (HAp, TCP), particle geometry, particle size, size distribution, and specific surface area are among the most important characteristics of CaP nanoparticles; the main polyester characteristics are its chemical structure, degradation rate, and intrinsic mechanical properties. On the other hand, weight or volume fraction of reinforcing particles determines the composition; while aggregation, agglomeration, and the orientation of anisotropic nanoparticles within the polymeric matrix influence the structure. Finally, interfacial interaction between the phases is usually determined by the surface properties of the reinforcing filler and usually can be improved by physical or chemical surface modification of the filler. Once again, we can answer this question: "why are polymer nanocomposites based on nano CaPs so attractive for bone tissue engineering applications?" First, there is the fact that the mechanical performance of nanometer-size reinforcement is superior to its microscale counterpart; mainly because of the smaller size of the fillers, leading to a dramatic increase in interfacial interactions as compared with the traditional composites. Bone-like CaP nanoparticles, due to their small dimensions, exhibit superior cell responses over their micron-sized counterpart. Current trends in CaP-based nanocomposites for bone regeneration applications are, therefore, to manipulate new nanocomposites having the main features of natural bone both in composition and structure at nanoscale. The physical, mechanical, and biological characterization of these new systems can be carried out by several techniques, which have been summarized in Figure 1.7 and discussed in the following sections.

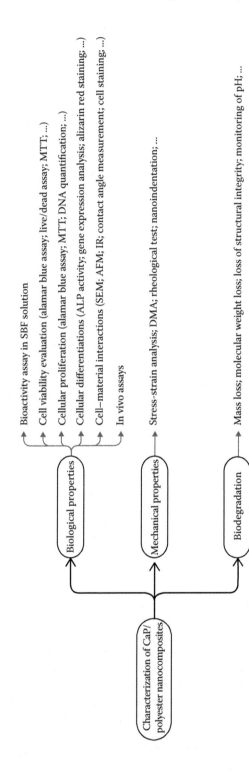

FIGURE 1.7 Different techniques for characterization of biomedical CaP/polyester nanocomposites.

1.5.1 Biological Characteristics

Although it is now well established that bioactive CaP ceramics can enhance cellular responses in vitro, but little has been known about the effect of nanophase CaP fillers embedded in the polyester matrix on the cellular processes. On the other hand, while a good number of in vivo studies exist for biodegradable polymers and bioactive ceramics alone, to our knowledge, in vivo assays for polymer/ceramic nanocomposites have just started. In particular, very few nano-CaP/polyester systems have been investigated in vivo up to now. However, the in vitro studies conducted on these nanocomposites can still provide reliable information that usually indicates their in vivo performance. As mentioned before, a common feature of bioactive CaP/polyester nanocomposites is their ability to develop an apatite layer after implantation, which is essential for bonding the scaffold to the surrounding tissue. Indeed, when a nanocomposite is claimed to be useful for bone repair, it always needs to be examined in terms of bioactive behavior [6,12,76]. A nanocomposite system that can demonstrate high bioactivity upon immersion in SBF solution (Section 1.3) should similarly have the ability to induce apatite formation in vivo [76]. In literature, there are a number of studies about bioactivity of polyester systems having CaP phase. As an example, Ni and Wang [77] prepared PHB/HAp composites containing 10, 20, and 30 vol.% of HAp for in vitro bioactivity evaluation using SBF solution. Results showed that a layer of bone-like apatite was formed within a short period on PHB/HAp composite after its immersion in SBF, demonstrating high in vitro bioactivity of the composite. Moreover, bioactivity of the composite could be tailored by varying the amount of HAp in the composite. Dynamic mechanical analysis (DMA) revealed that the storage modulus of PHB/HAp composite increased initially with immersion time in SBF, due to apatite formation on composite surface and decreased after prolonged immersion in SBF, indicating degradation of the composite in the simulated body environment. A typical apatite layer formed on the polyester nanocomposites made of PHB and 30 wt.% HAp nanoparticles after 30 days immersion in SBF is illustrated by scanning electron microscopy (SEM) in Figure 1.8.

According to Figure 1.8, while a dense mineral layer can be formed on the surface of HAp-filled nanocomposites, the unfilled PHB polymer (i.e., control) only shows a few of scattered particles on its surface. This clearly indicates that while neat PHB cannot be effectively bioactive, PHB/HAp nanocomposites have a great ability to induce the formation of minerals in vitro [6]. Recently, Kim and Koh [78] synthesized PCL/HAp composite microspheres with an aligned porous structure by freezing the droplets of HAp-containing PCL solutions in a poly(vinyl alcohol) aqueous solution. They showed that incorporation of HAp particles to the PCL polymer led to a considerable improvement in the in vitro bioactivity, which was assessed again by immersing the PCL/HAp composite microspheres in SBF. They reported that a number of apatite crystals could be precipitated on the surface of the porous PCL/HAp composite microspheres after soaking in the SBF only for 7 days.

The influence of the topographical and chemical structures on the biocompatibility and cellular response of polyester nanocomposites has been a focus of interest in recent years. Although CaP nanoparticles can form a homogeneous suspension with the solution of polyester prior to solidification, the amount of CaP nanoparticles that

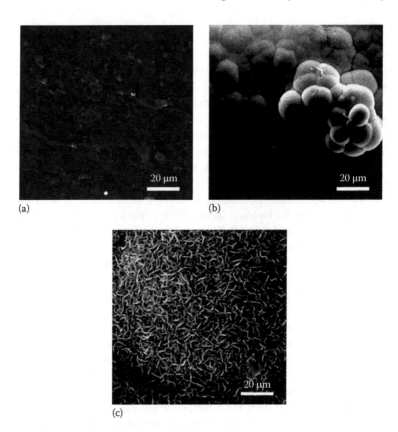

(a)   (b)

(c)

FIGURE 1.8 SEM micrographs of polymeric films after 30 days immersion in SBF for pure PHB (a), PHB/HAp nanocomposite containing 30 wt.% nanoparticles at low magnification (b), and high magnification (c). (Reprinted from Sadat-Shojai, M. et al., *Mater. Sci. Eng. C.*, 33, 2776, 2013. With permission.)

can actually appear on the surface of polymer matrix and interact with cells may not reflect the average value for the bulk. Cai et al. [72] investigated the role of exposed HAp nanoparticles in influencing mouse pre-osteoblastic MC3T3-E1 cell behavior on the surface of nanocomposites prepared by photocrosslinking of PCL diacrylate (PCLDA). They found that cell attachment, proliferation, and differentiation were significantly enhanced when HAp content was increased in crosslinked PCLDA/HAp nanocomposites due to more bioactive HAp, higher surface stiffness, and rougher topography. More exposed HAp on the surface of cut semicrystalline PCLDA/HAp nanocomposites resulted in improved hydrophilicity and significantly better cell attachment, proliferation, and differentiation compared with the original surface. Accordingly, their study demonstrated that HAp nanoparticles may not be fully exploited in polymer/HAp nanocomposites where the top polymer surface covers the particles. Hence, they suggested that removal of this polymer layer can generate more desirable surfaces and osteoconductivity for bone repair and regeneration. Very recently, we [6] dealt with the in vitro biological properties of solution-cast

PHB/HAp nanocomposites having different HAp concentrations and tried to explain the effects of HAp nanoparticles on cellular responses in terms of cell–material interactions. For this, we examined the influence of HAp nanoparticles embedded in PHB matrix on growth and metabolic activity of different cell lines (3T3 fibroblasts and MC3T3-El mouse preosteoblasts) using DNA quantification and Alamar Blue (AB) assay, respectively. Moreover, calcium deposition and ALP activity were used to reveal the effect of nanophase HAp on the differentiation of MC3T3-El (Figure 1.7). According to our results, there was a significant increase in metabolic activity of 3T3 fibroblasts on the surface of PHB/HAp nanocomposites from day 1 to day 4 and then from day 4 to day 7 for all composites containing different HAp concentrations. The increase in cell metabolic activity over the culture period clearly demonstrated that PHB/HAp specimens had high cell viability and cell attachment. The results also showed that greater metabolic activities were obtained for 5%, 15%, and 30% filled samples compared to the control (neat polymer) after 4 and 7 days of culture. For example, there was a more than twofold increase in the %AB reduction of the 15% filled sample compared to the control on day 4 of culture. The same increase, but with a lower magnitude, was observed at day 7 when cells are close to confluence. On the other hand, there was again a significant increase in AB reduction of MC3T3-El preosteoblasts for filled nanocomposites in comparison to the unfilled polymer at days 1, 4, and 7 of culture, of which the most pronounced increase was observed on day 4. For example, the metabolic activity of 15% filled sample was more than 2.5-fold of that of control. These data confirmed that HAp nanoparticles significantly improved the cellular activity of preosteoblasts. However, our results showed that while metabolic activity increased from day 1 to day 4 in all conditions, almost no increase in metabolic activity was observed from day 4 to day 7, except for the control sample. To examine whether the increase in cell metabolic activity can be a consequence of increased cell number, we measured cell proliferation using DNA quantification at the same time points over the culture period. Consistent with the AB results, we found that fibroblasts cultured on the filled nanocomposites showed more DNA content and hence more proliferation compared to the control sample. Additionally, a significant increase in DNA content was observed over the culture period, indicating that cells were alive and grew continuously in all groups. The 4-day DNA assay showed a pronounced increase in proliferation of MC3T3-El on the surface of both 15% and 30% filled samples when compared to the control. However, we did not find differences in cell proliferation among samples after 7 days, suggesting that the observed trends in AB assay at day 7 cannot completely account for the cell proliferation. By contrast, consistent with the trend observed in AB graph, a gradual increase in cell number was observed from day 1 to day 4 followed by a cell quiescence between the fourth and seventh days of culture. Presumably, the initially high proliferative rates of the cells resulted in their early confluence and subsequently their differentiation, a feature that was investigated using ALP and histological analyses. Under certain stimuli, the preosteoblasts may differentiate into premature osteoblasts and further into mature osteoblasts. This process, which is marked by the formation of mineralized nodules, indicates the ability of a material to promote bone formation. We used Alizarin Red staining to study the differentiation of mouse MC3T3-El cells (Figure 1.7). Our results indicated that a very significant increase in cell differentiation was observed in samples with 5, 15, and 30 wt.% HAp filler in comparison with the samples with 0, 1, and 5 wt.% HAp filler and plastic cell culture surface, after both 7 and 21 days of culture. Interestingly, while almost no detectable mineralized nodule was found on the unfilled sample (i.e., sample without HAp nanoparticles), nanocomposites with high filler contents exhibited a pronounced biomineralization on their surface, indicating that HAp nanoparticles efficiently induce cell differentiation in addition to cell proliferation. According to the results, the maximum mineralization was observed for 15% filled sample with more than tenfold increase at day 21 compared to the plastic surface. These observations also confirmed the AB and DNA results, where there was no increase in cell proliferation from day 4 to day 7, indicative of a transition from a proliferating to a differentiating state. To further confirm the results, we also measured ALP activity at different time points. According to the results, after 1 day of culture, ALP activity increased with increasing HAp content (up to 15%) and then decreased at 30% filler content. Moreover, an abrupt decrease in ALP activity was clearly observed between day 1 and day 4 or day 7, and the magnitude of difference became more pronounced with the increasing HAp concentration. ALP is an enzyme catalyzing the hydrolysis of phosphomonoesters to inorganic phosphate required for the maintenance of cellular metabolism. On day 1, the increased ALP activity of samples with higher filler contents represented more proliferation rate, which finally led to the more cell number on day 4 of culture, as also indicated by the DNA quantification. Interestingly, 15% filled sample, which exhibited the most cell number after 4 days of culture, had the highest ALP activity at day 1 with the most pronounced decrease in ALP expression between day 1 and day 4, resulting in high differentiation at days 7 and 21. By contrast, the cell numbers of unfilled sample (i.e., control) at both day 1 and day 4 were significantly lower than the filled samples, and there was no significant difference in ALP activities between days 1 and 4. According to the obtained results, we identified three distinct stages in the cellular response to PHB/HAp nanocomposites. The initial stage is characterized as cell proliferation, and preosteoblasts have a high level of metabolic activity and ALP, but still remain undifferentiated, as evidenced by the absence of mineralization. This stage is also marked by a significant increase in cell number. A sudden decrease in ALP activity is characterized as the second stage, which occurs at approximately the fourth day after culture. The final stage of MC3T3-E1 maturation begins at about the seventh day and is defined by an expression of the mineralized nodules associated with progressive increases in mineralization until 21 days after culture. Our results clearly demonstrate the positive effect of HAp nanoparticles by which both cell proliferation at the first stage and cell differentiation at the second and third stages were efficiently increased. Studies have found that some biological responses, for example, DNA synthesis, focal contact formation of cells, and cytoskeleton organization, can effectively be improved in the presence of bioactive HAp [72,79]. It is now well established that both surface texture (topography) and surface chemistry can alter cell behavior at many levels. Accordingly, to explain the observed cell responses in our study, we explored the surface morphology and surface topography of the prepared nanocomposites. SEM morphology examination revealed that the incorporation of HAp into the PHB matrix resulted in an increase in surface roughness. Moreover, the results clearly showed that HAp nanoparticles exposed on the surface significantly increased with the increasing HAp concentration. Therefore, we concluded that the increased cell response in both 3T3 and MC3T3 cell types was the result of the exposed HAp on the composite surface. Surface analysis was also carried out using atomic force microscopy to quantify the topography of the composite surface. The results showed that surface roughness parameters first changed nonsignificantly with HAp addition, then abruptly increased with the addition of HAp filler, and finally again diminished. This result indicated that the introduction of HAp nanoparticles into the semicrystalline PHB can roughen its surface, if the concentration of filler is appropriately chosen. This is a consequence of the fact that HAp nanoparticles affect the crystallization of PHB from its melt and probably from its solution during the solvent casting process [6]. As the nature of the crystalline structure should affect the surface characteristics, this may be the reason why the addition of HAp to PHB alters the surface roughness. From these results, it could be concluded that the increase in surface roughness and exposed HAp synergistically promoted cell proliferation and subsequent cell differentiation; composition with 15% HAp exhibited the best cell response because it had the highest surface roughness and a large amount of exposed HAp on its surface. Although composition with 30% HAp had a low surface roughness, but the high HAp exposed on the surface improved the cell processes, which was comparable to that of the 15% filled sample.

In another study [80], the in vitro osteogenic and inflammatory properties of PHBV were examined with various CaP-reinforcing phases: nanosized HAp; submicron-sized calcined HAp (cHAp); and submicron-sized β-TCP, using bioassays of cultured osteoblasts, osteoclasts, and macrophages. The study showed that the addition of a nanosized reinforcing phase to PHBV, while improving osteogenic properties, also reduced the proinflammatory response. Pro-inflammatory responses of macrophages to PHBV itself were shown to be very high, but the introduction of a reinforcing CaP phase markedly reduced this response, with the PHBV/HAp nanocomposite material yielding the greatest reduction. Moreover, cultures of osteoblasts were demonstrated to readily attach and mineralize on all the materials, with PHBV/HAp inducing the highest levels of mineralization. The improved biological performance of PHBV/HAp composites when compared with PHBV/cHA and PHBV/β-TCP composites was clearly a result of the nanosized reinforcing phase of PHBV/HAp and the greater surface presentation of mineral in the nanocomposites. Recently, Lao et al. [38] prepared PLGA fibrous composite scaffolds having HAp nanoparticles by the electrospinning process. According to their results, agglomerates gradually appeared and increased on the fiber surface along with increase in the HAp concentration. In vitro mineralization in the SBF solution revealed that the PLGA/HAp fibrous scaffolds had stronger biomineralization ability than the control PLGA scaffolds. They also assessed the cellular responses of the fibrous scaffolds of the control PLGA and PLGA with 5 wt.% HAp by in vitro culture of MC3T3-E1 cells. Results showed that both types of scaffolds could support cell proliferation, but the cells cultured on the PLGA/HAp fibers showed a more spreading morphology. Moreover, despite the similar level of cell viability and cell number at each time interval, cells cultured on the PLGA/HAp scaffolds showed significantly higher ALP activity than that on the control scaffolds by a factor of 60% at 7 days.

Results from these studies, taken together, suggest that the use of a carefully chosen reinforcing CaP phase with an optimized concentration can vastly improve the biological response to the polyester biomaterials. In particular, these findings clearly show that surface roughness and surface chemistry are the predominant parameters influencing the in vitro cell responses.

1.5.2 MECHANICAL CHARACTERISTICS

A common reason for adding fillers to organic polymers is to increase the mechanical strength of the resultant composite. Bone substitute materials, in particular, must have sufficient mechanical strength to be applicable as bone replacement and to support bone formation at the site of implantation in vivo. Mechanical properties of the substrate have also been demonstrated to have a profound impact on the cell behavior [81]. As mentioned before, the incorporation of CaP fillers into a polyester matrix will combine the osteoconductivity of CaP phase with the good mechanical properties and processability of polymers. As other composite systems, the mechanical properties of CaP-reinforced nanocomposites are expected to be strongly influenced by a number of factors, for example, geometry, crystallinity, size, and size distribution of nanoparticles, volume percentage of nanoparticles, polyester properties (e.g., its molecular weight and intrinsic strength), dispersion quality of nanoparticles in the polymer matrix, and state of the filler–matrix interface. For example, strength and modulus of composite systems generally increase, and deformability and impact strength usually decrease with decreasing particle size [75]. Moreover, the reinforcing effects of the filler increase with the anisotropy of particle [75,82,83]. In fact, particles can be differentiated by their degree of anisotropy (or aspect ratio); fillers with plate-like or fiber-like geometries reinforce polymers more than spherical particles, and the influence of particles with 3D complex shapes is expected to be even stronger. However, there seems to be little effort on the fabrication of polyester composites with the anisotropic CaP nanoparticles. Unfortunately, little work has been reported to evaluate the real effects of particle characteristics on the CaP-reinforced polyester nanocomposites, at least in the open literature.

Recently, we [6] examined the viscoelastic behavior of the neat PHB polymer and 15% HAp-filled PHB nanocomposite using DMA over the temperature range −70°C to 120°C. According to the results, the storage modulus was found to increase in PHB/HAp nanocomposite compared to the neat PHB, indicating that HAp has a strong reinforcing effect on the elastic properties of the polymer matrix. Indeed, the storage modulus reveals the capability of a material to store mechanical energy without dissipation; the higher the storage modulus, the harder the material is. Moreover, addition of HAp nanoparticles resulted in a small shift of glass transition temperature (determined from the maximum of the tan δ curve) to a higher temperature, as a result of the restrained mobility of PHB chains in the presence of filler. In addition, the transition peak dropped obviously, and a certain broadening was observed in the presence of HAp. The damping factor (i.e., tan δ) gives the fractional energy lost in a system due to deformation; a high value of tan δ often implies imperfections in the elasticity of a system. Accordingly, lower tan δ in filled nanocomposite suggests that when the stress is removed, the energy stored in deforming the material is recovered more quickly compared to the unfilled polymer. From these results, it can be clearly deduced that the addition of HAp nanoparticles increased the mechanical properties of the PHB matrix. From literature, it can be seen that some dense CaP-reinforced nanocomposites match cancellous bone characteristics and approach cortical bone characteristics. However, comparison of the mechanical properties of porous composite scaffolds with the mechanical properties of natural bone reveals the insufficient mechanical strength, toughness, and elastic modulus of these scaffolds, limiting their load-bearing applications. Moreover, sometimes by comparing the mechanical properties of the porous nanocomposites to those of porous pure polymer, only a slight increase in the mechanical strength can be revealed [8]. In other words, the reinforcing effects of CaP particles on stiffness and strength are sometimes below expectations; most probably because of three major reasons. First, this behavior can be attributed to the lack of interfacial interactions between the hydrophilic CaP fillers and the hydrophobic polyester matrix, resulting in poor filler dispersion and weak ceramic–polymer interface. In other words, the lack of strong adhesion between organic and inorganic phases will result in an early failure at the interface and thus in a decrease in the mechanical properties [84–86]. In addition, CaP particles may cause a significant reduction in the degree of crystallinity of the crystalline polymer matrix, which in turn lowers the matrix modulus. Thus, the positive influence on the modulus caused by the relatively rigid CaP filler can be offset by the negative effect caused by the reduction in matrix crystallinity. On the other hand, some filler particles may be excluded upon crystallization of the polymer matrix during the polymer solidification, resulting in filler agglomeration at the extremities of the spherulites. Not only would this reduce the effective filler modulus (since the shear modulus of agglomerated filler grains would be low), but would also facilitate internal voiding and debonding between the matrix and filler [87].

While it seems that we cannot effectively control the crystallization behavior of semicrystalline polyesters in the presence of CaP particles, but an improvement of the interfacial adhesion between particles and matrix is certainly possible, simply by surface modification of CaP particles at the nanosize range. This is usually achieved by grafting organic molecules (e.g., coupling agents) to the active hydroxyl groups (OH) on the CaP surface prior to composite processing. Surface treatment of inorganic phase can modify both particle–particle and particle–matrix interactions, and properties of the resulting composite are usually affected by the combined effect of both interactions [8,84–86]. However, because of the limited number of active OH groups on the CaP surface and their relatively low reactivity, there are only a few studies reporting the preparation of surface-functionalized CaP particles. In addition, the increase in interfacial bonding strength by the introduction of organic molecules may have an impact on degradation kinetics and cytotoxicity of the resulting composite, a feature which is unknown and remains to be investigated. Another concern is specific surface area of the nanoparticles, which must be taken into consideration during any surface treatment [75]. Recently, Li et al. [84] have tried to modify the surface of HAp particles by the ring-opening polymerization of LA. The modified HAp particles were then characterized by infrared spectroscopy and thermogravimetric analysis. They indicated that LA could be graft-polymerized onto the surface of HAp. According to the results, the modified HAp particles were well dispersed in the PLA matrix than the unmodified HAp particles, and the adhesion between HAp particles and PLA matrix was improved. As expected, the modified PLA/HAp composites showed superior mechanical properties compared to the unmodified PLA/HAp composite. In another study, Hong et al. [85] tried to graft PLLA onto the surface of the HAp nanoparticles in order to improve the bonding between HAp particles and PLLA, and hence to increase the mechanical properties of PLLA/HAp nanocomposites. They showed that PLLA molecules grafted on the HAp surfaces played an important role in improving the adhesive strength between the particles and the polymer matrix. At a low content of surface-grafted HAp, the PLLA/HAp nanocomposites exhibited higher bending strength and impact energy than the pure PLLA, and at a higher content of surface-grafted HAp, the modulus was remarkably increased. It implied that PLLA could be strengthened as well as toughened by surface-grafted HAp nanoparticles. These improvements can be ascribed first to the grafted PLLA molecules, which tie molecules between the fillers and the PLLA matrix, and second to the surface-grafted HAp particles, which are uniformly distributed in the composites and play the role of the heterogeneous nucleating agents in the crystallization of the PLLA matrix. Very recently, Diao et al. [86] used dodecyl alcohol to modify HAp nanoparticles through esterification reaction in order to improve the dispersibility of HAp in PLA/HAp nanocomposites prepared by melt blending. They reported that the surface modification of HAp nanoparticles with hydrophobic regents resulted in good dispersibility of HAp nanoparticles in the PLA matrix and improved interfacial interactions between PLA and HAp nanoparticles.

1.5.3 DEGRADATION

Degradation is a general process where the deterioration in the properties of material takes place due to different factors such as humidity, light, heat, and mechanical tensions [88]. As a consequence of degradation, the resulting smaller fragments do not contribute effectively to the mechanical properties, and a material completely fails when a sufficient deterioration occurs. Degradation of biomedical composite scaffolds under physiological environments, also called biodegradation, depends on several factors, such as composition, pore structure, scaffolds geometry, fluid flow, hydrophilicity, and pH of the surrounding media. The study of degradation of CaP-reinforced polyester scaffolds is an important area in bone tissue engineering, particularly since a better understanding of material degradation will ensure the effective bone regeneration. Ideally, the degradation kinetic of composite scaffolds should be precisely designed to allow cells to proliferate and secrete their own ECM while the scaffold gradually degrades leaving space for new cells. In other words, the physical support provided by the 3D scaffold must be maintained until the engineered bone tissue has sufficient mechanical integrity to support itself [8]. However, so far not enough attention has been given to the long-term in vitro and in vivo degradation of CaP/polyester nanocomposites as compared to the evaluation of their biological and mechanical properties, probably because of the complicated reactions involved in the degradation process.

It is known that among the common biodegradable polyesters, PGA has the fastest degradation rate, while the slowest degradation rate has been reported to belong to the PCL [8,41,42]. Indeed, polymer blends containing the large amounts of PGA (or PLGA) have been shown to degrade faster [89]. On the other hand, PCL may take several years (3 years or more) to fully degrade in vivo [90]. Similarly, PLLA has a very low resorption rate due to its high crystallinity leaving behind crystalline residues even after several years [91,92]. The degradation rate of most PHA polyesters is usually between those of PLLA and PGA. The degradation kinetic of polyesters is also governed by their crystallinity as the crystal segments are chemically more stable than amorphous segments. PLGA, for instance, has a wide range of degradation rates, depending on its molecular weight and composition (i.e., contents in L-LA and D-LA and/or GA units) and hence its degree of crystallinity [8]. It is well known that amorphous regions are preferentially degraded in semicrystalline polyesters like PHB; moreover, hydrolysis of amorphous polyesters like PDLLA is generally faster than the crystalline ones [8,56,93]. In fact, the amount of absorbed water strongly depends on the diffusion coefficients of chain fragments within the polymer matrix. Therefore, PGA has the fastest degradation rate because of its stronger acidity and more hydrophilicity compared to PLA, which is hydrophobic due to its methyl groups (Figure 1.5). Moreover, among PLA isomers, a polymer composed of L-lactic repeating units takes more than 5 years for total absorption, whereas only about 1 year is needed for amorphous PDLLA (stereochemistry influences crystallinity; better alignment of neighbors leads to higher crystallinity) [8].

In addition to the improvement in biological and mechanical properties of polyesters upon the addition of CaP particles, some researchers have also incorporated CaP particles to stabilize the pH of the environment surrounding polyesters and to control their degradation behavior. In fact, the possibility of counteracting the acidic degradation of polyesters at the polymer surface is another reason given for the use of CaP/polyester composites. In this manner, dissolved phosphate ions released from the CaP particles can buffer the acidity of the carboxylic end groups produced by the polyester chain cleavage. Consequently, the pH of the surrounding media remains more stable for the composites than for the pure polyesters, preventing the inflammatory response resulting from the acidic degradation products [8,64,65]. Furthermore, the inclusion of CaP phases can modify the surface and bulk properties of composite scaffolds by increasing the hydrophilicity and water absorption of the polymer matrix [8]. The chemical phenomena involved in the biodegradation of CaP-reinforced polyester scaffolds can be classified as follows: (1) hydrolysis reaction of the ester bonds; (2) acid dissociation of the carboxylic ($-COOH$) end groups; (3) dissolution of the CaP particles; and (4) buffering reactions by the dissolved phosphate ions [64]. According to this classification, the first step of the biodegradation is the diffusion of water into the scaffold, followed by chain cleavage of the polyester through the hydrolysis reaction between the ester bonds and water. Although water absorption often continues to increase during the entire degradation process, the water content reaches an abundant level in a few days and further absorption of water has little effect on the degradation rate [64]. The hydrolysis reaction produces hydroxyl alcohol and carboxylic acid end groups. The carboxylic end groups formed by chain cleavage have a high degree of acid disassociation to generate H^+ and are, therefore, able to catalyze the hydrolysis of other ester bonds. This phenomenon is called autocatalysis. During the autocatalyzed degradation, the polyester changes to oligomers and finally to monomers (e.g., lactic acid in the case of PLA) [37,56,64,93].

However, some experiments suggested that the rate of degradation in vivo may be faster than the in vitro rate of hydrolysis at the same temperature and pH [94,95]. In fact, the ester bonds are usually prone to both chemical and enzymatic hydrolysis, and hence enzymes secreted by the body's immune system can further catalyze the degradation reaction in vivo. As mentioned before, another phase of the composite, that is, CaP particles can also dissolve in water, producing calcium and phosphate ions. However, crystalline CaP phases have usually long degradation times both in vitro and in vivo, typically in the order of months or even years [8,19]. Moreover, the dissolution rate of CaP depends on the type, degree of the saturation, and pH of the solution, solid/solution ratio, and the composition and crystallinity of the CaP phase. For instance, crystalline and amorphous HAp structures, respectively, exhibit the slowest and the fastest degradation rate compared with some other phases (e.g., α-TCP or β-TCP) [8]. Although the solubility of CaP particles is rather poor, but the buffering reactions between PO_4^{3-} (resealed from CaP) and H^+ (released from COOH groups), an inverse analogy to the dissolution of phosphoric acid (H_3PO_4), can continuously lead to further dissolution of the CaP particles [64].

Although different factors have been suggested to affect the degradation kinetics of CaP/polyester composites (e.g., chemical composition, molecular mass, polydispersity, and configurational structure of polyester, processing history, environmental conditions, stress and strain, device size, porosity, and overall hydrophilicity), but the effect of various CaP with different phases and crystallinities on the biodegradation of polyesters in nanocomposites is under discussion and no conclusion can be made about their exact mechanisms on the basis of present literature. Recently, Pan et al. [64] have tried to present a model for biodegradation of composite materials made of polyesters and TCP using a set of differential equations. However, their model ignores the diffusion of the various reaction products out of the composite into the degradation media, and is, therefore, only valid for the early stage of degradation of the composite. More recently, Sultana and Khan [56] investigated the long-term in vitro degradation properties of scaffolds based on PHBV and HAp nanoparticles. For this, they fabricated 3D porous scaffolds using the emulsion-freezing/freeze-drying technique. According to the results, mass loss and molecular weight loss of PHBV along with the loss of structural integrity were observed during degradation. Their experiments also suggested that accelerated weight loss was observed for PHBV/HAp nanocomposite scaffolds as compared to the pure PHBV scaffold. Moreover, an increasing trend of crystallinity was observed during the initial period of degradation time, and the compressive properties decreased more than 40% after a 5-month in vitro degradation.

1.6   CONCLUSION AND OUTLOOK

From medicine and materials science perspective, the present challenge in bone tissue engineering is to design and fabricate bioactive and biodegradable 3D scaffolds of tailored mechanical stability and biodegradation kinetics, which are able to maintain their integrity for predictable times under load-bearing physiological conditions. As reviewed here, the bioactive and biodegradable man-made CaP/polyester nanocomposites are particularly attractive as bone tissue engineering scaffolds due to their excellent processability, bioactivity, adjustable biodegradation kinetics, and the possibility of biomolecule incorporation. The experimental examples summarized here represented some research efforts aimed at understanding the in vitro mechanical and biological performance of different CaP/polyester composites. The many possibilities for tailor-made biomimetic CaP/polyester nanocomposites have shown this class of composites to have a bright future as bone tissue engineering scaffolds. However, substantial research efforts are still required, in particular to address the following key challenges:

- To better understand the in vivo behavior of nano-CaP/polyester systems.
- Fabrication of polyester composites with the anisotropic CaP nanoparticles of complex geometries (e.g., nanofibers, dandelion structure, or plate-like particles) to additionally improve the mechanical strength of the resulting scaffolds.
- Evaluation of the real effects of particle characteristics on the composite performance.
- Surface modification of CaP particles by grafting new organic molecules and polymers to increase the interfacial bonding strength without impacting the degradation kinetics and biocompatibility of the final composite.
- To determine and describe the complicated effects of CaPs of different phases and crystallinities on the reactions involved in the biodegradation of CaP/polyester composites.
- Finally, to increase the mechanical integrity of currently available CaP/polyester nanocomposites to at least that of cancellous or cortical bone. Indeed, achieving the mechanical properties of the natural bone, for example by the development of new CaP geometries, not only improves the performance of current bone scaffolds, but also may allow replacing bigger sections of damaged bone tissue than what is possible today.

In addition to these challenges, a comprehensive study on the interactions between bone cells and surface of different CaP/polyester systems has yet to be conducted. This is particularly important as it has been proposed that surface texture and surface chemistry can alter cell behavior at many levels. Furthermore, incorporation of biomolecules into the nanocomposite scaffolds is important for determining the potential of the scaffold to further accelerate bone healing. Such studies would also determine some strategies to incorporate osteogenic cells into the porous nanocomposites. Moreover, development of biodegradable polyesters with new compositions (e.g., novel PHA copolymers) can also be another interesting challenge for future research.

REFERENCES

1. Capanna, R., Campanacci, D. A., Belot, N. et al. 2007. A new reconstructive technique for intercalary defects of long bones: The association of massive allograft with vascularized fibular autograft. Long-term results and comparison with alternative techniques. *Orthop. Clin. North Am.* 38: 51–60.
2. McGarvey, W. C. and Braly, W. G. 1996. Bone graft in hindfoot arthrodesis: Allograft vs autograft. *Orthopedics* 19: 389–394.
3. Petricca, S. E., Marra, K. G. and Kumta, P. N. 2006. Chemical synthesis of poly(lactic-co-glycolic acid)/hydroxyapatite composites for orthopaedic applications. *Acta Biomater.* 2: 277–286.

4. Bhumiratana, S., Grayson, W. L., Castaneda, A. et al. 2011. Nucleation and growth of mineralized bone matrix on silk-hydroxyapatite composite scaffolds. *Biomaterials* 32: 2812–2820.
5. Ben-David, D., Kizhner, T., Livne, E. and Srouji, S. 2010. A tissue-like construct of human bone marrow MSCs composite scaffold support in vivo ectopic bone formation. *J. Tissue Eng. Regen. Med.* 4: 30–37.
6. Sadat-Shojai, M., Khorasani, M.-T., Jamshidi, A. and Irani, S. 2013. Nano-hydroxyapatite reinforced polyhydroxybutyrate composites: A comprehensive study on the structural and in vitro biological properties. *Mater. Sci. Eng. C* 33: 2776–2287.
7. Sadat-Shojai, M., Khorasani, M.-T. and Jamshidi, A. 2015. 3-Dimensional cell-laden nano-hydroxyapatite/protein hydrogels for bone regeneration applications. *Mater. Sci. Eng. C* 49: 835–843.
8. Rezwan, K., Chen, Q., Blaker, J. and Boccaccini, A. R. 2006. Biodegradable and bioactive porous polymer/inorganic composite scaffolds for bone tissue engineering. *Biomaterials* 27: 3413–3431.
9. Tong, H.-W. and Wang, M. 2011. Electrospinning of poly (hydroxybutyrate-co-hydroxyvalerate) fibrous scaffolds for tissue engineering applications: Effects of electrospinning parameters and solution properties. *J. Macromol. Sci. B* 50: 1535–1558.
10. Badylak, S. F. 2005. Regenerative medicine and developmental biology: The role of the extracellular matrix. *Anat. Rec. (Part B: New Anat.)* 287: 36–41.
11. Duan, B. and Wang, M. 2010. Customized Ca–P/PHBV nanocomposite scaffolds for bone tissue engineering: Design, fabrication, surface modification and sustained release of growth factor. *J. R. Soc. Interface* 7: S615–S629.
12. Sadat-Shojai, M. 2010. *Hydroxyapatite: Inorganic Nanoparticles of Bone (Properties, Applications, and Preparation Methodologies).* Tehran, Iran: Iranian Students Book Agency (ISBA) (in Persian).
13. Teixeira, S., Rodriguez, M., Pena, P. et al. 2009. Physical characterization of hydroxyapatite porous scaffolds for tissue engineering. *Mater. Sci. Eng. C* 29: 1510–1514.
14. Seol, Y.-J., Kim, J. Y., Park, E. K., Kim, S.-Y. and Cho, D.-W. 2009. Fabrication of a hydroxyapatite scaffold for bone tissue regeneration using microstereolithography and molding technology. *Microelectron. Eng.* 86: 1443–1446.
15. Ogino, M., Ohuchi, F. and Hench, L. L. 1980. Compositional dependence of the formation of calcium phosphate films on bioglass. *J. Biomed. Mater. Res.* 14: 55–64.
16. Sadat-Shojai, M., Khorasani, M.-T., Dinpanah-Khoshdargi, E. and Jamshidi, A. 2013. Synthesis methods for nanosized hydroxyapatite with diverse structures. *Acta Biomater.* 9: 7591–7621.
17. Malmberg, P. and Nygren, H. 2008. Methods for the analysis of the composition of bone tissue, with a focus on imaging mass spectrometry (TOF-SIMS). *Proteomics* 8: 3755–3762.
18. Batchelar, D. L., Davidson, M. T., Dabrowski, W. and Cunningham, I. A. 2006. Bone-composition imaging using coherent-scatter computed tomography: Assessing bone health beyond bone mineral density. *Med. Phys.* 33: 904–915.
19. Murugan, R. and Ramakrishna, S. 2005. Development of nanocomposites for bone grafting. *Compos. Sci. Technol.* 65: 2385–2406.
20. O'Hare, P., Meenan, B. J., Burke, G. A. et al. 2010. Biological responses to hydroxyapatite surfaces deposited via a co-incident microblasting technique. *Biomaterials* 31: 515–522.
21. Habibovic, P., Kruyt, M. C., Juhl, M. V. et al. 2008. Comparative in vivo study of six hydroxyapatite-based bone graft substitutes. *J. Orthop. Res.* 26: 1363–1370.
22. Sadat-Shojai, M., Khorasani, M.-T. and Jamshidi, A. 2012. Hydrothermal processing of hydroxyapatite nanoparticles: A Taguchi experimental design approach. *J. Cryst. Growth* 361: 73–84.

23. Cai, Y., Liu, Y., Yan, W. et al. 2007. Role of hydroxyapatite nanoparticle size in bone cell proliferation. *J. Mater. Chem.* 17: 3780–3787.
24. Wang, Y., Liu, L. and Guo, S. 2010. Characterization of biodegradable and cytocompatible nano-hydroxyapatite/polycaprolactone porous scaffolds in degradation in vitro. *Polym. Degrad. Stab.* 95: 207–213.
25. Dong, Z., Li, Y. and Zou, Q. 2009. Degradation and biocompatibility of porous nano-hydroxyapatite/polyurethane composite scaffold for bone tissue engineering. *Appl. Surf. Sci.* 255: 6087–6091.
26. Wang, L. and Nancollas, G. H. 2009. Pathways to biomineralization and biodemineralization of calcium phosphates: The thermodynamic and kinetic controls. *Dalton Trans.* 15: 2665–2672.
27. Li, B., Guo, B., Fan, H. and Zhang, X. 2008. Preparation of nano-hydroxyapatite particles with different morphology and their response to highly malignant melanoma cells in vitro. *Appl. Surf. Sci.* 255: 357–360.
28. Kamakura, S., Sasano, Y., Shimizu, T. et al. 2002. Implanted octacalcium phosphate is more resorbable than β-tricalcium phosphate and hydroxyapatite. *J. Biomed. Mater. Res.* 59: 29–34.
29. Zhou, H., Nabiyouni, M., Lin, B. and Bhaduri, S. B. 2013. Fabrication of novel poly (lactic acid)/amorphous magnesium phosphate bionanocomposite fibers for tissue engineering applications via electrospinning. *Mater. Sci. Eng. C* 33: 2302–2310.
30. Combes, C. and Rey, C. 2010. Amorphous calcium phosphates: Synthesis, properties and uses in biomaterials. *Acta Biomater.* 6: 3362–3378.
31. Ma, Z., Chen, F., Zhu, Y.-J., Cui, T. and Liu, X.-Y. 2011. Amorphous calcium phosphate/poly (D,L-lactic acid) composite nanofibers: Electrospinning preparation and biomineralization. *J. Colloid Interface Sci.* 359: 371–379.
32. Sadat-Shojai, M. 2009. Preparation of hydroxyapatite nanoparticles: Comparison between hydrothermal and solvo-treatment processes and colloidal stability of produced nanoparticles in a dilute experimental dental adhesive. *J. Iran. Chem. Soc.* 6: 386–392.
33. Sadat-Shojai, M., Atai, M. and Nodehi, A. 2011. Design of experiments (DOE) for the optimization of hydrothermal synthesis of hydroxyapatite nanoparticles. *J. Braz. Chem. Soc.* 22: 571–582.
34. Kostopoulos, L. and Karring, T. 1994. Guided bone regeneration in mandibular defects in rats using a bioresorbable polymer. *Clin. Oral Implants Res.* 5: 66–74.
35. Gogolewski, S., Jovanovic, M., Perren, S., Dillon, J. and Hughes, M. 1993. Tissue response and in vivo degradation of selected polyhydroxyacids: Polylactides (PLA), poly(3-hydroxybutyrate)(PHB), and poly (3-hydroxybutyrate-co-3-hydroxyvalerate) (PHB/VA). *J. Biomed. Mater. Res.* 27: 1135–1148.
36. Chen, G.-Q. and Wu, Q. 2005. The application of polyhydroxyalkanoates as tissue engineering materials. *Biomaterials* 26: 6565–6578.
37. Lee, B. N., Kim, D. Y., Kang, H. J. et al. 2012. In vivo biofunctionality comparison of different topographic PLLA scaffolds. *J. Biomed. Mater. Res. A* 100: 1751–1760.
38. Lao, L., Wang, Y., Zhu, Y., Zhang, Y. and Gao, C. 2011. Poly (lactide-co-glycolide)/hydroxyapatite nanofibrous scaffolds fabricated by electrospinning for bone tissue engineering. *J. Mater. Sci. Mater. Med.* 22: 1873–1884.
39. Köse, G. T., Korkusuz, F., Korkusuz, P. et al. 2003. Bone generation on PHBV matrices: An in vitro study. *Biomaterials* 24: 4999–5007.
40. Kumarasuriyar, A., Jackson, R., Grøndahl, L. et al. 2005. Poly (β-hydroxybutyrate-co-β-hydroxyvalerate) supports in vitro osteogenesis. *Tissue Eng.* 11: 1281–1295.
41. Hutmacher, D. W. 2000. Scaffolds in tissue engineering bone and cartilage. *Biomaterials* 21: 2529–2543.
42. Seal, B., Otero, T. and Panitch, A. 2001. Polymeric biomaterials for tissue and organ regeneration. *Mat. Sci. Eng. R* 34: 147–230.

43. Jiang, L., Zhang, J. and Wolcott, M. P. 2007. Comparison of polylactide/nano-sized calcium carbonate and polylactide/montmorillonite composites: Reinforcing effects and toughening mechanisms. *Polymer* 48: 7632–7644.
44. Kim, K., Yu, M., Zong, X. et al. 2003. Control of degradation rate and hydrophilicity in electrospun non-woven poly (D, L-lactide) nanofiber scaffolds for biomedical applications. *Biomaterials* 24: 4977–4985.
45. Aslan, S., Calandrelli, L., Laurienzo, P., Malinconico, M. and Migliaresi, C. 2000. Poly (D, L-lactic acid)/poly (ε-caprolactone) blend membranes: Preparation and morphological characterisation. *J. Mater. Sci.* 35: 1615–1622.
46. Maglio, G., Migliozzi, A., Palumbo, R., Immirzi, B. and Volpe, M. G. 1999. Compatibilized poly (ε-caprolactone)/poly (l-lactide) blends for biomedical uses. *Macromol. Rapid Commun.* 20: 236–238.
47. Kuo, S. W., Huang, C. F., Tung, Y. C. and Chang, F. C. 2006. Effect of bisphenol A on the miscibility, phase morphology, and specific interaction in immiscible biodegradable poly (ε-caprolactone)/poly (L-lactide) blends. *J. Appl. Polym. Sci.* 100: 1146–1161.
48. Pitt, G., Gratzl, M., Kimmel, G., Surles, J. and Sohindler, A. 1981. Aliphatic polyesters II. The degradation of poly (DL-lactide), poly (ε-caprolactone), and their copolymers in vivo. *Biomaterials* 2: 215–220.
49. Doi, Y., Kitamura, S. and Abe, H. 1995. Microbial synthesis and characterization of poly (3-hydroxybutyrate-co-3-hydroxyhexanoate). *Macromolecules* 28: 4822–4828.
50. Anderson, A. J. and Dawes, E. A. 1990. Occurrence, metabolism, metabolic role, and industrial uses of bacterial polyhydroxyalkanoates. *Microbiol. Rev.* 54: 450–472.
51. Fukada, E. and Ando, Y. 1986. Piezoelectric properties of poly-β-hydroxybutyrate and copolymers of β-hydroxybutyrate and β-hydroxyvalerate. *Int. J. Biol. Macromol.* 8: 361–366.
52. Misra, S. K., Nazhat, S. N., Valappil, S. P. et al. 2007. Fabrication and characterization of biodegradable poly (3-hydroxybutyrate) composite containing bioglass. *Biomacromolecules* 8: 2112–2119.
53. Zhao, Y., Zou, B., Shi, Z., Wu, Q. and Chen, G.-Q. 2007. The effect of 3-hydroxybutyrate on the in vitro differentiation of murine osteoblast MC3T3-E1 and in vivo bone formation in ovariectomized rats. *Biomaterials* 28: 3063–3073.
54 Reusch, R. N. 1995. Low molecular weight complexed poly (3-hydroxybutyrate): A dynamic and versatile molecule in vivo. *Can. J. Microbiol.* 41: 50–54.
55. Doyle, C., Tanner, E. and Bonfield, W. 1991. In vitro and in vivo evaluation of polyhydroxybutyrate and of polyhydroxybutyrate reinforced with hydroxyapatite. *Biomaterials* 12: 841–847.
56. Sultana, N. and Khan, T. H. 2012. In vitro degradation of PHBV scaffolds and nHA/PHBV composite scaffolds containing hydroxyapatite nanoparticles for bone tissue engineering. *J. Nanomater.* 2012: 1–12.
57. Luzier, W. D. 1992. Materials derived from biomass/biodegradable materials. *Proc. Natl. Acad. Sci.* 89(3): 839–842.
58. Holland, S., Jolly, A., Yasin, M. and Tighe, B. 1987. Polymers for biodegradable medical devices: II. Hydroxybutyrate-hydroxyvalerate copolymers: Hydrolytic degradation studies. *Biomaterials* 8: 289–295.
59. Chaikof, E. L., Matthew, H., Kohn, J. et al. 2002. Biomaterials and scaffolds in reparative medicine. *Ann. NY Acad. Sci.* 961: 96–105.
60. Kim, H.-W., Knowles, J. C. and Kim, H.-E. 2005. Hydroxyapatite porous scaffold engineered with biological polymer hybrid coating for antibiotic Vancomycin release. *J. Mater. Sci. Mater. Med.* 16: 189–195.
61. LeGeros, R. Z. and LeGeros, J. P. 1999. Dense hydroxyapatite. In *An Introduction to Bioceramics*, eds. L. L. Hench and J. Wilson, pp. 139–180. Singapore: Word Scientific.

62. Hench, L. L. 1999. Bioactive glasses and glasses-ceramics. In *Bioceramics-Applications of Ceramic and Glass Materials in Medicine*, ed. J. F. Shackelford, 37–64. Switzerland: Trans Tech Publication.

63. Kim, H.-W., Lee, E.-J., Kim, H.-E., Salih, V. and Knowles, J. C. 2005. Effect of fluoridation of hydroxyapatite in hydroxyapatite-polycaprolactone composites on osteoblast activity. *Biomaterials* 26: 4395–4404.

64. Pan, J., Han, X., Niu, W. and Cameron, R. E. 2011. A model for biodegradation of composite materials made of polyesters and tricalcium phosphates. *Biomaterials* 32: 2248–2255.

65. Li, H. and Chang, J. 2005. pH-compensation effect of bioactive inorganic fillers on the degradation of PLGA. *Compos. Sci. Technol.* 65: 2226–2232.

66. Alexandre, M. and Dubois, P. 2000. Polymer-layered silicate nanocomposites: Preparation, properties and uses of a new class of materials. *Mat. Sci. Eng. R* 28: 1–63.

67. Filová, E., Suchý, T., Sucharda, Z. et al. 2014. Support for the initial attachment, growth and differentiation of MG-63 cells: A comparison between nano-size hydroxyapatite and micro-size hydroxyapatite in composites. *Int. J. Nanomed.* 9: 3687–3706.

68. Heo, S. J., Kim, S. E., Wei, J. et al. 2009. Fabrication and characterization of novel nano- and micro-HA/PCL composite scaffolds using a modified rapid prototyping process. *J. Biomed. Mater. Res. A* 89: 108–116.

69. Balik, K., Suchy, T., Sucharda, Z. et al. 2008. Effect of nano/micro particles of calcium phosphates on the mechanical properties of composites based on polysiloxane matrix reinforced by polyamide. *Ceram. Silik.* 52: 205–300.

70. Webster, T. J., Ergun, C., Doremus, R. H., Siegel, R. W. and Bizios, R. 2000. Enhanced functions of osteoblasts on nanophase ceramics. *Biomaterials* 21: 1803–1810.

71. Jack, K. S., Velayudhan, S., Luckman, P. et al. 2009. The fabrication and characterization of biodegradable HA/PHBV nanoparticle–polymer composite scaffolds. *Acta Biomater.* 5: 2657–2667.

72. Cai, L., Guinn, A. S. and Wang, S. 2011. Exposed hydroxyapatite particles on the surface of photo-crosslinked nanocomposites for promoting MC3T3 cell proliferation and differentiation. *Acta Biomater.* 7: 2185–2199.

73. Kim, S. E., Choi, H. W., Lee, H. J. et al. 2008. Designing a highly bioactive 3D bone-regenerative scaffold by surface immobilization of nano-hydroxyapatite. *J. Mater. Chem.* 18: 4994–5001.

74. Sun, F., Koh, K., Ryu, S.-C., Han, D.-W. and Lee, J. 2012. Biocompatibility of nanoscale hydroxyapatite-embedded chitosan films. *B Korean Chem. Soc.* 33: 3950–3956.

75. Moczo, J. and Pukanszky, B. 2008. Polymer micro and nanocomposites: Structure, interactions, properties. *J. Ind. Eng. Chem.* 14: 535–563.

76. Kokubo, T. and Takadama, H. 2006. How useful is SBF in predicting in vivo bone bioactivity? *Biomaterials* 27: 2907–2915.

77. Ni, J. and Wang, M. 2002. In vitro evaluation of hydroxyapatite reinforced polyhydroxybutyrate composite. *Mater. Sci. Eng. C* 20: 101–109.

78. Kim, M.-J. and Koh, Y.-H. 2013. Synthesis of aligned porous poly (ε-caprolactone) (PCL)/hydroxyapatite (HA) composite microspheres. *Mater. Sci. Eng. C* 33: 2266–2272.

79. Ribeiro, N., Sousa, S. and Monteiro, F. 2010. Influence of crystallite size of nanophased hydroxyapatite on fibronectin and osteonectin adsorption and on MC3T3-E1 osteoblast adhesion and morphology. *J. Coll. Interface Sci.* 351: 398–406.

80. Cool, S., Kenny, B., Wu, A. et al. 2007. Poly (3-hydroxybutyrate-co-3-hydroxyvalerate) composite biomaterials for bone tissue regeneration: In vitro performance assessed by osteoblast proliferation, osteoclast adhesion and resorption, and macrophage proinflammatory response. *J. Biomed. Mater. Res. A* 82: 599–610.

81. Rehfeldt, F., Engler, A. J., Eckhardt, A., Ahmed, F. and Discher, D. E. 2007. Cell responses to the mechanochemical microenvironment: Implications for regenerative medicine and drug delivery. *Adv. Drug Deli. Rev.* 59: 1329–1339.

82. Sadat-Shojai, M., Atai, M., Nodehi, A. and Khanlar, L. N. 2010. Hydroxyapatite nanorods as novel fillers for improving the properties of dental adhesives: Synthesis and application. *Dent. Mater.* 26: 471–482.

83. Sadat-Shojai, M., Atai, M. and Nodehi, A. 2013. Method for production of biocompatible nanoparticles containing dental adhesive. US Patent 8,357,732.

84. Li, J., Lu, X. and Zheng, Y. 2008. Effect of surface modified hydroxyapatite on the tensile property improvement of HA/PLA composite. *Appl. Surf. Sci.* 255: 494–497.

85. Hong, Z., Zhang, P., He, C. et al. 2005. Nano-composite of poly (L-lactide) and surface grafted hydroxyapatite: Mechanical properties and biocompatibility. *Biomaterials* 26: 6296–6304.

86. Diao, H., Si, Y., Zhu, A., Ji, L. and Shi, H. 2012. Surface modified nano-hydroxyapatite/poly (lactide acid) composite and its osteocyte compatibility. *Mater. Sci. Eng. C* 32: 1796–1801.

87. Bergmann, A. and Owen, A. 2003. Hydroxyapatite as a filler for biosynthetic PHB homopolymer and P (HB–HV) copolymers. *Polym. Int.* 52: 1145–1152.

88. Pandey, J. K., Raghunatha Reddy, K., Pratheep Kumar, A. and Singh, R. 2005. An overview on the degradability of polymer nanocomposites. *Polym. Degrad. Stab.* 88: 234–250.

89. Dunn, A. S., Campbell, P. G. and Marra, K. G. 2001. The influence of polymer blend composition on the degradation of polymer/hydroxyapatite biomaterials. *J. Mater. Sci. Mater. Med.* 12: 673–677.

90. Sun, H., Mei, L., Song, C., Cui, X. and Wang, P. 2006. The in vivo degradation, absorption and excretion of PCL-based implant. *Biomaterials* 27: 1735–1740.

91. Hasırcı, V., Lewandrowski, K., Gresser, J., Wise, D. and Trantolo, D. 2001. Versatility of biodegradable biopolymers: Degradability and an in vivo application. *J. Biotechnol.* 86: 135–150.

92. Bergsma, J., Rozema, F., Bos, R. et al. 1995. In vivo degradation and biocompatibility study of in vitro pre-degraded as-polymerized polylactide particles. *Biomaterials* 16: 267–274.

93. Li, S. 2006. Degradation of biodegradable aliphatic polyesters. In *Scaffolding in Tissue Engineering*, ed. P. X. Ma and J. Elisseeff, 335–352. Taylor & Francis: Boca Raton, FL.

94. Yeo, A., Rai, B., Sju, E., Cheong, J. and Teoh, S. 2008. The degradation profile of novel, bioresorbable PCL–TCP scaffolds: An in vitro and in vivo study. *J. Biomed. Mater. Res. A* 84: 208–218.

95. Tracy, M., Ward, K., Firouzabadian, L. et al. 1999. Factors affecting the degradation rate of poly (lactide-co-glycolide) microspheres in vivo and in vitro. *Biomaterials* 20: 1057–1062.

2 Biodegradable Nanocomposites for Imaging, Tissue-Repairing, and Drug-Delivery Applications

Congming Xiao

CONTENTS

2.1 INTRODUCTION

Biomaterial science is an interdisciplinary field. During its development, various kinds of newly emerging concepts such as self-assembly and nanotechnology have been introduced into this field. As a result, *biomaterial* has been redefined again and again [1,2]. By taking the advantages of nanotechnology and biodegradable polymers, biodegradable nanocomposites (BNCs) are prepared and applied as biomaterials. Most BNCs are employed as matrices of drug release, scaffolds of tissue repairing, or carriers of imaging agents. In order to make the status, basic concepts, and methods of BNCs easy to understand, a series of questions and answers is presented.

2.1.1 WHAT ARE THE KEY COMPONENTS FOR DEVELOPING BNCs?

Biodegradable polymeric and inorganic substances are two kinds of components utilized to generate biodegradable polymer-based nanocomposites. Both natural and synthetic polymers are biodegradable [3–5]. To be a good candidate for biomedical application, an available or synthetic polymer must possess excellent biocompatibility and biofunctionality [6]. Usually, polymers are used as the dispersing matrix or surface coating. Inorganic substances constitute another phase of BNCs and exhibit their individual function. They are summarized in Table 2.1.

It can be anticipated that polymers and inorganic substances can be combined in numerous ways. Then, how can BNCs be formed and what are the details of the obtained system?

2.1.2 WHAT ARE THE GENERAL APPROACHES TO PREPARING BNCs?

Biodegradable nanocomposites are obtained through physical or chemical combination [12–15] of inorganic and polymeric components. Accordingly, the particles may be conjugated with the polymer chains or dispersed in the polymer matrix (Figure 2.1). Both the inorganic nanoparticles and the polymers can be formed in situ or prepared in advance. Therefore, there are a variety of strategies for developing BNCs.

A simple and effective method to disperse inorganic particles in polymer is solution blending and subsequent solvent evaporation or emulsion encapsulation. The polymers applied for the encapsulation process are pre-made and obtained via polymerization of monomer in the dispersion media. The encapsulation efficiency of the emulsion process can be modulated by varying the emulsion system, such as mini-, micro-, or double ones [14,15]. In addition,

---

TABLE 2.1
Possible Polymeric and Inorganic Components for BNC

Polymers		Inorganic Nanoparticles [7–11]	
Natural	**Synthetic [4]**	**Substances**	**Intrinsic Properties**
Polysaccharides:	Polyesters: $[R-CO-O]_n$	Hydoxyapatite: $Ca_{10}(PO_4)_6(OH)_2$	Bioactive
	Polycarbonates: $[R-O-CO-O]_n$	Ferroferric oxide: Fe_3O_4	Superparamagnetic
	Polyanhydrides: $[R-CO-O-CO]_n$	Quantum dot	Fluorescent
Protein-based polymers: $[NH-CRR'-CO]_n$	Polyurethanes: $[R-NH-CO-O]_n$	Gold	Optical, sensing
	Polyethers: $[R-O]_n$	Silica	Biocompatible
	Polyaminoacids: $[NH-CHR-CO]_n$	Carbon nanotube	Photothermal

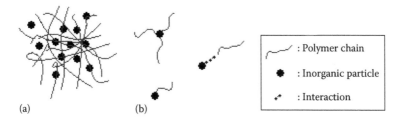

(a)   (b)

⌐⁓	: Polymer chain
●	: Inorganic particle
⸰⁺	: Interaction

FIGURE 2.1 Morphology of biodegradable nanocomposites: (a) dispersed and (b) conjugated.

the electrostatic interaction between charged inorganic nanoparticles, acting as seeds, and oppositely charged polyelectrolytes makes the layer-by-layer (LbL) technique useful for the development of BNCs [14]. On the other hand, the self-assembly of polymers is also adopted to prepare BNCs. It is found that the hierarchical self-assembly of protein is useful for bottom-up engineering of a wide array of composites, and quantum dots (QDs) can be introduced at different stages of the self-assembly process to controllably vary the morphology of the composites [16]. It is also found that the LbL assembly between a pair of polyelectrolytes is an effective approach to fabricate BNCs. Magnetic alginate microspheres are prepared via the emulsification/internal gelation technique and utilized as substrates. Then, the multilayer composite microspheres are obtained through the alternating LbL assembly of a water-soluble chitosan derivative and alginate [17]. These composites are all prepared through physical process, and the inorganic particles are preformed.

The inorganic particles can also be formed via physical approach during generating composites, which may avoid the tendency of nanoparticles to form agglomerate. The sol–gel processing of nanoparticles within polymer results in the formation of an interpenetrating network between inorganic and organic components, that is, a well-dispersed and stable composite can be obtained in this way. Besides, another promising methodology is the in situ growth of nanoparticles in a polymer matrix, which can be preformed or formed simultaneously via suitable reactions, such as reduction and decomposition, of their respective precursors [15]. Interestingly, the in situ formation of magnetic particles can be conducted easily and rapidly under mild conditions. Alginate-g-poly(vinyl alcohol) (PVA) is physically crosslinked with ferrous ions to form microparticles through emulsification/internal gelation, and the microparticles are transformed into ferromagnetic microparticles via a self-oxidation procedure within minutes [18]. The aforementioned physical fabrication processes of BNCs are illustrated in Figure 2.2.

The chemical approach, that is, coupling the two components via covalent linkage, is an effective strategy to achieve nanocomposites, which provide good dispersion stability of inorganic nanoparticles in the polymer matrices [12,15]. Generally, it is carried out through different reactions between the active sites on the inorganic particles and the reactive groups contained on the polymer chains. The common reactions between functional groups, such as amine and carboxyl groups, are available. On the other hand, Click chemistry, including copper (I)-catalyzed

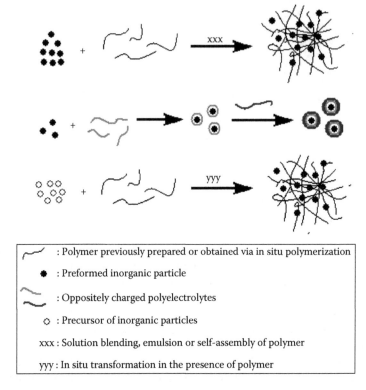

: Polymer previously prepared or obtained via in situ polymerization

: Preformed inorganic particle

: Oppositely charged polyelectrolytes

: Precursor of inorganic particles

xxx : Solution blending, emulsion or self-assembly of polymer

yyy : In situ transformation in the presence of polymer

FIGURE 2.2   Formation of physical biodegradable nanocomposites.

alkeyne-azide cycloaddition, thiol-ene reaction, and Diels–Alder reaction, has been paid growing attention for chemically forming BNCs recently [13,19]. The reactions between the polymer and inorganic nanoparticles are usually classified as graft-to and graft-from strategies. Graft-to strategy means functional-group-terminated polymers react with an appropriate surface of the particles (a), while graft-from implies polymer chains are grown from an initiator-immobilized surface of the particles (b) [12,15]. In fact, several steps may be involved in either strategy. The chemical approaches are briefly shown in Figure 2.3.

Evidently, both physical and chemical ways have their individual advantages and shortcomings. There is room for improving the preparation method. For example, one-pot methodology is presented to synthesize PVA/ZnO QD nanocomposites, which does not need the steps of separation and purification of QDs [20]. In addition, both components of BNCs are probably all polymeric ones. Nevertheless, what should be taken seriously is that the targeted nanocomposites are for biomedical applications. No matter what strategy is adopted for preparation, the obtained nanocomposite should meet the basic requirements, such as biocompatibility, of biomedical applications. Consequently, the next question is, what are the potential applications of BNCs?

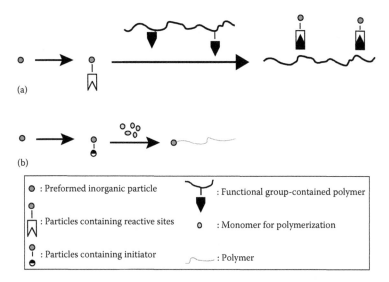

(a)

(b)

◉ : Preformed inorganic particle	: Functional group-contained polymer
: Particles containing reactive sites	o : Monomer for polymerization
: Particles containing initiator	: Polymer

FIGURE 2.3 Formation of chemical biodegradable nanocomposites. (a) Graft-to strategy and (b) graft-from way.

2.2 WHAT ARE THE COMMON APPLICATIONS OF BNCs?

The applications of BNCs have focused on three fields, including drug delivery, tissue repairing, and imaging. Recently, the development of BNCs has resulted in the formation of a new sub discipline, named nanomedicine.

2.2.1 HOW CAN BNCs BE APPLIED TO TISSUE REPAIRING?

Hydroxyapatite (HA) has excellent biocompatibility, bioactivity, and osteoconductivity, but its mechanical properties are poor [8]. Biodegradable polymers possess structural continuity and design flexibility [21]. By combining the advantages of both components, BNCs containing HA nanoparticles are suitable for orthopedic reconstruction. Poly(propylene fumarate) (PPF) is a biodegradable unsaturated polyester. It is subjected to a radical crosslinking reaction with N-vinyl pyrrolidone in the presence of HA nanoparticles to form a thermoset nanocomposite. The in vivo femoral bone repair, which has been carried out on a rabbit animal model, indicates that the HA/PPF nanocomposite is both biocompatible and osteocompatible [8].

Bone tissue engineering (BTE) is an attractive alternative to bone tissue reconstruction. One of the prerequisites for BTE is the design of an ideal scaffold. Such a 3D material should resemble as much as possible the morphology of natural bone. Natural bone is actually a nanocomposite of HA and collagen. Thus, nanocomposites made of HA and polymers have being developed as the template for BTE [22]. To develop tissue-engineered bone substitute that can mimic the structural, mechanical, and biological properties of natural bone, a composite composed of polyvinyl alcohol (PVA), collagen, and HA nanoparticles is prepared.

The nanostructure and composition of this composite are similar to that of bone and can be applied as a scaffold for BTE [23]. Polygalacturonic acid (PgA) is de-esterified pectin, a plant polysaccharide, and can form complex with chitosan in solution since they are electrostatically complementary. Accordingly, PgA/chitosan/HA nanocomposite is synthesized through in situ mineralization and shows higher mechanical properties than those of binary ones [24]. Mechanical properties, biocompatibility, and tunable biodegradability are critical for a nanocomposite for BTE. In order to develop such a kind of nanocomposites, fumarate-based copolyesters are in situ polymerized with HA. The experimental results show that the nanocomposites are mechanically favorable, bioactive, and biodegradable, and they are regarded as a promising candidate for orthopedic applications [25]. By taking advantage of the formability of polymer and the bioactivity of HA, a triblock copolymer of L-lactide and ε-caprolactone is mixed with HA nanoparticles to fabricate nanocomposite scaffold by using solution casting, gas foaming, and salt leaching techniques. The resultant nanocomposite is thought to be a good bone substitute [26]. In addition, other biodegradable polymers such as aliphatic polyesters are also utilized to prepare nanocomposites with tunable properties for tissue engineering [27].

BNC scaffolds can be considered analogues of extracellular matrix (ECM). The artificial ECMs possessing biocompatibility, controlled biodegradability and porosity, and surface adhesion capability are reliable alternatives in the regeneration of new tissue. They are not only used for BTE, but also suitable for reconstructing cartilage, vascular, neural, bladder, and intraocular lens [28–30]. All components of the nanocomposites are cellulose, and their derivatives are particularly suitable for creating artificial blood vessel [30]. The compositions and roles of BNCs in tissue reconstruction are outlined in Figure 2.4.

2.2.2 How Can BNCs Be Applied to Drug Delivery?

Due to the enhanced permeability and retention effect, nanosized drug-delivery systems (NDDS) exhibit improved therapeutic properties and reduced adverse effects. NDDS hold great promise for delivering drug to the desired site of action. In fact, some NDDS have been approved for clinical applications.

The surface plasmon resonance effect of gold nanoparticles offers BNCs light responsiveness. By taking advantage of the biocompatibility of hydrogels and the inherent properties of inorganic nanoparticles, the obtained BNCs can exhibit some

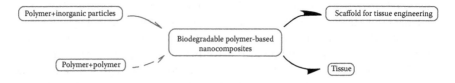

FIGURE 2.4 Tissue-repairing application of biodegradable nanocomposites.

interesting characteristics and are biocompatible simultaneously. κ-Carrageenan, a kind of water-soluble sulfated polysaccharide, has the ability to form thermo-reversible hydrogel. Accordingly, gold nanoparticles with variable shapes blend with κ-carrageenan to form hydrogel nanocomposites. The release of model drug from the nanocomposites follows either a diffusion or a polymer relaxation mechanism, which is modulated with the morphology of gold nanoparticles. In the incorporation of nano-gold, κ-carrageenan hydrogel/Au is a potentially remotely controlled light-triggered NDDS [31]. Besides gold nanoparticles, carbon nanotube and superpara-magnetic iron oxide nanoparticles (SPION) are promising candidates to combine with various conventional or stimuli-responsive hydrogels for constructing remotely controlled NDDS [32,33]. Application of a high-frequency alternating magnetic field (AMF) to nanocomposite containing SPION results in uniform heating within the nanocomposite. Polymer or copolymer of N-isopropylacrylamide (NIPAM) is negative temperature sensitive. Magnetic NIPAM-based hydrogel nanocomposite, which is prepared by crosslinking NIPAM with tetra(ethylene glycol) dimethacry-late in the presence of SPION, will collapse when it is subjected to AMF due to a rise in temperature. As a result, the imbibed drug is released [34]. Though poly(N-isopropylacrylamide) is not biodegradable, this is a way to trigger the on-demand pulsatile drug release. Actually, there are several temperature-responsive natural polymers such as gelatin, collagen, methylcellulose (MC), and hydroxypropylcel-lulose (HPC) [35]. The hydrogel nanocomposites obtained from these polymers belong to real BNCs indeed.

BNCs obtained from all polymeric components show favorable processability, excellent biocompatibility, and controllable biodegradability. They are promising candidates for the development of NDDS. A nanocomposite is prepared through electrostatic interaction between γ-polyglutamic acid and polyethylenimine (PEI). The ability to protect pDNA, cell viability, and transfection efficiency of the polypeptide-based BNCs are evaluated, and the results demonstrate that the system is effective for in vivo gene delivery [36]. A composite nanogel containing anticancer drug is synthesized to accomplish deep tumor penetration. The nano-gel, which is prepared from N-lysinal-N-succinyl chitosan, NIPAM, and bovine serum albumin, has core-shell structure. Such a nanogel shows pH sensitivity. The variation of physiological conditions triggers the swelling-shrinking of the nanogel and leads to the controlled release of anticancer drug [37]. In view of their individual advantages, a ternary bionanocomposite composed of PVA, cel-lulose crystals (CNC), and poly(D,L-lactide-co-glycolide) (PLGA) nanoparticles is prepared by simply mixing PLGA nanoparticles that are loaded with fluores-cein isothiocynate–labelled bovine serum albumin with PVA and CNC. PVA/CNC/PLAG is considered an effective NDDS for therapeutic application [38].

As mentioned in Section 2.2, incorporation of inorganic nanoparticles usually makes polymer responsive to environmental stimuli. By combining inorganic par-ticles with smart polymers, a multi responsive composite can be formed. Triple-responsive MC/Fe-Alg-g-PVA/PVA/Fe$_3$O$_4$ hydrogel composite is prepared by physical crosslinking and in situ self-oxidation. The obtained composite microgels show pH-, temperature-, and magnetism-sensitive release behavior [39]. Due to the intrinsic

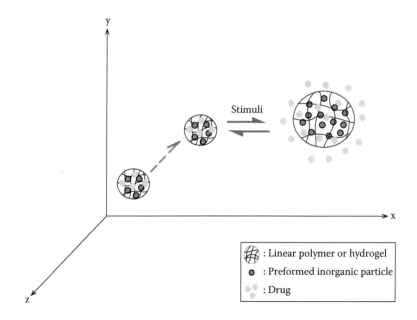

FIGURE 2.5   Drug-delivery application of biodegradable nanocomposites.

properties of inorganic nanoparticles, BNCs are usually sensitive to the environmental stimuli, which exhibits responsive drug delivery, as shown in Figure 2.5.

2.2.3 How Can BNCs Be Applied to Imaging?

Noninvasive diagnosis and real-time monitoring of therapy become more and more important in practical biomedical applications. In other words, imaging technologies are essential for the development of biomaterials science [40,41]. Particularly, many inorganic nanoparticles exhibit optical and magnetic characteristics, which enable them to engineer BNCs for imaging tissue response, visualizing tissue integration, or tracking cells and other purposes.

In view of the advantages such as excellent temporal and spatial resolution, rapid in vivo acquisition of images, and long effective imaging window, magnetic resonance imaging (MRI) has received growing attention recently. Usually, contrast agents are applied to enhance MRI at tissue, cellular, or molecular levels. SPION is an effective contrast agent for MRI. For in vivo applications, it is necessary for SPION to be well dispersed in water, which is generally achieved by coating it with biocompatible hydrophilic dextran or encapsulating with biocompatible amphiphlic poly(ethylene glycol)-b-poly(ε-caprolactone) (PEG-b-PCL) [42,43]. The gadolinlium diethylenetriaminepentaacetic acid (Gd-DTPA) chelate is also extensively utilized as a contrast agent for MRI, but its imaging time is short and its specificity to target organs is poor. Thus, BNCs containing Gd-DTPA are prepared and show favorable potential in tumor diagnosis. Gd-DTPA-contained BNCs can be obtained through forming complex with dextran or polylysine derivative as well as conjugating with human serum albumin nanoparticles [44].

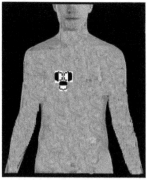 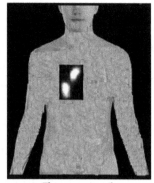

Contrast agent   Fluorescent probe

FIGURE 2.6   Roles of biodegradable nanocomposites played in imaging.

Due to unique properties such as high sensitivity, high selectivity, convenience, diversity, and nondestructive character, fluorescent nanocomposites have been widely applied in biological imaging. Generally, fluorescent nanocomposites can be obtained by embedding inorganic composition inside a polymeric matrix or covalently attaching onto the surface of polymeric nanoparticles [45]. For example, QDs are attractive fluorescent probes for in vitro and in vivo imaging. In order to acquire biocompatibility, biostability, and suitable surface functions, QDs are modified with various strategies such as PEGylation coating or capping with amphiphilic polymers [46]. The emerging fluorescent BNCs may provide new imaging agents with unique properties.

In a word, BNCs are applied to enhance the contrast of related tissues or to exhibit fluorescent patterns (Figure 2.6).

2.2.4   HOW CAN BNCS BE APPLIED TO THERANOSTICS?

Now that nanomaterials are a good tool for imaging or individual drug delivery, they are considered good candidates for application in diagnosis and therapy at the same time, which in turn has led to the development of new nanomaterials for theranostics [9]. A theranostics system integrates the therapeutic and diagnostic functions in a same entity, which provides the possibility to monitor in real time drug release and distribution, to detect diseases, and to assess the effectiveness of treatment promptly [47]. Polymer-based systems for theranostics have been extensively explored during the last decade [48].

SPION, docetaxel (Dtxl) or paclitaxel (PTX), and arginine-glycine-asparatic acid (RGD) or prostate stem cell antigen (PSCA) are MRI contrast agent, anticancer drugs, and tumor-targeting substances, respectively. SPION and Dtxl or PTX are encapsulated with poly(lactide-co-glycolide) (PLGA) by using emulsion-evaporation method. Subsequently, RGD or PSCA is conjugated on the surface of the nanoparticles via functional poly(ethylene glycol) (PEG). The obtained nanocomposites are promising multifunctional BNCs for both cancer therapy and MRI [49,50]. The combination between SPION and polymer can be in chemical way as well. SPION is covalently bonded with doxorubicin (DOX), an antitumor drug,

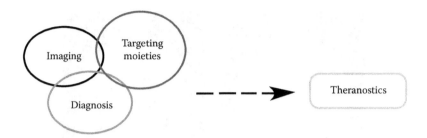

FIGURE 2.7   Formation of merging field for biodegradable nanocomposites.

and PEG via pH-sensitive acylhydrazone linkages. The formulated nanocomposite shows pH-sensitive release and magnetic targeting behavior and is promising for synergistic MRI diagnosis and tumor therapy [51]. Magnetic mesoporous silica nanoparticles (MMSNs) can be directed to the targeted sites. By conjugating MMSNs with tansactivator protein (TAT), nanoparticles can be developed for nuclear-targeted drug delivery. Considering TAT is positively charged at physiological pH, which may lead to undesired side effects, nanoparticles are decorated with a chitosan derivative to temporarily shield the positive charge of TAT. The stability of the nanoparticles is enhanced, and their circulation time in blood is prolonged. As a result, a kind of BNCs for targeting delivery is obtained. In addition, the embedded Fe_3O_4 offers these BNCs the possibility to be used as contrast agent for MRI simultaneously [52].

Nanoparticles such as upconversion nanoparticles and QDs exhibit unique optical characteristics and are useful for bioimaging. By coupling with folic acid or RGD onto PEGylated and doxorubicin-loaded nanoparticles, these nanocomposites show targeted cancer therapy and cell imaging [53]. Integration of magnetic and luminescent properties of inorganic particles, the biocompatibility and stability of polymer, and the targeting capability of specific ligands lead to a multifunctional BNC with tailored properties, which is a promising platform for simultaneous therapy, diagnosis, and real-time monitoring. A chitosan-based nanocomposite is prepared by coating ferroferric oxide nanoparticles with carboxymethyl chitosan (CMCS), subsequently doping with QDs via LbL assembly between CMCS and QDs, and then conjugating with folate. Due to its high drug-loading efficiency, low cytotoxicity, and favorable cell compatibility, such a BNC is a potential candidate for targeted drug delivery and cellular imaging [54].

It is thus clear that the combination of magnetic response and luminescent property enables BNCs to be applied for a new biomedical application, theranostics (Figure 2.7).

2.3   IS THERE ANYTHING TO CONSIDER ABOUT BNCs?

The main goal of designing and preparing BNCs is to explore their biomedical applications. Therefore, the safety of BNCs is a very important issue due to the possible hazard of BNCs to human health and their accumulation in the body [47,55]. Because no exact biocompatibility criteria have been established [56], it is necessary to study the interactions of BNCs and biological systems in detail [57]. Every aspect involved, such as careful purification at the stage of preparing inorganic nanoparticles, release possibility and degree of inorganic nanoparticles from BNCs, and safety evaluation of BNCs for various biomedical applications, should be paid much attention.

Indeed, nanotechnology makes the development of BNCs robust, but the adverse effects of nanomaterials are usually ignored. One should take a lesson from the past development of BNCs, that is, considerable investigation should be taken before introducing a new concept into the biomedical field.

Certainly, the story of BNCs is far from complete. The information for this chapter was acquired from the literatures published 2008–2014. Consequently, the state of the art should be renewed once the progress is reported.

REFERENCES

1. Jandt KD. Revolutions and trends in biomaterials science—A perspective. *Adv Eng Mater* 2007, 9: 1035–1050.
2. Williams DF. On the nature of biomaterials. *Biomaterials* 2009, 30: 5897–5902.
3. Nair LS, Laurencin CT. Biodegradable polymers as biomaterials. *Prog Polym Sci* 2007, 32: 762–798.
4. Ulery BD, Nair LS, Laurencin CT. Biomedical applications of biodegradable polymers. *J Polym Sci Part B: Polym Phys* 2011, 49: 832–864.
5. Tian HY, Tang ZH, Zhuang XL, Chen XS, Jing XB. Biodegradable synthetic polymers: Preparation, functionalization and biomedical application. *Prog Polym Sci* 2012, 37: 237–280.
6. Vert M. Not any new functional polymer can be for medicine: What about artificial biopolymer? *Macromol Biosci* 2011, 11: 1653–1661.
7. Gao JH, Gu HW, Xu B. Multifunctional magnetic nanoparticles: Design, synthesis and biomedical applications. *Acc Chem Res* 2009, 42: 1097–1107.
8. Jayabalan M, Shalumon KT, Mitha MK, Ganesan K, Epple M. Effect of hydroxyapatite on the biodegradation and biomechanical stability of polyester nanocomposites for orthopaedic applications. *Acta Biomater* 2010, 6: 763–775.
9. Barreto JA, O'Malley W, Kubeil M, Graham B, Stephan H, Spiccia L. Nanomaterials: Applications in cancer imaging and therapy. *Adv Mater* 2011, 23: H18–H40.
10. Gaharwar AK, Kishore V, Rivera C, Bullock W, Wu CJ, Akkus O, Schmit G. Physically crosslinked nanocomposites from silicate-crosslinked PEO: Mechanical properties and osteogenic differentiation of human mesenchymal stem cell. *Macromol Sci* 2012, 12: 779–793.
11. Xue XJ, Wang F, Liu XG. Emerging functional nanomaterials for therapeutics. *J Mater Chem* 2011, 21: 13107–13127.
12. Li DX, He Q, Li JB. Smart core/shell nanocomposites: Intelligent polymers modified gold nanoparticles. *Adv Colloid Interface Sci* 2009, 149: 28–38.
13. Erathodiyil N, Ying JY. Functionalization of inorganic nanoparticles for bioimaging applications. *Acc Chem Res* 2011, 44: 925–935.
14. Ladj R, Bitar A, Eissa MM, Fessi H, Mugnier Y, Le Dantec R, Elaissari A. Polymer encapsulation of inorganic nanoparticles for biomedical applications. *Int J Pharm* 2013, 458: 230–241.
15. Kango S, Kalia S, Celli A, Njuguna J, Habibi Y, Kumar R. Surface modification of inorganic nanoparticles for development of organic-inorganic nanocomposite: A review. *Prog Polym Sci* 2013, 38: 1232–1261.

16. Majithia R, Patterson J, Bondos SE, Meissner KE. On the design of composite protein-quantum dot biomaterials via self-assembly. *Biomacromolecules* 2011, 12: 3629–3637.
17. Xiao CM, Sun F. Fabrication of distilled water-soluble chitosan/alginate functional multilayer composite microspheres. *Carbohydr Polym* 2013, 98: 1366–1370.
18. Ma PP, Xiao CM, Li L, Shi HS, Zhu MZ. Facile preparation of ferromagnetic alginate-g-poly(vinyl alcohol) microparticles. *Euro Polym J* 2008, 44: 3886–3889.
19. Thanh NTK, Green LAW. Functionalisation of nanoparticles for biomedical applications. *Nano Today* 2010, 5: 213–230.
20. Gong XH, Tang CY, Pan L, Hao ZH, Tsui CP. Characterization of poly(vinyl alcohol) (PVA)/ZnO nanocomposites prepared by a one-pot method. *Composites Part B* 2014, 60: 144–149.
21. We GB, Ma PX. Nanostructured biomaterials for regeneration. *Adv Funct Mater* 2008, 18: 3568–3582.
22. Chiara G, Letizia F, Lorenzo F, Edoardo S, Diego S, Stefano S, Eriberto B, Barbara Z. Nanostructured biomaterials for tissue engineered bone tissue reconstruction. *Int J Mol Sci* 2012, 13: 737–757.
23. Asran AS, Henning S, Michler GH. Polyvinyl alcohol-collagen-hydroxyapatite biocomposite nanofibrous scaffold: Mimicking the key features of natural bone at the nanoscale level. *Polymer* 2010, 51: 868–876.
24. Verma D, Katti KS, Katti DR, Mohanty B. Mechanical response and multilevel structure of biomimetic hydroxyapatite/polygalacturonic/chitosan nanocomposites. *Mater Sci Eng C* 2008, 28: 399–405.
25. Victor SP, Muthu J. Bioactive, mechanically favorable, and biodegradable copolymer nanocomposites for orthopedic applications. *Mater Sci Eng C* 2014, 39: 150–160.
26. Torabinejad B, Mohammadi-Rovshandeh J, Davachi SM, Zamanian A. Synthesis and characterization of nanocomposite scaffold based on triblock copolymer of L-lactide, ε-caprolactone and nano-hydroxyapatite for bone tissue engineering. *Mater Sci Eng C* 2014, 39: 199–210.
27. Armentano A, Dottori M, Fortunati E, Mattioli S, Kenny JM. Biodegradable polymer matrix nanocomposites for tissue engineering. *Polym Degrad Stab* 2010, 95: 2126–2146.
28. Zhang LJ, Webster TJ. Nanotechnology and nanomaterials: Promises for improved tissue regeneration. *Nano Today* 2009, 4: 66–80.
29. Annaka M, Mortensen K, Matsuura T, Ito M, Nochioka K, Ogata N. Organic-inorganic nanocomposite gels as an in situ gelation biomaterial for injectable accommodative intraocular lens. *Soft Matter* 2012, 8: 3185–3196.
30. Pooyan P, Kim IT, Jacob KI, Tannenbaum R, Garmestani H. Design of a cellulose-based nanocomposite as a potential polymeric scaffold in tissue engineering. *Polymer* 2013, 54: 2105–2114.
31. Salgueiro AM, Daniel-d-Silva AL, Fateixa S, Trindade T. κ-Carrageenan hydrogel nanocomposites with release behavior mediated by morphological distinct Au nanofillers. *Carbohydr Polym* 2013, 91: 100–109.
32. Campkell SB, Hoare T. Externally addressable hydrogel nanocomposites for biomedical applications. *Curr Opin Chem Eng* 2014, 4: 1–10.
33. Satarkar NS, Biswal D, Hilt JZ. Hydrogel nanocomposites: A review of applications as remote controlled biomaterials. *Soft Matter* 2010, 6: 2364–2371.
34. Satarkar NS, Hilt JZ. Magnetic hydrogel nanocomposites for remote controlled pulsatile drug release. *J Control Release* 2008, 130: 246–251.
35. Liu TY, Hu SH, Liu DM, Chen SY, Chen IW. Biomedical nanoparticles carriers with combined thermal and magnetic responses. *Nano Today* 2009, 4: 52–65.

36. Tripathi SK, Goyal R, Ansari KM, Ram KR, Shukla Y, Chowdhuri DK, Gupta KC. Polyglutamic acid-based nanocomposites as efficient non-viral gene carriers in vitro and vivo. *Euro J Pharm Biopharm* 2011, 79: 473–484.
37. Ju CY, Mo R, Xue JW, Zhang L, Zhao ZK, Xue LJ, Ping QN, Zhang C. Sequential intra-intercellular nanoparticles delivery system for deep tumor penetration. *Angew Chem Int Ed* 2014, 53: 6253–6258.
38. Resclgnano N, Fortunati E, Montesano S, Emiliani C, Kenny JM, Martino S, Armentano I. PVA bio-nanocomposite: A new take-off using cellulose nanocrystals and PLGA nanoparticles. *Carbohydr Polym* 2014, 99: 47–58.
39. Xiao CM, Ma PP, Geng NN. Multi-responsive methylcellulose/Fe-alginate-g-PVA/PVA/Fe_3O_4 microgels for immobilizing enzyme. *Polym Adv Technol* 2011, 22: 2649–2652.
40. Appel AA, Anastasio MA, Larson JC, Brey EM. Imaging challenges in biomaterials and tissue engineering. *Biomaterials* 2013, 34: 6615–6630.
41. Koo H, Huh MS, Ryu JH, Lee D-E, Sun IC, Choi K, Kim K, Kwon IC. Nanoprobes for biomedical imaging in living systems. *Nano Today* 2011, 6: 204–220.
42. Lu J, Ma SL, Sun JY, Xia CC, Liu C, Wang ZY, Zhao XN et al. Manganese ferrite nanoparticles micellar nanocomposites as MRI contrast agent for liver imaging. *Biomaterials* 2009, 30: 2919–2928.
43. Cheng D, Hong GB, Wang WW, Yuan RX, Ai H, Shen J, Liang BL, Gao JM, Shuai XT. Nonclustered magnetite nanoparticle encapsulated biodegradable polymeric micelles with enhanced properties for in vivo tumor imaging. *J Mater Chem* 2011, 21: 4796–4804.
44. Watcharin W, Schmiethals C, Pleli T, Kőberle V, Korkusuz H, Huebner F, Zeuzem S et al. Biodegradable human serum albumin nanoparticles as contrast agents for the detection of hepatocellular carcinoma by magnetic resonance imaging. *Euro J Pharm Biopharm* 2014, 87: 132–141.
45. Chen MJ, Yin MZ. Design and development of fluorescent nanostructures for bioimaging. *Prog Polym Sci* 2014, 39: 365–395.
46. Hezinger AFE, Tessmar J, Göpferich A. Polymer coating of quantum dots—A powerful tool toward diagnostics and sensorics. *Euro J Pharm Biopharm* 2008, 68: 138–152.
47. Mura S, Couvreur P. Nanotheranostics for personalized medicine. *Adv Drug Deliv Rev* 2012, 64: 1394–1416.
48. Krasia-Christoforou T, Georgiou TK. Polymeric theranostics: Using polymer-based systems for simultaneous imaging and therapy. *J Mater Chem B* 2013, 1: 3002–3025.
49. Ling Y, Wei K, Luo Y, Gao X, Zhong SZ. Dual docetaxel/superparamagnetic iron oxide loaded nanoparticles for both targeting magnetic resonance imaging and cancer therapy. *Biomaterials* 2011, 32: 7139–7150.
50. Schleich N, Sibret P, Danhier P, Ucakar B, Laurent S, Muller RN, Jérôme C, Gallez B, Préat V, Danhier F. Dual anticancer drug/superparamagnetic iron oxide-loaded PLAG-based nanoparticles for cancer therapy and magnetic resonance imaging. *Int J Pharm* 2013, 447: 94–101.
51. Zhu LJ, Wang DL, Wei X, Zhu XY, Li JQ, Tu CL, Su Y, Wu JL, Zhu BS, Yan DY. Multifunctional and pH-sensitive superparamagnetic iron oxide nanocomposites for targeted drug delivery and MRI imaging. *J Control Release* 2013, 169: 228–238.
52. Li ZH, Dong K, Huang S, Ju EG, Liu Z, Yin ML, Ren JS, Qu XG. A smart nanoassembly for multistage targeted drug delivery and magnetic resonance imaging. *Adv Funct Mater* 2014, 24: 3612–3620.
53. Wang C, Cheng L, Liu Z. Drug delivery with upconversion nanoparticles for multifunctional targeted cancer cell imaging and therapy. *Biomaterials* 2011, 32: 1110–1120.

54. Shen JM, Tang WJ, Zhang XL, Chen T, Zhang HX. A novel carboxymethyl chitosan-based folate/Fe$_3$O$_4$/CdTe nanoparticles for targeted drug delivery and cell imaging. *Carbohydr Polym* 2012, 88: 239–249.

55. Chatterjee K, Sarkar S, Rao KJ, Paria S. Core/shell nanoparticles in biomedical applications. *Adv Colloid Interface Sci* 2014, 209: 8–39.

56. Naahidi S, Jafari M, Edalat F, Raymond K, Khademhosseini A, Chen P. Biocompatibility of engineered nanoparticles for drug delivery. *J Control Release* 2013, 166: 182–194.

57. Gautam A, van Veggel FCJM. Synthesis of nanoparticles, their biocompatibility, and toxicity behavior for biomedical applications. *J Mater Chem B* 2013, 1: 5186–5200.

3 Electrospun Nanostructures as Biodegradable Composite Materials for Biomedical Applications

Elena Pâslaru (Stoleru), Bogdănel S. Munteanu, and Cornelia Vasile

CONTENTS

3.1 INTRODUCTION

Various blends and composites have been developed during the past few years in order to free some of the polymers from renewable resources disadvantages, such as poor mechanical properties, or to offset the high price of synthetic biodegradable polymers (Yu et al. 2006). Electrospun fibers have exceptional properties, such as high specific surface area, and can be easily designed to have enhanced mechanical properties, biocompatibility, and cellular response, making them appealing to be used in composites materials applicable in the medical field (Baptista et al. 2013).

Electrospinning is a fascinating fiber fabrication technique that gained attention during the past decade due to the ability to produce nanoscale materials (Bhardwaj and Kundu 2010; Ding et al. 2002; Pham et al. 2006).

3.2 ELECTROSPINNING PRINCIPLES

The basic electrospinning setup consists of three major components: a high-voltage power supply, an electrically conducting spinneret, and a collector separated at a defined distance (Figure 3.1).

The basic principle of the electrospinning method is as follows: an electric voltage is applied at the tip of a capillary/needle, which contains the polymer solution with a specific surface tension, and the grounded fiber collector in order to facilitate the ejection of the charged jet toward the collector. Sessile and pendant droplets of polymer solutions acquire stable shapes when they are electrically charged by applying an electrical potential difference between the droplet and a flat plate, if the potential is not too high. These stable shapes result only from equilibrium of the electric forces and surface tension in the cases of inviscid, Newtonian, and viscoelastic liquids. It is widely assumed that when the critical potential has been reached and any further increase will destroy the equilibrium, the liquid body acquires a conical shape referred to as Taylor's cone. Such deformation is attributed to two main reasons: (1) electrostatic repulsion between the surface charges of the droplet and (2) Coulombic forces exerted by the external electric field applied. The polymeric solution jet moves toward the fiber collector with simultaneous evaporation of the solvent molecules, leading to the deposition of a mat of nanofibers on the collector surface. This system is known as a simple nozzle or *monoaxial* (Figure 3.1) due to the fact that it employs only one capillary containing the polymer solution to be electrospun.

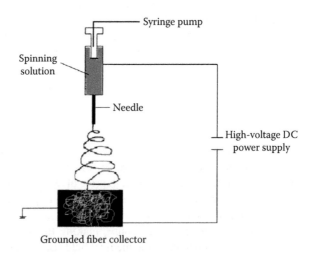

FIGURE 3.1 Basic electrospinning setup (mono-axial).

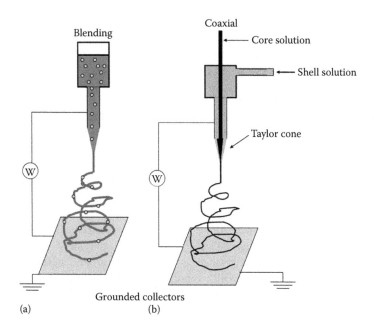

FIGURE 3.2 Schematic representations of various configurations of solution blending (a) and coaxial (b) electrospinning.

Moreover, there are other electrospinning configurations, such as blending (Figure 3.2a) and multiple electrospinning (Theron et al. 2005), core-shelled electrospinning (Sun et al. 2003), and blow-assisted electrospinning, which combines the process of electrospinning with air blowing around the spinneret (Hsiao et al. 2012).

Coaxial configuration (see Figure 3.2b) is much versatile and useful for a wide range of applications. This configuration involves two coaxial capillaries that permit simultaneous electrospinning of two polymer solutions into core–shell structured nanofiber. In this case, two separate polymer solutions flow through two different capillaries, which are coaxial with smaller capillary inside a larger capillary. The greatest advantage of coaxial electrospinning is its versatility in the type (hydrophilic or hydrophobic) and size (ranging from 100 nm to 300 μm) of fibers it can produce (Beck et al. 2011).

Electrospinning has been used to fabricate fibers with different structures and morphologies, such as single fibers with different composition and structures (blending and core–shell composite fibers) and fiber assemblies (fiber bundles, membranes, and scaffolds) (Cui et al. 2010). Using coaxial electrospinning, composite nanofibers with a core–shell structure can be produced.

Despite electrospinning's relative ease of use, there are a number of processing parameters that can greatly affect fiber formation and structure. Grouped in order of relative impact to the electrospinning process, these parameters are applied voltage, polymer flow rate, and capillary–collector distance (Sill and von Recum 2008).

The *strength of the applied electric field* controls the formation of fibers from several microns in diameter to tens of nanometers. Suboptimal field strength could lead to bead defects in the spun fibers or even failure in jet formation (Boland et al. 2005; Jeun et al. 2007; Llorens et al. 2013).

Polymer flow rate also has an impact on fiber size and additionally can influence fiber porosity as well as fiber shape (Inami et al. 2013; Milleret et al. 2011; Pillay et al. 2013; Zargham et al. 2012).

While playing a much smaller role, *the distance between capillary tip and collector* can also influence fiber size by one or two orders of magnitude. Additionally, this distance can dictate whether the end result is electrospinning or electrospraying (Martins et al. 2008; Sill and von Recum 2008; Yu et al. 2011; Zhang et al. 2009).

In addition to the processing parameters, a number of solution parameters play an important role in fiber formation, structure, and morphology (Sill and von Recum 2008). In relative order of their impact on the electrospinning process, these include polymer concentration (Correia et al. 2014; Frenot and Chronakis 2003; Tan et al. 2007), solvent volatility (Mondal 2014), and solvent conductivity (Luo et al. 2012).

A number of *biodegradable* electrospinnable polymers are available: poly(hydroxyalkanoates) (Chanprateep 2010), poly(propylene carbonate) (PPC) (Luinstra and Borchardt 2012), poly(hydroxybutyrate-co-hydroxyvalerate) (Kulkarni et al. 2010), methoxy poly(ethylene glycol) (Podaralla et al. 2012), poly lactic-co-glycolic acid (PLGA) (Makadia and Siegel 2011), and polycaprolactone (Muñoz-Bonilla et al. 2013).

3.3   ELECTROSPINNING APPLICATIONS

The biomedical field is one of the important application areas that utilize the technique of electrospinning, such as filtration and protective material, electrical and optical applications, sensors, nanofiber-reinforced composites, etc.

Although studies on the in vivo feasibility of electrospun nanofibers in bone reconstruction and tissue engineering progress are currently in the early stages, recent reports of electrospun nanofibers with new compositions targeted for bone as well as some processing tools to design 3D scaffolding and tissue engineering have highlighted the potential use of electrospun materials in bone tissue engineering (Jang et al. 2009).

3.3.1   TISSUE ENGINEERING

Tissue engineering (tissue regeneration) is an interdisciplinary field that makes use of scaffolds to provide support for cells to regenerate new *extra cellular matrix* (ECM), which has been destroyed by disease, injury, or congenital defects without stimulating any immune response (Agarwal et al. 2008). The ECM is the noncellular component that not only provides essential physical scaffolding for the cellular constituents but also initiates crucial biochemical and biomechanical cues that are required for tissue morphogenesis, differentiation, and homeostasis (Frantz et al. 2010). It separates different tissues, forms a supportive meshwork around cells, and provides anchorage to the cells. It is made up of proteins and glycosaminoglycans (GAGs), which are carbohydrate polymers (Agarwal et al. 2008).

The structural and functional properties of natural ECMs are crucial for the proliferation, differentiation, and migration of cells. As a consequence, there is an increasing tendency to design scaffold materials, as applied in tissue regeneration approaches, according to the characteristics of ECM. The nanoscale architecture of the ECM influences the adhesion and orientation of cells, while the release of biomolecules from the ECM regulates cellular proliferation and differentiation (Sun et al. 2014). Consequently, the scaffolds used for tissue regeneration should provide more than only physical support for cells. An appropriate architecture has to be combined with the release of biomolecules in the design process of scaffolds in order to obtain the optimal cellular behavior. Thus, the scaffold should have high porosity (Rnjak-Kovacina et al. 2011) with proper pore size distribution and large surface area. Biodegradability is often required with the degradation rate matching the rate of new-tissue formation. The scaffold must possess the required mechanical and structural integrity to prevent the pores of the scaffold from collapsing during new-tissue formation (Gholipour Kanani and Hajir Bahrami 2010). Finally, the scaffold should be nontoxic to cells and biocompatible, promoting cell adhesion, proliferation, and migration.

Tissue engineering scaffolds have been prepared using a multitude of different techniques, such as gas foaming, emulsion freeze drying, and rapid prototyping (Park et al. 2013). Recently, electrospinning has attracted a lot of attention due to its relative simplicity regarding the generation of fibrous scaffolds with nanoscale dimensions. In general, the electrospinning process shows excellent promise for tissue engineering and regenerative medicine as the nanofibers have 3D porous structure and high surface area similar to ECM, providing sites for cell attachment and consequently a high cell density. The electrospun nanofiber scaffolds have controllable morphology (diameter, composition, structure, alignment) and mechanical properties. Electrospun nanofibers can be used as carriers for sustained drug/gene/growth factor delivery and can be used as substrates for regulating cell behaviors, including morphology, proliferation, migration, and differentiation (Ma et al. 2013).

In recent years, the biomedical field has paid much attention to the production, processing, and applications of *polyhydroxyalkanoates*, which are natural polymers synthesized by a wide variety of microorganisms such as soil bacteria, blue–green algae, and genetically modified plants, the most common type being the *poly(hydroxybutyrate)* (PHB). Ultrafine fibers of PHB, poly(hydroxybutyrate-co-hydroxyvalerate) (PHBV), and their blends have been produced using chloroform as a solvent system. The indirect cytotoxicity evaluation with mouse fibroblasts indicated that these mats posed no threat to the cells (Sombatmankhong et al. 2006). By adding DMF to the PHB/chloroform solution, the electrospinning process for the PHB polymer becomes more stable, allowing complete polymer crystallization during the jet travelling between the tip and the grounded collector (Correia et al. 2014).

Blends of PHB and various polymers were studied. Nanofibers of poly(3-hydroxybutyric acid) and poly(propylene carbonate) (1,1,1,3,3,3 hexafluoro-2-propanol and 2,2,2 trifluoroethanol used as solvents) supported the growth and proliferation of human dermal fibroblasts and keratinocytes with normal morphology, while having good tensile properties (Nagiah et al. 2013). Also, PHB and dodecylbenzene sulfonic acid (DBSA) doped polyaniline in chloroform/trifluoroethanol mixture with possible use as scaffolds for tissue engineering (Fryczkowski and Kowalczyk 2009).

Blend composition has important influence on adhesion and proliferation. Cell culture experiments with a human kerocytatine cell line (HaCaT) and dermal fibroblast on the electrospun PHB and polyvinyl alcohol (PVA)/PHB miscible blend nanofibers (using 1,1,1,3,3,3-hexafluoro-2-propanol as solvent) showed maximum adhesion and proliferation on pure PHB. However, the addition of 5 wt.% PVA to PHB inhibited growth of HaCaT cells but not of fibroblasts. On the contrary, adhesion and proliferation of HaCaT cells were promoted on PVA/PHB (50/50) fibers, which inhibited the growth of fibroblasts. The hydrolytic degradation of PHB was accelerated with increasing PVA fraction (Asran et al. 2010).

To improve cell compatibility, the surface of poly(3-hydroxyalkanoate) (PHA) was *functionalized* by introducing epoxy groups on the fiber through two different methodologies: (1) preliminary chemical conversion of double bonds of unsaturated PHAs into epoxy groups, followed by electrospinning of epoxy-functionalized PHAs blended with nonfunctionalized PHAs; and (2) electrospinning of nonfunctionalized PHAs, followed by glycidyl methacrylate grafting polymerization under UV irradiation. The latter approach generated a higher density of epoxy groups on the fiber surface. Further, epoxy groups can be chemically modified via the attachment of a peptide sequence such as Arg-Gly-Asp (RGD) to obtain biomimetic scaffolds. Human mesenchymal stromal cells exhibited a better adhesion on the latter scaffolds than that on nonfunctionalized PHA mats (Ramier et al. 2014).

Highly porous fibers were prepared by *water bath electrospinning* (using a water bath collector) (Pant et al. 2011b) of pure poly(ε-caprolactone) (PCL) and its blends with methoxy poly(ethylene glycol) (MPEG). In vitro cytotoxicity assessment of the fiber mats (using mouse osteoblasts [MC3T3-E1] as reference cell lines) indicated that the porous electrospun mat containing amount of MPEG was nontoxic to the cell. Cell culture results showed that porous fibrous mats were good in promoting cell attachment and proliferation (Pant et al. 2011a).

There are studies concerning composite nanofibers from electrospun *natural polymers*. Hyaluronic acid (HA) and collagen were dissolved in a sodium hydroxide (NaOH)/*N,N*-dimethyl formamide (DMF) solvent mixture at a concentration of 10 wt.% and successfully electrospun into a nanofiber web with a *soft, fluffy structure* by the combined effects of numerous minijet evolutions and their subsequent vertical growth. By the simultaneous deposition of salt particulates as a porogen during electrospinning and subsequent chemical crosslinking and salt leaching, a water-swellable HA-based scaffold retaining a macroporous and nanofibrous geometry was produced. The cytocompatibility tests using bovine chondrocytes cultured on the scaffolds revealed that cellular adhesion and proliferation were enhanced in proportion to the content of collagen, and the seeded chondrocytes maintained the roundness characteristic of a chondroblastic morphology (Kim et al. 2008).

Different from the conventional electrospinning process, which involves a positively charged conductive needle and a grounded fiber collector (i.e., positive voltage electrospinning), pseudo-negative voltage electrospinning, with grounded needle and positively charged collector, was investigated for making ultrafine

PHBV fibers. High applied voltages facilitated the formation of large-diameter fibers during positive voltage electrospinning but small-diameter fibers during pseudo-negative voltage electrospinning. Additionally, protein adsorption and hence cell adhesion can be enhanced when the substrate (scaffold) is selected such that it bears opposite charges with respect to the polarity of a particular kind of protein. Positive voltage electrospinning and negative voltage electrospinning (including pseudo-negative voltage electrospinning) can produce suitably charged fibrous scaffolds that favor tissue regeneration, which facilitates cell–scaffold interactions and provides another useful aid in the tissue engineering of various human body tissues (Tong and Wang 2011).

3.3.1.1 Growth Factors

Macromolecular bioactive agents such as anionic polysaccharides (i.e., heparin, HA, and DNA) and growth factors play important roles in harnessing and controlling cellular functions in tissue regeneration. Ideal tissue engineering scaffolds should not only mimic the topography and compositions of ECM, but also be integrated with macromolecular bioactive agents in order to finely modulate the cell migration, proliferation, and differentiation (Zhu and Marchant 2011).

Composite nanofibers from electrospun *natural and synthetic polymer hybrids* are extensively used for the purpose of constructing biomimetic cellular scaffolds (Gunn and Zhang 2010) as they combine key characteristics of the constituents on the nanoscale, which are important for cell functions such as adhesion, migration, proliferation, and differentiation. Due to the dissimilarity in the chemical structures, the two types of polymers are often poorly miscible in solution, which results in composite nanofibers with different microphase-separated structures because of phase separation phenomenon in the spinning solution (Stoyanova et al. 2014) and rapid solidification. Phase separation is usually observed in blend nanofibers with major (matrix) and minor constituents, which affects the mechanical properties as a result of the inhomogeneity (Del Gaudio et al. 2011).

Gelatin is a proteinaceous material prepared by hydrolytic degradation of naturally occurring collagen. Because of its biodegradability, biocompatibility, and cell affinity, it is a good candidate for use in the field of tissue engineering. The electrospun gelatin membranes have been successfully prepared for various applications (Zhan and Lan 2012). The nanofibrous scaffolds of gelatin mimic not only the topography but also chemical composition of ECM and could support the growth of various cells (Zhang et al. 2005).

Phase separation has significant impact on cell adhesion and proliferation behaviors for *gelatin/polycaprolactone* (PCL) (50/50 wt./wt.) electrospun nanofibers. The more homogeneous fibers (without phase separation), obtained by adding acetic acid (0.2% relative to trifluoroethanol) in the initial gelatin/PCL/trifluoroethanol, provided superior cytocompatibility over the nonhomogeneous fibers obtained from gelatin/PCL/trifluoroethanol solution (Feng et al. 2014).

The presence of gelatin in the *gelatin/nylon-6* composite nanofibers improved the adhesion, viability, and proliferation properties of osteoblast cells (analyzed by an in vitro cell compatibility test). No component partitioning was observed in the composite mat indicating good phase miscibility of gelatin with nylon-6 in the common solvent (formic acid/acetic acid). Also, the formation of a strong hydrogen bond between gelatin and nylon-6 might be the cause of the increased thermal degradation temperature of the two polymers in composite mats (Pant and Kim 2013).

Core–shell fibrous scaffolds composed of gelatin-coated PCL were fabricated by coaxial electrospinning. The presence of PCL in the core section of the core–shell fibers significantly enhanced both the morphological stability and mechanical strength of the fibrous membranes (Zhao et al. 2007). In another study, the outer gelatin layer was crosslinked by exposing the membranes in glutaraldehyde vapor. The core–shell fibers could effectively immobilize two types of agents (FITC-labeled bovine serum albumin [FITC–BSA] or FITC–heparin) under mild conditions. Furthermore, vascular endothelial growth factor (VEGF) could be conveniently impregnated into the fibers through specific interactions with the adsorbed heparin in the outer cationized gelatin layer. Sustained release of bioactive VEGF could be achieved for more than 15 days (Lu et al. 2009). By optimizing the glutaraldehyde/gelatin feed ratio, other authors have found that the mechanical strength of the hydrated, crosslinked core–shell fibrous scaffolds was significantly enhanced because of the presence of hydrophobic PCL in the core region of the fibers. Results of cell culture studies suggested that the crosslinked, core–shell fibrous scaffolds were nontoxic and capable of supporting fibroblast adhesion and proliferation (Zhao et al. 2007).

3.3.1.2 Cardiovascular Tissue Engineering

Electrospinning has applications in the area of cardiovascular tissue engineering. Bioresorbable vascular grafts were produced from electrospun nanofibers of collagen and other biopolymers. These bioresorbable grafts have compositions that allow for the in situ remodeling of the structure, with the eventual replacement of the graft with completely autologous tissue (Sell et al. 2009).

Developing scaffolds that can maintain their mechanical integrity while exposing to cells, at long-term cyclic mechanical strains, is especially necessary in cardiovascular applications. To combine mechanical properties with cell viability, double-layered small-diameter tubular scaffolds containing both melt-spun macrofibers (<200 μm diameter) and electrospun submicron fibers (>400 nm in diameter) were produced by electrospinning of nanofibers on top of the melt-spun microfibers. The tubes were fabricated from an elastomeric bioresorbable 50:50 poly(L-lactide-co-e-caprolactone) copolymer having dimensions of 5 mm in diameter and porosity of over 75%. For electrospinning, two different solvents were used: acetone and 1,1,1,3,3,3-hexafluoro-2-propanol. The melt-spun monofilaments were wound up directly after extrusion on a rotating Teflon-coated mandrel and were removed, while maintaining its shape, as a tube, after collection once they had cooled to room temperature. Melt-spun tubes were further used as the base mandrel for the collection of electrospun PLCL nanofibers. The two obtained layers were well bonded together and were not separable with manual manipulation. Micro- and nanocombined structures can be advantageous, since the nanolayer can mimic the ECM, whereas the microlayer will provide larger pores, which facilitate superior cell infiltration.

That electrospun structures can promote cell proliferation and that the effect of any residual solvent on cell behavior are not significantly detrimental (Chung et al. 2010).

A critical design requirement for small-diameter (<6 mm) bioengineered vascular grafts is the formation of a continuous monolayer of endothelial cells (ECs) on the lumen of the construct by seeding endothelial progenitor cells on the lumen surface of the vascular graft prior to implantation. Therefore, an ideal bioengineered vascular graft should possess a continuous monolayer of ECs that functions similar to the native endothelium while remaining adherent under physiological flow conditions. The endothelium in native vessels is composed of ECs aligned with the direction of blood flow in straight vessel segments. To study the effect of electrospun scaffold orientation and fibers diameter on EC morphology, alignment, and structural protein organization, scaffolds consisting of a polymer blend of type I collagen and PCL were electrospun onto a grounded stationary tissue culture polystyrene rotating substrate. Subsequently, primary human umbilical vein ECs were seeded onto the scaffolds. It was found that ECs on electrospun scaffolds formed confluent monolayers and alignment of cells was found to systematically increase as a function of increased fiber orientation, leading to a fully aligned endothelium on the most aligned scaffolds. ECs on fully aligned scaffolds displayed greater levels of adherence to the scaffolds under physiological shear stress as compared to those on random and semi-aligned scaffolds (Whited and Rylander 2014).

3.3.1.3 Bone Tissue Regeneration

An ideal material for bone repair must be biocompatible and bioactive, able to initiate osteogenesis, and should have a composition and structural properties similar to bone. From the biological perspective, the natural bone matrix is a combination of organic and inorganic nanocomposite materials and consists of a naturally occurring polymer and a biological mineral. It is composed of approximately 70 wt.% inorganic crystals (mainly hydroxyapatite, HA) and 30 wt.% organic matrix (mainly Type I collagen). Structurally, it is hierarchically organized from macro- and micro- to nanoscale, where the basic building blocks are the plate-like HA nanocrystals well aligned onto the collagen nanofibers (Abdal-hay et al. 2014).

Implants intended for bone tissue regeneration were obtained based on nanofibrous 3D scaffolds of bioresorbable poly-ε-caprolactone mimicking the fibrillar architecture of bone matrix. Layer-by-layer nano-immobilization of the growth factor bone morphogenetic protein 2 (BMP-2) in association with chitosan or poly-L-lysine over the nanofibers is described. The osteogenetic potential of the scaffolds coated with layers of chitosan and BMP-2 was demonstrated in vitro and in vivo in mouse calvaria, through enhanced osteopontin gene expression and calcium phosphate biomineralization (Ferrand et al. 2014).

New biodegradable mats were successfully obtained by functional PVA/gelatin blend fiber mats containing biphasic calcium phosphate (BCP) nanoparticles for bone regeneration. The addition of BCP was found to have increased fiber diameter, tensile strength, osteoblast cell adhesion, proliferation, and protein expression. In vivo bone formation was examined using rat models, and increased bone formation was observed for the 50% BCP-loaded electrospun PVA/gelatin blends within 2 and 4 weeks (Linh et al. 2013).

3.3.2 Releasing Systems (Drug-Delivery Systems)

The principle of controlled drug release therapy involves the delivery of a certain amount of drug, over a specified period of time, with a predictable and controllable rate (Vasile et al. 2014b). Due to the high surface area to volume ratio, the electrospun polymer nanofibers provide a useful pathway for delivery of water-insoluble drug. The drug releasing profile can be finely tailored by controlling not only the fibers' composition but also the morphology of nanofibers (Baptista et al. 2013).

Polymer nanofibers obtained through electrospinning have been proposed for a variety of applications for various release systems. Compared with other dosage forms, several advantages of using electrospun polymer nanofibers have been recognized. Therapeutic compounds can be conveniently incorporated into the carrier polymers using electrospinning; the drug release profile can be finely tailored by a modulation on the morphology, porosity, and composition of the nanofibrous membrane. The very small diameter of the nanofibers can provide short diffusion passage length (Ji et al. 2011), and the high surface area is helpful to a mass transfer and efficient drug release (Zamani et al. 2013).

To achieve drug release from nanofibers, two basic delivery designs are known: matrices and reservoirs (Sirc et al. 2012; Vasile et al. 2014a).

In the *matrix-type structure*, drug is dispersed through the monoaxial electrospun polymeric solution (*blend electrospinning*) and released based on solid-state diffusion or a desorption mechanism, while in *reservoir-type structure*, the drug is enclosed in polymeric nanofibers, forming so-called *core–shell* structure (drug-loaded core covered with polymer shell), which is made by *coaxial electrospinning* process. Blend electrospinning *simply entraps* bioactive agents within ultrafine fibers by dispersing them into polymer solution directly, whereby the main disadvantages of this method are *severe burst release* effect and the reduction of effective lifetime (Jiang et al. 2014) while the shell layer from the core–shell structure serves as a barrier to prevent the premature release of the core contents (Jiang et al. 2014).

Nonwoven mats made through coaxial electrospinning combine advantageous characteristics from each of the constituent materials. Various drugs and bioactive agents such as antibiotics, DNA, proteins, or growth factors can be directly incorporated into core protected by the shell layer and released over a long time period. As drug carriers, fibrous structure produced by coaxial electrospinning can potentially provide a better therapeutic effect and reduced toxicity. Also, for core–shell nanofibers, overall drug loading is lower than blend fibers as shell polymers do not contain any drug (Maleki et al. 2013).

3.3.2.1 Blend *Encapsulation*

Two kinds of drugs can be simultaneously encapsulated by *blend electrospinning* into polymer electrospun nanofibers. A co-delivery system based on the electrospun poly(lactic-co-glycolic acid) (PLGA)/*mesoporous silica nanoparticles* (MSNs) composite mat was designed for the co-encapsulation and prolonged release of one hydrophilic and one hydrophobic drug simultaneously. The MSNs were chosen to load the hydrophobic model drug fluorescein (FLU) and hydrophilic model drug rhodamine B (RHB). Both model drugs RHB and FLU maintained sustained delivery with controllable release kinetics during the releasing period. A higher concentration of PLGA in the composite resulted in thicker fibers with slower (more sustained) release kinetics of the two drugs. The fiber diameters increased significantly after release of drugs as a result of the relaxation of polymer chain. Although the polymer chain relaxed, the releases of the two drugs still maintained sustained release kinetics from composite mats. It was speculated that the drug release might be mainly dominated by diffusion and the relaxation of polymer chain was favor for diffusion (Song et al. 2012).

Curcumin from *Curcuma longa* L., which is also known as turmeric, has antioxidant, anti-inflammatory, and anti-tumor properties. The in vitro evaluations suggested that curcumin-incorporated zein nanofibers showed sustained release of curcumin and maintained its free radical scavenging ability while providing the structure for the attachment and growth of fibroblast as cell culture surfaces (Dhandayuthapani et al. 2012). In another work, curcumin (0.5–1.5 wt.%) was incorporated into the silk fibroin solution and electrospun to obtain curcumin-incorporated silk nanofibers with diameters between 50 and 200 nm. The SNFs and CSNFs were thermally stable up to ca 350°C as evidenced by TGA. The glass transition temperature (Tg) of SNFs (168°C) increased to 184°C in the case of CSNFs as confirmed by DSC. The percentage in vitro cumulative release of curcumin at the end of the 10th day for 0.5, 1, and 1.5 wt.% formulations was 82%, 84%, and 80%, respectively (Elakkiya et al. 2014).

Chitosan-ethylenediamine tetraacetic acid/polyvinyl alcohol nanofiber mats containing extracts from fruit hull of *Garcinia mangostana* (GM) (1, 2, and 3 wt.% α-mangostin) exhibited antioxidant and antibacterial activity. During the wound healing test, the mats accelerated the rate of healing when compared to the control (gauze-covered). The mats maintained 90% of their content of α-mangostin for 3 months (Charernsriwilaiwat et al. 2013).

Sandwich-structured electrospun membranes, with PLGA/collagen for the surface layers and PLGA/drugs (vancomycin, gentamicin, and lidocaine) for the core layer were obtained. The biodegradable nanofibrous membranes released high concentrations of vancomycin and gentamicin for 4 and 3 weeks, respectively, and lidocaine for 2 weeks. The antibacterial activity of the released vancomycin and gentamicin ranged from 30% to 100% and 37% to 100%, respectively. In addition, results indicated that the nanofibrous membranes were functionally active in responses in human fibroblasts, which make them candidates for biodegradable biomimetic nanofibrous extracellular membranes for long-term drug delivery of various pharmaceuticals (Chen et al. 2012).

Alpha-tocopherol, the main component of a group of compounds known as vitamin E, is a powerful antioxidant that can scavenge free radicals and the main fat-soluble vitamin responsible for protecting cell membranes against peroxidation (Ji et al. 2014; Lima et al. 2014). Vitamin E was encapsulated into chitosan coatings (Stoleru et al. in press) and poly(lactic acid) (PLA) nanofibers (Munteanu et al. 2014) by monaxial electrospinning to obtain multifunctional antimicrobial and antioxidative materials. It was noticed that vitamin E addition into chitosan matrix leads to changes in polymer's rheological properties, which further influences the electrospraying process and deposited coating morphology (as noticed in Figure 3.3).

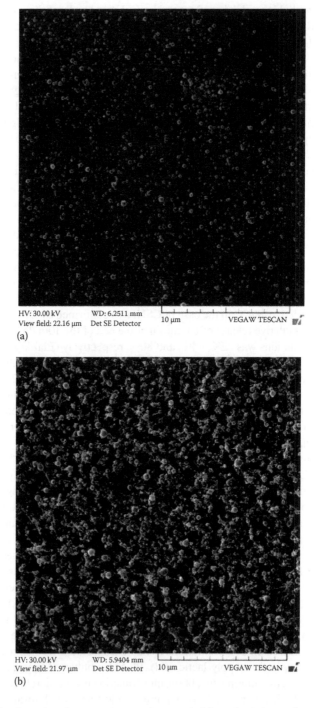

FIGURE 3.3 Scanning electron micrographs recorded for polyethylene substrate coated by electrospraying with chitosan (a) and chitosan/3 wt% vitamin E blend (b).

The obtained materials have both antibacterial and antioxidative properties, which are maintained even after subjecting the samples to desorption in harsh environment.

3.3.2.2 Coaxial *Encapsulation*

Coaxial electrospinning is an alternative approach to encapsulate drugs or biologically active compounds inside polymer nanofibers (Braghirolli et al. 2014). In a typical process, two or more polymer liquids are forced by an electrostatic potential to eject out through *different coaxial capillary channels (needles)*, resulting in a core–shell-structured composite nanofiber. As long as the shell fluid is able to be processed along with electrospinning, the core fluid can either be or not be electrospinnable.

Compared with coaxial electrospinning, blend electrospinning is assumed to be relatively easy to perform, but biomolecules may lose their bioactivity due to conformational changes in the organic solution environment (Ji et al. 2011). As coaxial electrospinning utilizes two separate channels for the different solutions (i.e., the organic polymer and biological solutions), it is hypothesized to be beneficial in maintaining the functional activity of biomolecules with an *effective protection of easily denatured biological agents* from the electrostatic field and organic solvent of shell solutions. Also, there is the possibility *to wrap all substances in the core regardless of drug–polymer interactions.* Hence, drugs, proteins, growth factors, and even genes can be incorporated into nanofibers by dissolving them in the core solutions. A drawback of the coaxial electrospinning comes from the differences in the conductivities and viscosities of the two solutions, which make it difficult to find the parameters for stable electrospinning in order to form a uniform fibrous structure.

The shell polymer, after the electrospinning, acts as a barrier to control the release of the loaded molecules. However, the limitation of loading capacity still remains due to the prerequisite of using an additional polymer as additive to achieve the minimum viscosity of the core solution required for viscous drag by the shell solution being drawn by the electrostatic force (Tiwari and Venkatraman 2012).

In wound healing applications, when the shell polymer is biodegraded and absorbed by human body, the drug or other therapeutic agents within the fibers will release and play a desired role. The very small diameter of the nanofibers allows the absorption to be accomplished in a short period of time. In this way, a controlled release of additives and physical caring for the wound can be achieved at the same time. On the other hand, the shell of nanofibers can provide temporal protection for certain bioactive substances such as growth factors, which need to be protected for a while prior to playing roles in the early application of wound healing (Huang et al. 2006).

Core–shell electrospinning requires the viscosity ratio between the core and shell solutions to be above a threshold to have sufficient viscous drag, as suggested by various studies (Reznik et al. 2006). Thus, a sufficiently high viscosity of the outer fluid, together with a low value of the inner/outer solution interfacial tension, is essential to develop a compound cone in steady state. Otherwise, for large values of the interfacial tension or low viscosity, the viscous drag exerted by the outer solution on the inner solution surface is unable to overcome the cohesive force of the surface tension, so the inner meniscus remains quasi-spherical and no double cone is developed (Diaz et al. 2006).

Drug/polycaprolactone (PCL) nanofibers in the form of core–shell structure with two model drugs as core (low molecular weight *gentamycin sulfate* and *resveratrol*) presented a smooth drug release for both the drug-loaded nanofibers with no burst release. No other carrying agent, such as a high molecular weight polymer, except for the respective solvents, was mixed with the drugs in making the cores, although the pure drug solutions alone cannot be made into any fiber. Gentamycin sulfate is an antibiotic that can inhibit or kill bacteria, and resveratrol is a natural antioxidant found in a wide variety of plants, which can be used to keep blood vessels open and pliable as well as to prevent blood platelets from aggregation or clumping together (Huang et al. 2006).

The core–shell nanostructure of the poly(lactide-co-glycolide)/tetracycline hydrochloride (TCH) core/shell nanofibers showed sustained drug release and *suppressed the burst release in comparison with the nanofibers* produced by monoaxial (blend) electrospinning (Maleki et al. 2013). The loading dosage of the tetracycline had no obvious effect on the morphology of the tetracycline hydrochloride loaded PVA/soybean protein isolate/zirconium (Tet–PVA/SPI/ZrO$_2$) nanofibers, but antimicrobial activity increased rapidly with increasing tetracycline content when tetracycline content was below 6 wt.%. The Tet–PVA/SPI/ZrO$_2$ nanofibrous membrane exhibited an effective and sustainable inhibition on the growth of *Staphylococcus aureus* (Wang et al. 2014a).

The feed rates of the core and the sheath strongly affect the stability and porous density of the core/shell (PEG/salicylic acid—core)/(PLA—shell), significantly influencing their salicylic acid (SA) release characteristics. At a lower ratio of feed rates of the core and the sheath, better stable core/sheath structures of nanofibers with higher porous density on the surface were formed resulting in a sustained release of SA over 5 days. Nonporous fibers showed a lower amount of drug release because the drug was embedded inside the core layer of the nonporous sheath layer. SA release from porous core/sheath nanofibers can be described based on a 1D Fickian diffusion mechanism, indicating that drug diffusion is a predominant factor in drug release. A cytotoxicity test suggested that the porous core/sheath nanofibers were nontoxic and supported cell attachment (Nguyen et al. 2012).

A fibro-porous wound dressing with antibacterial activity was fabricated from polycaprolactone (PCL) solution containing crude extract of biophytum sensitivum (BS), a potential antibacterial herbal drug. The release characteristics by total immersion method in phosphate buffer and acetate buffer displayed an increase in drug release with time. The PCL/BS nanofiber mats exhibited antibacterial activity against *S. aureus* and *Escherichia coli* (Namboodiri and Parameswaran 2013).

A modified coaxial process using *shell fluids comprising only solvent* was used to produce ketoprofen-loaded cellulose acetate nanofibers. With a sheath-to-core flow rate ratio of 2:10, the nanofibers prepared from the coaxial process had a smaller average diameter, narrower size distribution, more uniform structures, and smoother surface morphologies than those generated from single fluid (monoaxial) electrospinning. In addition, the coaxial fibers provided a better zero-order drug release profile. The core electrospinnable cellulose acetate solutions were prepared by dissolving cellulose acetate and ketoprofen in an acetone/dimethylacetamide/ethanol mixture, while the same mixture (4:1:1 by volume) was used as the sheath fluid. Throughout modified coaxial electrospinning, the sheath solvent (1) facilitates the formation of Taylor's cone due to lower surface tension of the core fluid; (2) surrounds the straight thinning jet of the core polymer solution, retarding evaporation of solvent from the core fluid while the sheath solvent itself evaporates to the atmosphere; and (3) follows the core fluid when entering the instability region. In the instability regions, where most of the solvents evaporate, the sheath solvent can retard the premature evaporation of core jet solvents, and hence keep the jet in a fluid state for longer (Yu et al. 2012). The same group obtained ketoprofen (KET)-loaded zein nanofibers using unspinnable dilluted 1% (w/v) zein solution as sheath fluid and electrospinnable zein/ketoprofen solutions as core fluid. In vitro dissolution tests showed that the nanofibers coated with blank zein did not exert any initial burst release effect and can enable linear drug release over a period of 16 h via a diffusion mechanism (Yu et al. 2013).

There are many studies concerning the enhancement of the biological functionality of electrospun scaffolds by incorporating *biomolecules* during electrospinning.

Polycaprolactone-based nanofibrous scaffolds with incorporated protein were produced via either the blend or the coaxial electrospinning technique. BSA was used as a model protein to determine release profiles, while alkaline phosphatase was used to determine protein activity after the electrospinning process. Coaxial electrospinning resulted in uniform fiber morphology with a core–shell structure, and a homogeneous protein distribution throughout the core of the fibers. In contrast, blend electrospinning formed bead-like fibers with a heterogeneous protein distribution in the fibers. The coaxial scaffold exhibited more sustained release profiles than the comparative blend scaffold, and the additive poly(ethyleneglycol) (PEG) in the coaxial scaffold accelerated protein release. Both electrospinning processes decreased the biological activity of the incorporated protein, but coaxial electrospinning showed up to 75% preservation of the initial biological activity and was demonstrated to be superior to blend electrospinning for the preparation of nanofibrous scaffolds with a uniform fibrous structure and protein distribution and sustained protein release kinetics as well as high preservation of the protein activity (Ji et al. 2010).

The *release behavior of different proteins* depends on the type of the protein and the morphology of the polymer/protein nanofibers. Poly(lactide-co-glycolic acid) (PLGA)/ lysozyme and PLGA/ gelatin showed slow initial release (by incubating the fibers in 2 mL of phosphate buffer saline pH 7.4) while PLGA/BSA released much faster. The differences in release behavior of the different proteins can be explained on the basis of partitioning effects. BSA, being more hydrophobic than lysozyme and gelatin, partitions more readily into the PLGA shell. This leads to the redistribution of the BSA into the PLGA and thus leads to faster release. Some monolithic fibers, in which protein is directly dissolved in the polymer solution (PLGA in a mixture of chloroform and DMF at a ratio of 80: 20), do not show such control over burst release and more than 30% of lysozyme was released in the first 24 h compared with about 5% for lysozyme–PLGA and about 7% for (lysozyme + PVA)–PLGA core–shell fibers (Tiwari and Venkatraman 2012).

Nanofibers with a core–sheath structure encapsulating BSA as a model protein for hydrophilic bioactive agents were prepared through emulsion electrospinning by incorporating *in the same solvent* the continuous phase of the dissolved polymer (poly(lactic-co-glycolic acid)) and the protein in the form of separated phase. The obtained scaffolds demonstrated a sustained release profile of BSA within 14 days and good biocompatibility of the scaffolds for NIH-3T3 fibroblast cells. *The core–sheath structure formation can be associated with the immiscibility of the organic and aqueous phases* during the electrospinning process and the fast solidification of the jet, which would prevent the two fluids from mixing significantly. Spherically shaped emulsion particles (or droplets) suffer substantial elongation when subjected to the process of electrospinning and are considerably elongated. As the organic solvent evaporates faster than water, the viscosity of the matrix surrounding the emulsion particles increases rapidly determining high rate elongation of the particles. In the same time, the aqueous phase droplets migrate to the center of the jet because of the viscosity gradient. Finally, solidification of the emulsion jets and hence formation of the composite nanofibers with a core–sheath structure (Norouzi et al. 2013) occur. Similar electrospun nanofibers with a core–shell were obtained from a homogeneous solution of poly(ethylene oxide) (PEO) and chitosan oligosaccharide (CS) using a conventional single-nozzle electrospinning setup. Because of the poor miscibility, the two polymers separate into a core–shell structure (PEO as core, CS as shell) (Zhang and Nie 2012). Other authors reported polyvinylpyrrolidone (PVP)/poly(vinylidene fluoride) (PVDF) core–shell nanofiber mats electrospun from the homogeneous blending solutions with the core–shell structure achieved by the thermal-induced phase separation (Wang et al. 2014b).

3.3.2.3   *Core–Shell*–Type Nanofibers for Encapsulate Drugs or Proteins Obtained by Emulsion Electrospinning

Emulsion electrospinning incorporates two phases, that is, the continuous/matrix phase of the dissolved polymer in organic solvent and the separated/isolation phase of emulsion particles/droplets with micro/nano size. The emulsion particles are stabilized by means of surfactants/emulsifiers embedded in the polymer matrix (Badawi and El-Khordagui 2014). The aim of using emulsion electrospinning is to fabricate *core–shell*–type nanofibers, which had the potential to encapsulate drugs or proteins in the core part of nanofibers (Li et al. 2009). The releasing behavior is controlled by the fiber structure and morphology by the diffusion mechanism caused by the concentration gradient and degradation of the polymer (Xiong et al. 2005).

Antimicrobial nanofibers were prepared by solubilizing an antimicrobial essential oil (eugenol; 0.75–1.5 wt.%) in surfactant micelles to form eugenol-containing microemulsions, which were further mixed with PVA and electrospun. Addition of loaded micelles or microemulsions resulted in irregular shaped nanofibrous structures with rough and patchy surfaces and broader fiber size distribution. While pure PVA nanofibers had a smooth surface with no visible inclusions inside the fibers, the nanofibers containing microemulsions had visible patches of microemulsion homogeneously dispersed throughout the fibers. Also, they had increased surface roughness due to the presence of subcutaneous microemulsion droplets, which allow for a rapid release of the encapsulated compound (Kriegel et al. 2009).

Cinnamaldehyde (CA), a volatile essential oil that eradicates pathogens nonspecifically, was incorporated (0.5% and 5.0%) into chitosan/poly(ethylene oxide) (PEO) solutions that were electrospun into nanofibers (approximately 50 nm diameter). The 5% CA mats released a statistically higher amount of CA liquid (approximately five times more) than the 0.5% CA mats. In time-dependent cytotoxicity studies, the intrinsic antibacterial activity of chitosan along with the quick release of CA enabled high inactivation rates against *E. coli* and *Pseudomonas aeruginosa* (Rieger and Schiffman 2014).

A newer encapsulation method involves the embedding of the volatile compounds in electrospun nanofibers, by emulsification of the volatile compound in a spinnable polymer solution (Ramamoorthy and Rajiv 2014). A highly volatile fragrance, (R)-(+)-limonene, was encapsulated into a PVA fibrous matrix by emulsion electrospinning. Subsequent to limonene dispersion in the aqueous PVA solution, the mixture was ultrasonicated to achieve a droplet diameter of about 1.1 ± 0.2 μm for the surfactant-free PVA/limonene emulsions. The nanofibers had a bead and displayed a sustained, slow release of volatiles over this long time interval (Camerlo et al. 2013).

ACKNOWLEDGMENT

The authors acknowledge the support given by the International Atomic Energy Agency through research project No. RO 17689.

REFERENCES

Abdal-hay, A., Vanegas, P., Hamdy, A.S., Engel, F.B., Lim, J.H. 2014. Preparation and characterization of vertically arrayed hydroxyapatite nanoplates on electrospun nanofibers for bone tissue engineering. *Chemical Engineering Journal* 254:612–622.

Agarwal, S., Wendorff, J.H., Greiner, A. 2008. Use of electrospinning technique for biomedical applications. *Polymer* 49:5603–5621.

Asran, A.Sh., Razghandi, K., Aggarwal, N., Michler, G.H., Groth, T. 2010. Nanofibers from blends of polyvinyl alcohol and polyhydroxy butyrate as potential scaffold material for tissue engineering of skin. *Biomacromolecules* 11:3413–3421.

Badawi, M.A., El-Khordagui, L.K. 2014. A quality by design approach to optimization of emulsions for electrospinning using factorial and D-optimal designs. *European Journal of Pharmaceutical Sciences* 58:44–54.

Baptista, A.C., Ferreira, I., Borges, J.P. 2013. Electrospun fibers in composite materials for medical applications. *Journal of Composites and Biodegradable Polymers* 1:56–65.

Beck, R., Gutterres, S., Pohlmann, A. 2011. *Nanocosmetics and Nanomedicines*. Berlin, Germany: Springer.

Bhardwaj, N., Kundu, S.C. 2010. Electrospinning: A fascinating fiber fabrication technique. *Biotechnology Advances* 28(3):325.

Boland, E.D., Coleman, B.D., Barnes, C.P., Simpson, D.G., Wnek, G.E., Bowlin, G.L. 2005. Electrospinning polydioxanone for biomedical applications. *Acta Biomaterialia* 1:115–123.

Braghirolli, D.I., Steffens, D., Pranke, P. 2014. Electrospinning for regenerative medicine: A review of the main topics. *Drug Discovery Today* 19:743–753.

Camerlo, A., Vebert-Nardin, C., Rossi, R.M., Popa, A.M. 2013. Fragrance encapsulation in polymeric matrices by emulsion electrospinning. *European Polymer Journal* 49:3806–3813.

Chanprateep, S. 2010. Current trends in biodegradable polyhydroxyalkanoates. *Journal of Bioscience and Bioengineering* 110:621–632.

Charernsriwilaiwat, N., Rojanarata, T., Ngawhirunpat, T., Sukma, M., Opanasopit, P. 2013. Electrospun chitosan-based nanofiber mats loaded with *Garcinia mangostana* extracts. *International Journal of Pharmaceutics* 452:333–343.

Chen, D.W., Hsu, Y.-H., Liao, J.-Y., Liu, S.-J., Chen, J.-K., Ueng, S.W.-N. 2012. Sustainable release of vancomycin, gentamicin and lidocaine from novel electrospun sandwich-structured PLGA/collagen nanofibrous membranes. *International Journal of Pharmaceutics* 430:335–341.

Chung, S., Ingle, N.P., Montero, G.A., Kim, S.H., King, M.W. 2010. Bioresorbable elastomeric vascular tissue engineering scaffolds via meltspinning and electrospinning. *Acta Biomaterialia* 6:1958–1967.

Correia, D.M., Ribeiro, C., Ferreira, J.C.C., Botelho, G., Ribelles, J.L.G., Lanceros-Mendez, S., Sencadas, V. 2014. Influence of electrospinning parameters on poly(hydroxybutyrate) electrospun membranes fiber size and distribution. *Polymer Engineering and Science* 54:1608–1617.

Cui, W., Zhou, Y., Chang, J. 2010. Electrospun nanofibrous materials for tissue engineering and drug delivery. *Science and Technology of Advanced Materials* 11:014108 (11pp).

Del Gaudio, C., Ercolani, E., Nanni, F., Bianco, A. 2011. Assessment of poly(ε-caprolactone)/poly(3-hydroxybutyrate-co-3-hydroxyvalerate) blends processed by solvent casting and electrospinning. *Materials Science and Engineering: A* 528:1764–1772.

Dhandayuthapani, B., Anila, M., Ravindran, G.A., Yutaka, N., Venugopal, K., Yasuhiko, Y., Maekawal, T., Sakthikumar, D. 2012. Hybrid fluorescent curcumin loaded zein electrospun nanofibrous scaffold for biomedical applications. *Biomedical Materials* 7 (2012) 045001 (16pp) DOI: 10.1088/1748–6041/7/4/045001.

Diaz, J.E., Barrero, A., Marquez, M., Loscertales, I.G. 2006. Controlled encapsulation of hydrophobic liquids in hydrophilic polymer nanofibers by co-electrospinning. *Advanced Functional Materials* 16:2110–2116.

Ding, B., Kim, H.-Y., Lee, S.-C., Shao, C.-L., Lee, D.-R., Park, S.-J., Kwag, G.-B., Choi, K.-J. 2002. Preparation and characterization of a nanoscale poly(vinyl alcohol) fiber aggregate produced by an electrospinning method. *Journal of Polymer Science: Part B: Polymer Physics* 40:1261–1268.

Elakkiya, T., Malarvizhi, G., Rajiv, S., Natarajan, T.S. 2014. Curcumin loaded electrospun *Bombyx mori* silk nanofibers for drug delivery. *Polymer International* 63:100–105.

Feng, B., Duan, H., Fu, W., Cao, Y., Zhang, W.J., Zhang, Y. 2014. Effect of inhomogeneity of the electrospun fibrous scaffoldsof gelatin/polycaprolactone hybrid on cell proliferation. *Journal of Biomedical Materials Research Part A* 103:431–438.

Ferrand, A., Eap, S., Richert, L., Lemoine, S., Kalaskar, D., Demoustier-Champagne, S., Atmani, H. et al. 2014. Osteogenetic properties of electrospun nanofibrous pcl scaffolds equipped with chitosan-based nanoreservoirs of growth factors. *Macromolecular Bioscience* 14:45–55.

Frantz, C., Stewart, K.M., Weaver, V.M. 2010. The extracellular matrix at a glance. *Journal of Cell Science* 123:4195–4200.

Frenot, A., Chronakis, I.S. 2003. Polymer nanofibers assembled by electrospinning. *Current Opinion in Colloid and Interface Science* 8:64–75.

Fryczkowski, R., Kowalczyk, T. 2009. Nanofibres from polyaniline/polyhydroxybutyrate blends. *Synthetic Metals* 159:2266–2268.

Gholipour Kanani, A., Hajir Bahrami, S. 2010. Review on electrospun nanofibers scaffold and biomedical applications. *Trends in Biomaterials and Artificial Organs* 24:93–115.

Gunn, J., Zhang, M. 2010. Polyblend nanofibers for biomedical applications: Perspectives and challenges. *Trends in Biotechnology* 28:189–197.

Hsiao, H.-Y., Huang, C.-M., Liu, Y.-Y., Kuo, Y.-C., Chen, H. 2012. Effect of air blowing on the morphology and nanofiber properties of blowing-assisted electrospun polycarbonates. *Journal of Applied Polymer Science* 124:4904–4914.

Huang, Z.-M., He, C.-L., Yang, A., Zhang, Y., Han, X.-J., Yin, J., Wu, Q. 2006. Encapsulating drugs in biodegradable ultrafine fibers through co-axial electrospinning. *Journal of Biomedical Materials Research* 77A:169–179.

Inami, T., Tanimoto, Y., Ueda, M., Shibata, Y., Hirayama, S., Yamaguchi, M., Kasai, K. 2013. Morphology and *in vitro* behavior of electrospun fibrous poly (D,L-lactic acid) for biomedical applications. *Advances in Materials Science and Engineering* 2013:ID 140643, 6 pages.

Jang, J.-H., Castano, O., Kim, H.-W. 2009. Electrospun materials as potential platforms for bone tissue engineering. *Advanced Drug Delivery Reviews* 61:1065–1083.

Jeun, J.-P., Kim, Y.-H., Lim, Y.-M., Choi, J.-H., Jung, C.-H., Kang, P.H., Nho, Y.-C. 2007. Electrospinning of poly(L-lactide-co-D, L-lactide). *Journal of Industrial Engineering Chemistry* 13:592–596.

Ji, H.-F., Sun, Y., Shen, L. 2014. Effect of vitamin E supplementation on aminotransferase levels in patients with NAFLD, NASH, and CHC: Results from a meta-analysis. *Nutrition* 30:986–991.

Ji, W., Sun, Y., Yang, F., van den Beucken, J.J.J.P., Fan, M., Chen, Z., Jansen, J.A.. 2011. Bioactive electrospun scaffolds delivering growth factors and genes for tissue engineering applications. *Pharmaceutical Research* 28:1259–1272.

Ji, W., Yang, F., van den Beucken, J.J.J.P., Bian, Z., Fan, M., Chen, Z., Jansen, J.A. 2010. Fibrous scaffolds loaded with protein prepared by blend or coaxial electrospinning. *Acta Biomaterialia* 6:4199–4207.

Jiang, H., Wang, L., Zhu, K. 2014. Coaxial electrospinning for encapsulation and controlled release of fragile water-soluble bioactive agents. *Journal of Controlled Release* 193:296–303.

Kim, T.G., Chung, H.J., Park, T.G. 2008. Macroporous and nanofibrous hyaluronic acid/collagen hybrid scaffold fabricated by concurrent electrospinning and deposition/leaching of salt particles. *Acta Biomaterialia* 4:1611–1619.

Kriegel, C., Kit, K.M., McClements, D.J., Weiss, J. 2009. Nanofibers as carrier systems for antimicrobial microemulsions. Part I: Fabrication and characterization. *Langmuir* 25:1154–1161.

Kulkarni, S.O., Kanekar, P.P., Nilegaonkar, S.S., Sarnaik, S.S., Jog, J.P. 2010. Production and characterization of a biodegradable poly(hydroxybutyrate-co-hydroxyvalerate) (PHB-co-PHV) copolymer by moderately haloalkali tolerant *Halomonas campisalis* MCM B-1027 isolated from Lonar Lake, India. *Bioresource Technology* 101:9765–9771.

Li, X., Su, Y., Zhou, X., Mo, X. 2009. Distribution of Sorbitan Monooleate in poly(l-lactide-co-ε-caprolactone) nanofibers from emulsion electrospinning. *Colloids and Surfaces B: Biointerfaces* 69:221–224.

Lima, M.S.R., Dimenstein, R., Ribeiro K.D.S. 2014. Vitamin E concentration in human milk and associated factors: A literature review. *Jornal de Pediatria (Rio J)* 90(5):440–448.

Linh, N.T.B., Lee, K.-H., Lee, B.-T. 2013. Functional nanofiber mat of polyvinyl alcohol/gelatin containing nanoparticles of biphasic calcium phosphate for bone regeneration in rat calvaria defects. *Journal of Biomedical Materials Research A* 101A:2412–2423.

Llorens, E., Armelin, E., Pérez-Madrigal, M.del M., del Valle, L.J., Alemán, C., Puiggalí, J. 2013. Nanomembranes and nanofibers from biodegradable conducting polymers. *Polymers* 5:1115–1157.

Lu, Y., Jiang, H., Tu, K., Wang, L. 2009. Mild immobilization of diverse macromolecular bioactive agents onto multifunctional fibrous membranes prepared by coaxial electrospinning. *Acta Biomaterialia* 5:1562–1574.

Luinstra, G.A., Borchardt, E. 2012. Material properties of poly(propylene carbonates). *Advances in Polymer Science* 245:29–48.

Luo, C.J., Stride, E., Edirisinghe, M. 2012. Mapping the influence of solubility and dielectric constant on electrospinning polycaprolactone solutions. *Macromolecules* 45:4669–4680.

Ma, B., Xie, J., Jiang, J., Shuler, F.D., Bartlett, D.E. 2013. Rational design of nanofiber scaffolds for orthopedic tissue repair and regeneration. *Nanomedicine (Lond)* 8:1459–1481.

Makadia, H.K., Siegel, S.J. 2011. Poly lactic-co-glycolic acid (PLGA) as biodegradable controlled drug delivery carrier. *Polymers (Basel)* 3:1377–1397.

Maleki, M., Latifi, M., Amani-Tehran, M., Mathur, S. 2013. Electrospun core–shell nanofibers for drug encapsulation and sustained release. *Polymer Engineering and Science* 53:1770–1779.

Martins, A., Reis, R.L., Neves, N.M. 2008. Electrospinning: Processing technique for tissue engineering scaffolding. *International Materials Reviews* 53(5):257–274.

Milleret, V., Simona, B., Neuenschwander, P., Hall, H. 2011. Tuning electrospinning parameters for production of 3d-fiber-fleeces with increased porosity for soft tissue engineering applications. *European Cells and Materials* 21:286–303.

Mondal, S. 2014. Influence of solvents properties on morphology of electrospun polyurethane nano fiber mats. *Polymers Advanced Technology* 25:179–183.

Muñoz-Bonilla, A., Cerrada, M.L., Fernández-García, M., Kubacka, A., Ferrer, M., Fernández-García, M. 2013. Biodegradable polycaprolactone-titania nanocomposites: Preparation, characterization and antimicrobial properties. *International Journal of Molecular Sciences* 14:9249–9266.

Munteanu, B.S., Aytac Z., Pricope G.M., Uyar T., Vasile C. 2014. Polylactic acid (PLA)/Silver-NP/VitaminE bionanocomposite electrospun nanofibers with antibacterial and antioxidant activity. *Journal of Nanoparticle Research* 16:2643 (12 pages).

Nagiah, N., Ramanathan, G., Uma, T.S., Madhavi, L., Anitha, R., Natarajan, T.S. 2013. Synthesis of blended fibers of poly(3-hydroxybutyric acid) and poly(propylene carbonate) scaffolds for tissue engineering. *Advances in Polymer Technology* 32:21370–21375. DOI: 10.1002/adv.21370.

Namboodiri, A.G., Parameswaran, R. 2013. Fibro-porous polycaprolactone membrane containing extracts of biophytum sensitivum: A prospective antibacterial wound dressing. *Journal of Applied Polymer Science* 129:2280–2286.

Nguyen, T.T.T., Ghosh, C., Hwang, S.-G., Chanunpanich, N., Park, J.S. 2012. Porous core/sheath composite nanofibers fabricated by coaxial electrospinning as a potential mat for drug release system. *International Journal of Pharmaceutics* 439:296–306.

Norouzi, M., Soleimani, M., Shabani, I., Atyabi, F., Ahvazf, H.H., Rashidi, A. 2013. Protein encapsulated in electrospun nanofibrous scaffolds for tissue engineering applications. *Polymer International* 62:1250–1256.

Pant, H.R., Baek, W., Nam, K.T., Seo, Y.A., Oh, H.J., Kim, H.Y. 2011a. Fabrication of polymeric microfibers containing rice-like oligomeric hydrogel nanoparticles on their surface: A novel strategy in the electrospinning process. *Materials Letters* 65:1441–1444.

Pant, H.R., Kim, C.S. 2013. Electrospun gelatin/nylon-6 compositenanofibers for biomedical applications. *Polymer International* 62:1008–1013.

Pant, H.R., Neupane, M.P., Pant, B., Panthi, G., Oh, H.-J., Lee, M.H., Kim, H.Y. 2011b. Fabrication of highly porous poly (ε-caprolactone) fibers for novel tissue scaffoldvia water-bath electrospinning. *Colloids and Surfaces B: Biointerfaces* 88:587–592.

Park, S.H., Park, D.S., Shin, J.W., Kang, Y.G., Kim, H.K., Yoon, T.R., Shin, J.W. 2013. Scaffolds for bone tissue engineering fabricated from two different materials by the rapid prototyping technique: PCL versus PLGA. *Journal of Materials Science: Materials in Medicine* 23:2671–2678.

Pham, Q.P., Sharma, U., Mikos, A.G. 2006. Electrospinning of polymeric nanofibers for tissue engineering applications: A review. *Tissue Engineering* 12:1197–1211.

Pillay, V., Dott, C., Choonara, Y.E., Tyagi, C., Tomar, L., Kumar, P., du Toit, L.C., Ndesendo, V.M.K. 2013. A review of the effect of processing variables on the fabrication of electrospun nanofibers for drug delivery applications. *Journal of Nanomaterials* 2013:ID 789289, 22 pages.

Podaralla, S., Averineni, R., Alqahtani, M., Perumal, O. 2012. Synthesis of novel biodegradable methoxy poly(ethylene glycol)-zein micelles for effective delivery of curcumin. *Molecular Pharmaceutics* 9:2778–2786.

Ramamoorthy, M., Rajiv, S. 2014. L-Carvone-loaded nanofibrous membrane as a fragrance delivery system: Fabrication, characterization and in vitro study. *Flavour and Fragrance Journal.* 29:334–339.

Ramier, J., Boubaker, M.B., Guerrouache, M., Langlois, V., Grande, D., Renard, E. 2014. Novel routes to epoxy functionalization of PHA-based electrospun scaffolds as ways to improve cell adhesion. *Journal of Polymer Science Part A: Polymer Chemistry* 52:816–824.

Reznik, S.N., Yarin, A.L., Zussman, E., Bercovicini, L. 2006. Evolution of a compound droplet attached to a core–shell nozzle under the action of a strong electric field. *Physics of Fluids* 18:062101. DOI: 10.1063/1.2206747.

Rieger, K.A., Bircha, N.P., Schiffman, J.D. 2013. Designing electrospun nanofiber mats to promote wound healing—A review. *Journal of Materials Chemistry B* 1:4531–4541.

Rieger, K.A., Schiffman, J.D. 2014. Electrospinning an essential oil: Cinnamaldehyde enhances the antimicrobial efficacy of chitosan/poly(ethylene oxide) nanofibers. *Carbohydrate Polymers* 113:561–568.

Rnjak-Kovacina, J., Wise, S.G., Li, Z., Maitz, P.K.M., Young, C.J., Wang, Y. 2011. Tailoring the porosity and pore size of electrospun synthetic human elastin scaffolds for dermal tissue engineering. *Biomaterials* 32:6729–6736.

Sell, S.A., McClure, M.J., Garg, K., Wolfe, P.S., Bowlin, G.L. 2009. Electrospinning of collagen/biopolymers for regenerative medicine and cardiovascular tissue engineering. *Advanced Drug Delivery Reviews* 61:1007–1019.

Sill, T.J., von Recum, H.A. 2008. Electrospinning: Applications in drug delivery and tissue engineering. *Biomaterials* 29:1989–2006.

Sirc, J., Kubinova, S., Hobzova, R., Stranska, D., Kozlik, P., Bosakova, Z., Marekova, D., Holan V., Sykova, E., Michalek, J. 2012. Controlled gentamicin release from multi-layered electrospun nanofibrous structures of various thicknesses. *International Journal of Nanomedicine* 7:5315–5325.

Sombatmankhong, K., Suwantong, O., Waleetorncheepsawat, S., Supaphol, P. 2006. Electrospun fiber mats of poly(3-hydroxybutyrate), poly(3-hydroxybutyrate-co-3-hydroxyvalerate), and their blends. *Journal of Polymer Science Part B: Polymer Physics* 44:2923–2933.

Song, B., Wu, C., Chang, J. 2012. Controllable delivery of hydrophilic and hydrophobic drugs from electrospun poly(lactic-co-glycolic acid)/mesoporous silica nanoparticles composite mats. *Journal of Biomedical Materials Research Part B* 100B:2178–2186.

Stoleru, E., Munteanu, B.S., Dumitriu, R.P., Coroaba, A., Drobotă, M., Fras Zemljic, L., Pricope, G.M., Vasile, C. Polyethylene materials with multifunctional surface properties. *Iranian Polymer Journal*, in press.

Stoyanova, N., Paneva, D., Mincheva, R., Toncheva, A., Manolova, N., Dubois, P., Rashkov, I. 2014. Poly(l-lactide) and poly(butylene succinate) immiscible blends: From electrospinning to biologically active materials. *Materials Science and Engineering: C* 41:119–126.

Sun, B., Long, Y.Z., Zhang, H.D., Li, M.M., Duvail, J.L., Jiang, X.Y., Yin, H.L. 2014. Advances in three-dimensional nanofibrous macrostructures *via* electrospinning. *Progress in Polymer Science* 39:862–890.

Sun, Z., Zussman, E., Yarin, A.L., Wendorff, J.H., Greiner, A. 2003. Compound core–shell polymer nanofibers by co-electrospinning. *Advanced Materials* 15:1929–1932.

Tan, S., Xianwei, H., Wu, B. 2007. Some fascinating phenomena in electrospinning processes and applications of electrospun nanofibers. *Polymer International* 56:1330–1339.

Theron, S.A., Yarin, A.L., Zussman, E., Kroll, E. 2005. Multiple jets in electrospinning: Experiment and modelling. *Polymer* 46:2889–2899.

Tiwari, S.K., Venkatraman, S. 2012. Electrospinning pure protein solutions in core–shell fibers. *Polymer International* 61:1549–1555.

Tong, H.-W., Wang, M. 2011. Electrospinning of poly(hydroxybutyrate-cohydroxyvalerate) fibrous tissue engineering scaffolds in two different electric fields. *Polymer Engineering and Science* 51:1325–1338.

Vasile, C., Nistor, M.T., Cojocariu, A.M. 2014a. Nanosize polymeric drug carrier systems. In *Nanotechnology and Drug Delivery*, Vol. 1: *Nanoplatforms in Drug Delivery*, ed. J.L. Arias, pp. 81–142. Boca Raton, FL: CRC Press.

Vasile, C., Oprea, A.M., Nistor, M.T., Cojocariu, A.M. 2014b. Drug delivery and release from polymeric. In *Nanomaterials in Nanotechnology and Drug Delivery*, Vol. 1: *Nanoplatforms in Drug Delivery*, ed. J.L. Arias, pp. 28–81. Boca Raton, FL: CRC Press.

Wang, H., Li, Y., Jiang, S., Zhang, P., Min, S., Jiang, S. 2014a. Synthesis, antimicrobial activity, and release of tetracycline hydrochloride loaded poly(vinyl alcohol)/soybean protein isolate/zirconium dioxide nanofibrous membranes. *Journal of Applied Polymer Science* 131:40903–40911.

Wang, M., Fang, D., Wang, N., Jiang, S., Nie, J., Yu, Q., Ma, G. 2014b. Preparation of PVDF/PVP core–shell nanofibers mats *via* homogeneous electrospinning. *Polymer* 55:2188–2196.

Whited, B.M., Rylander, M.N. 2014. The influence of electrospun scaffold topography on endothelial cell morphology, alignment, and adhesion in response to fluid flow. *Biotechnology and Bioengineering* 111:184–195.

Xiong, X.Y., Tam, K.C., Gan, L.H. 2005. Release kinetics of hydrophobic and hydrophilic model drugs from pluronic F127/poly(lactic acid) nanoparticles. *Journal of Controlled Release* 103:73–82.

Yu, D.G., Branford-White, C., White, K., Chatterton, N.P., Zhu, L.M., Huang, L.Y., Wang, B. 2011. A modified coaxial electrospinning for preparing fibers from a high concentration polymer solution. *eXPRESS Polymer Letters* 5(8):732–741.

Yu, D.-G., Chian, W., Wang, X., Li, X.-Y., Li, Y., Liao, Y.-Z. 2013. Linear drug release membrane prepared by a modified coaxial electrospinning process. *Journal of Membrane Science* 428:150–156.

Yu, D.G., Yu, J.H., Chen, L., Williams, G.R., Wang, X. 2012. Modified coaxial electrospinning for the preparation of high-quality ketoprofen-loaded cellulose acetate nanofibers. *Carbohydrate Polymers* 90:1016–1023.

Yu, L., Dean, K., Li, L. 2006. Polymer blends and composites from renewable resources. *Progress in Polymer Science* 31:576–602.

Zamani, M., Prabhakaran, M.P., Ramakrishna, S. 2013. Advances in drug delivery via electrospun and electrosprayed nanomaterials. *International Journal of Nanomedicine* 8:2997–3017.

Zargham, S., Bazgir, S., Tavakoli, A., Rashidi, A.S., Damerchely, R. 2012. The effect of flow rate on morphology and deposition area of electrospun Nylon 6 nanofiber. *Journal of Engineered Fibers and Fabrics* 7:42–49.

Zhan, J., Lan, P. 2012. The review on electrospun gelatin fiber scaffold. *Journal of Research Updates in Polymer Science* 1:59–71.

Zhang, J., Nie, J. 2012. Transformation of complex internal structures of poly(ethylene oxide)/chitosan oligosaccharide electrospun nanofibers. *Polymer International* 61:135–140.

Zhang, X., Reagan, M.R., Kaplan, D.L. 2009. Electrospun silk biomaterial scaffolds for regenerative medicine. *Advanced Drug Delivery Reviews* 61(12):988–1006.

Zhang, Y.Z., Ouyang, H.W., Lim, C.T., Ramakrishna, S., Huang, Z.M. 2005. Electrospinning of gelatin fibers and gelatin/PCL composite fibrous scaffolds. *Journal of Biomedical Materials Research Part B* 72B:156–165.

Zhao, P.C., Jiang, H.L., Pan, H., Zhu, K.J., Chen, W. 2007. Biodegradable fibrous scaffolds composed of gelatin coated poly(e-caprolactone) prepared by coaxial electrospinning. *Journal of Biomedical Materials Research Part A* 83:372–382.

Zhu, J., Marchant, R.E. 2011. Design properties of hydrogel tissue-engineering scaffolds. *Expert Review of Medical Devices* 8:607–626.

4 Starch-Based Nanocomposites for Biomedical Applications

Fernando G. Torres and Diego Arce

CONTENTS

4.1 STARCH: MOLECULAR STRUCTURE, GELATINIZATION, THERMOPLASTIC STARCH

4.1.1 NATIVE STARCH

Starch is a polysaccharide enzymatically produced by plants as an energy source in the form of discrete granules [1]. It is the main energy reserve in higher plants, and it is stored in tubers, seeds, roots, and stems over long periods of time, allowing the formation of large granular structures [2]. Corn, wheat, cassava, and potato starch are the most industrially important sources of starch. Other sources used to obtain starch are rice, banana, taro, and chestnuts, among others.

Starch granules are formed by two types of complex carbohydrate polymers: amylose and amylopectin [3]. Amylose makes up around 10%–30% of the granule, while amylopectin covers the remaining 70%–90% [4,5]. Amylose is a linear polymer formed by long chains of $\alpha(1–4)$-linked D-glucose units with a degree of polymerization in a range of 300–10,000 depending on its botanical origin [6]. Amylopectin is an extremely high-molecular-weight polymer. It has the same backbone structure of amylose, but with many α(1–6)-linked branch points [7]. The different structures of amylose and amylopectin can be observed in Figure 4.1.

4.1.2 STARCH GELATINIZATION

Using the right amount of water and heat, starch can be processed as a thermoplastic in order to produce films, foams, and sheets. During this process, a variety of chemical and physical reactions take place, such as water diffusion, granular expansion, gelatinization, decomposition, melting, and crystallization. Gelatinization is considered the most important reaction because it is the basis for the transition of starch to a thermoplastic [8].

Gelatinization occurs when starch is heated in the presence of water. The starch granules swell irreversibly and leach amylose losing birefringence [8]. This phenomenon causes the disruption of the crystalline structure of starch [9–12]. The temperature at which gelatinization takes place depends on the type of starch. In general, this process takes place at around 70°C under atmospheric pressure [11,13–15]. Some studies have indicated that the gelatinization temperature is influenced by the molecular structure of amylopectin, the amylose-amylopectin ratio, the crystalline structure of the starch granule, the presence of other minor constituents, and the maturity of the starch source [16–21].

Torres et al. [22] reported the gelatinization temperature of 22 varieties of starch obtained from Andean crops such as sweet potato, corn, potato, and cassava, among others. The gelatinization temperature of the starches studied ranges between 60.1°C and 73.5°C. Other studies report the gelatinization temperature of different species of potato starches [23] and cornstarches [24] in the ranges 68.9–70.8°C and 66.3–69.0°C, respectively.

4.1.3 MODIFIED STARCH

Native starch has some limitations for industrial applications, such as its low shear stress resistance, thermal resistance, thermal decomposition, and high retrogradation. In order to overcome these limitations, native starch is modified by physical and chemical methods [25]. In general, modified starches exhibit better paste clarity, stability, and increased resistance to retrogradation [26]. Crosslinking and substitution are used in chemical starch modification to produce modified starches for specific applications [27].

Different treatments for starch modification have been applied. Some of these treatments include self-association, complexation with salts, grafting, covalent crosslinking, and others [28–30]. The treatments applied for the modification of starches vary according to the application in which starch would be used. For example, Singh et al. [31] listed some types of starch modifications for food applications, such as pre-gelatinization, enzymatic hydrolysis, oxidation/bleaching, pyroconversion, and others, describing their properties and specific applications.

Regarding the field of biomedical applications, different types of modified starches, such as cadexomer iodine (CI), oxidized starch (OS), and hydroxyethyl (HES) are being used [32–44].

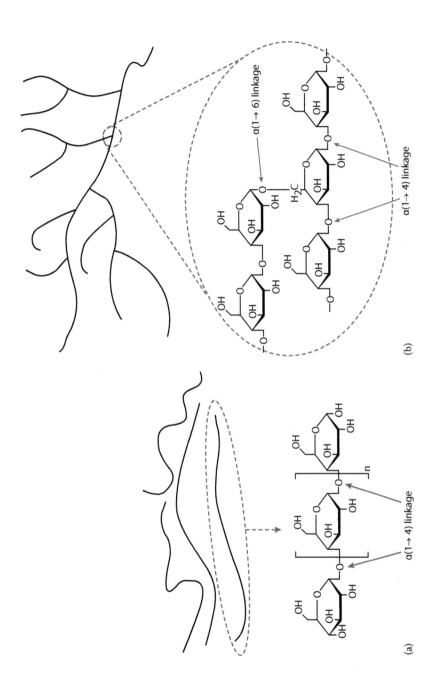

FIGURE 4.1 Molecular structure of starch: (a) amylose and (b) amylopectin. (Reproduced from Xie, F. et al., *Progr. Polym. Sci.*, 38, 1590, 2013. With permission.)

Cadexomer iodine is a hydrophilic starch crosslinked with epichlorohydrin and iodine arranged in the form of small beads [32]. In comparison with other iodophores, there is no chemical bonding between the iodine and the modified starch [33]. Instead, iodine is physically immobilized in the microsphere's matrix [32]. CI has a highly absorptive capacity; 1 g of CI can absorb up to 7 g of fluid [33]. One application of CI as a biomaterial is for wound-dressing applications. The starch matrix swells when CI is applied to an exudative wound, increasing the size of its micropores and slowly releasing iodine into the wound. This results in a sustained level of iodine in the wound bed [34]. Several studies have found that CI is an effective debriding and antiseptic agent for chronic wounds, such as venous leg ulcers [36–40].

The production of OS is achieved by the reaction of starch and an oxidizing agent under a controlled temperature and pH. OS characteristics include low-viscosity, high-stability, film-forming ability, and binding properties [41,42]. OS is used as a surface-sizing agent and as a coating binder in the paper industry [43]. In order to improve the mechanical properties of OS-based films, blends of OS and other polymers, such as polymethylcellulose, polyethylene, and polyvinyl alcohol (PVA), have been prepared [9]. Also, Wang et al. [44] used OS to produce electrospun PVA-OS fibers.

Hydroxyethyl starch (HES) is obtained by hydrolysis and subsequent hydroxyethylation of amylopectin. HES is usually produced by the reaction of starch with ethylene oxide at temperatures below 50°C in aqueous slurries in the presence of a swelling inhibiting salt [45]. Different types of HES are used as plasma expanders for the treatment of hypovolemia and arterial perfusion disorders, as well as for preoperative autologous blood donation and acute normovolaemic hemodilution [46].

4.2 STARCH AS BIOMATERIAL: BIOCOMPATIBILITY OF STARCH-BASED PRODUCTS AND STARCH-BASED PRODUCTS FOR BIOMEDICAL APPLICATIONS

Starch-based polymers have some advantages that make them suitable as medical polymer materials [47–52]:

- Good biocompatibility of starch
- Biodegradability and nontoxicity of starch products
- Acceptable mechanical properties of starch-based products

4.2.1 BIOCOMPATIBILITY

Biocompatibility is defined as the ability of a material to perform with an appropriate host response in a specific situation [53]. Williams [54] described three important characteristics that must be considered for a material to be biocompatible:

- Biocompatibility depends not only on the materials but also on the situation in which the material is used.
- Many applications require that the material react with the tissues instead of being ignored by them.
- Some applications require that the material degrade over time.

According to Marques et al. [55], biocompatibility is an inherent property of structures derived from organic polymers such as starch-based materials. The biocompatibility of starch-based products is due to the presence of major biocompatible structural components such as starch polymer molecules and products obtained from partial hydrolysis.

Because of its biocompatibility, starch-based materials have been used in several biomedical applications [56–63]. Studies carried out by Torres et al. [10] confirmed the biocompatibility of native starch products. They used starches from 17 different Andean crops in order to prepare films for cell seeding. Their results confirmed the in vitro biocompatibility of starch films with 3T3 fibroblast cells. Figure 4.2 shows the proliferation of 3T3 fibroblast cell lines after 3 days in a control flask and in an Andean potato starch film. The cells showed similar morphology among the different types of films and the control group.

Marques et al. [47] performed cytotoxicity and cell adhesion tests in two different blends of cornstarch—starch/ethylene vinyl alcohol (SEVA-C) and starch/cellulose acetate (SCA)—and their respective composites with hydroxyapatite (HA). Their results showed that those materials could be used in the future in applications for bone replacement/fixation and tissue engineering scaffolding due to their good cytocompatibility.

Mendes et al. [48] performed an extensive biocompatibility evaluation of the same materials (SEVA-C and SEVA-C reinforced with hydroxyapatite). They performed in vitro and in vivo assays. Their results concluded that these materials did not show

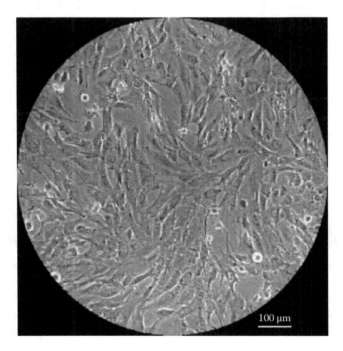

FIGURE 4.2 Proliferation of 3T3 fibroblast cell line after 3 days in a potato starch film. (Reproduced from Jenkins, P.J. et al., *Starch/Starke*, 45, 417, 1993. With permission.)

relevant toxicity in short- and long-term testing and also induced a satisfactory tissue response. Starch/polyaniline composites were tested using cytotoxicity assays [62]. The authors reported that the biocompatibility of the composites increased with a higher content of starch. Other studies tested the biocompatibility of starch-coated PbSe nanoparticles [63]. The results concluded that the coating was biocompatible and nontoxic.

4.2.2 BIOMEDICAL APPLICATIONS

Several biomedical applications have been developed over the last few years using starch-based biomaterials, including starch-based scaffolds for tissue engineering, drug-delivery systems, and starch-based hemostatic agents.

Several starch-based biodegradable polymers have been developed for bone tissue engineering [64–66]. Starch-based biodegradable bone cements can provide immediate structural support and degrade from the site of application [64]. Moreover, they can be combined with bioactive particles, which induce the growth of new bone in the cement–bone interface [65].

Starch-based biodegradable polymers can also be used as bone tissue engineering scaffolds [66]. A scaffold is an important component in the engineering of hard tissues in the biomedical field. It should allow the flow of an appropriate culture media, providing nutrients to the cells and removing the metabolites resulting from the cells activity [67]. Ideally, scaffolds must be designed using a polymer with an adequate degradation rate that is in phase with the formation of new tissue [68]. Starch has been used for the development of bone tissue engineering scaffolds [67–74]. Several processing methodologies have been developed in this area, such as injection molding, extrusion using blowing agents, compression molding, solvent casting, particle leaching, and rapid prototyping [67,69]. The processing technique must allow for the preparation of 3D scaffolds with controlled porosity and adequate pore sizes, as well as tissue-matching mechanical properties and an appropriate biological response [68]. Figure 4.3 shows the development of a starch-based scaffold fabricated by a rapid prototyping method [69].

Starch–polycaprolactone (SPCL) composites have been used as scaffolds. Neves et al. [67] studied the production of porous structures from starch-poly(ethylene vinyl alcohol) and starch-poly(lactic acid) for the development of scaffolds. They found

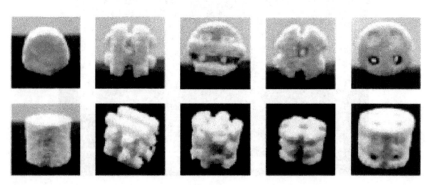

FIGURE 4.3 Starch-based scaffold fabricated by rapid prototyping. (Reproduced from Yang, J. et al., *Coll. Surf. B Biointerf.*, 115, 368, 2014. With permission.)

that SPCL scaffolds exhibit adequate porosity and mechanical properties to support cell adhesion and proliferation [72,74]. These studies also showed that tissue ingrowth could occur with the implantation of SPCL scaffolds [68,72]. The degradation analysis on these starch-based scaffolds has shown that they are susceptible to enzymatic degradation [72].

Santos et al. [73] reported the study of the growth of endothelial cells (ECs) on tissue-engineered scaffolds of SPCL. This was performed in order to assure the viability of the scaffold upon implantation and examine the interaction between ECs and SPCL fiber meshes. The results confirmed the cell compatibility and potential suitability of these scaffolds for the vascularization process in bone tissue engineering.

Salgado et al. [70] evaluated the in vivo endosseous response of starch-based scaffolds implanted in rats. They concluded that these starch-based scaffolds were well integrated in the defect site and surrounding marrow, indicating their good biocompatibility. The biomaterials exhibited a favorable bony response and a very early bone formation.

Darwish et al. [71] reported the fabrication of maxillofacial bone plates using green cornstarch composites. Glycerol plasticized starch was reinforced with pseudostem banana fibers at different weight fractions. Their experimental results showed that increasing the weight fraction of the banana fibers progressively improved the mechanical properties, reaching a maximum value at 50 wt.% fibers. Furthermore, incorporating banana fibers into the thermoplastic starch matrix improved the thermal properties of the composite.

Many studies have reported the use of starch as a biomaterial to develop drug-delivery systems [75–78]. Several reports describe the use of chemically modified starches for drug-delivery systems. Epichlorohydrin-crosslinked high amylose starch has been used for the controlled release of drugs [76]. A complex of amylose, butan-1-ol, and an aqueous dispersion of ethylcellulose has been used to coat pellets containing salicylic acid to treat colon disorders [77]. Kost and Shefer [78] used crosslinked starch for entrapment and controlled release of bioactive molecules such as salicylic acid.

Starch graft copolymers have also been used as drug-delivery systems. Simi and Abraham [79] grafted fatty acid on starch using potassium persulfate as catalyst in order to produce starch nanoparticles loaded with indomethacin, as model drug. Shaikh et al. [80] prepared acrylic monomers-starch graft copolymers by means of a ceric ion initiation method and used paracetamol as a model drug. Their results indicated that the graft copolymers may be useful to overcome the stomach's harsh environment and can be used as excipients in colon-targeting matrices.

Starch-based biodegradable polymers, in the form of microspheres or hydrogels, are suitable for drug-delivery systems [81,82] offering a device with no need for surgical removal after drug depletion [64]. The unique properties of starch-based hydrogels, such as hydrophilicity, permeability, biocompatibility, and similarity to soft biological systems, make them useful for various biomedical applications [83]. The 3D structure of starch-based hydrogels enables them to absorb and store plenty of water, without showing an important decrease in mechanical properties [64]. For these reasons, starch-based hydrogels have received growing interest for biomedical applications.

Polyvinyl alcohol/starch-blend hydrogels can be prepared by chemical crosslinking. Membranes synthesized by crosslinking of cornstarch and PVA with glutaraldehyde have shown adequate mechanical strength [84]. The resulting hydrogel membrane can be used as artificial skin, which can be used to deliver directly various nutrients, healing factors, and medications onto the site of action [85]. Shalviri et al. [86] prepared hydrogels by crosslinking starch with varying levels of xanthan gum and sodium trimetaphosphate. Their results suggested that such hydrogels can be potentially used as a film-forming material in controlled release formulations. Reis et al. [81] also prepared hydrogels by means of a crosslinking polymerization technique.

Elvira et al. [87] developed a range of starch-based biodegradable hydrogels. These materials were produced by free radical polymerization by mixing a solid and a liquid component. It was possible to produce both thermoplastic and cross-linked hydrogels, which could be used for multiple biomedical applications. Some of the hydrogels exhibited the most desirable kinetic behavior to be used as controlled release carrier. These hydrogels were also pH sensitive, degradable, and presented interesting swelling characteristics, which might allow for their application on a range of biomedical applications.

An investigation into the development of natural-based hemostatic with 50:50 chitosan–rice starch volume ratios showed reasonable properties for bleeding control due to its acceptable physical properties, fast blood absorption rate, and low hemoglobin leakage. Furthermore, with lower production cost and some superior properties over the available commercial products, the hemostatic agent has a potential to be commercialized and implemented for medical applications in the near future [88].

4.3   STARCH-BASED NANOCOMPOSITES

Starch has been used to develop a variety of composite bionanomaterials. For these nanocomposites, starch has been used as a matrix or as reinforcement.

4.3.1   STARCH AS MATRIX

With the incorporation of nano-reinforcements in a starch matrix, the resulting nanocomposites generally show improvement in some of their properties, such as mechanical properties (yield strength and Young´s modulus), thermal stability, moisture resistance, oxygen barrier property, and biodegradation rate. The improvement is due to the homogeneous dispersion of the aggregated nano-reinforcement and the strong interface adhesion, which contributes to the formation of a rigid nanocomposite network and influences the molecular and crystalline structures in the matrix. Also, conventional organomodifiers are used to increase hydrophobicity, resulting in reduced compatibility with the hydrophilic starch matrix [7].

Some factors that influence the improvement of starch matrix characteristics [7] are

- Plasticizer(s)/additive(s) used during preparation
- Starch source of the matrix
- Chemical modification of native starch
- Presence of other polymer(s) in the nanocomposite
- Processing and annealing conditions used during preparation
- Nano-reinforcement aspect ratio/surface area, chemistry, and mechanical properties

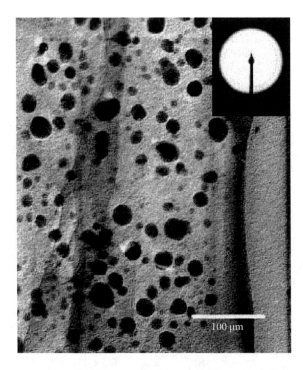

100 μm

FIGURE 4.4   TEM image of silver nanoparticles embedded in a soluble starch matrix. (Reproduced from Vigneshwaran, N. et al., *Carbohydr. Res.*, 341, 2012, 2006. With permission.)

As an example, starch was used as a macromolecular matrix on a study reported by Konwarh et al. [89]. They investigated the differential templating attributes of starch under ambient aging and sonication for biomimetically generated silver nanoparticles. Chang et al. [90,91] found that chitin/chitosan nanoparticles could be uniformly dispersed in a starch matrix at low loading levels, resulting in improved properties. However, when the nano-reinforcement addition was high, conglomeration or aggregation occurred. Figure 4.4 shows a TEM image of silver nanoparticles embedded in a soluble starch matrix [92].

Chung et al. used a starch solution as a matrix to develop a starch–clay nanocomposite. They measured the improvement of properties and found that the elastic modulus of the matrix and strength increased 35% and 30% compared to the unfilled starch matrix, and the nanocomposite did not experience a decrease in elongation at break. They also noticed that increasing the amount of water decreased the elastic modulus of both pure starch and starch nanocomposites. The change was less pronounced in the nanocomposites, suggesting that the addition of clay to form nanocomposites can improve the stability of starch-based products during transportation and storage [93].

Grande et al. [94] reported the development of a nanocomposite based on starch and bacterial cellulose (BC) nanofibrils. BC is an example of a self-assembled material formed by a coherent network of nanofibers of cellulose secreted by

Gluconacetobacter bacteria. Taking advantage of this characteristic, they used a bioinspired bottom-up technique to produce self-assembled starch-based nanocomposites. Figure 4.5 shows environmental scanning electron microscopy (ESEM) micrographs of BC-potato starch (a) and BC-cornstarch (b) nanocomposites showing the starch covering layer, and some uncovered nanofibrils (white arrows).

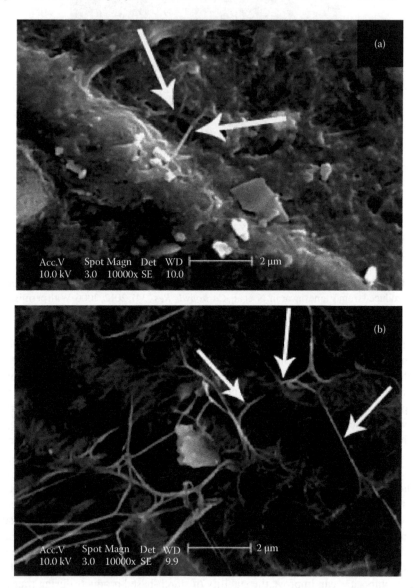

FIGURE 4.5 ESEM micrograph of (a) BC-potato starch and (b) BC-corn starch nanocomposite showing the starch covering layer, and some uncovered nanofibrils (white arrows). (Reproduced Grande, C.J. et al., *Mat. Sci. Eng. C*, 29, 1098, 2009. With permission.)

4.3.2 STARCH AS REINFORCEMENT

Starch nanoparticles can be produced by different routes. According to the production route, one can obtain crystalline or amorphous starch nanoparticles [95]. Hydrolysis of starch leads to the development of crystalline nanoparticles (nanocrystals), while regeneration and mechanical treatment of starch lead to the production of both amorphous and crystalline nanoparticles. The size of the nanoparticles and other relevant properties of the nanocomposites (such as tensile strength and elongation at break) depend on the production method used for their processing [95]. Figure 4.6 shows TEM images of starch nanoparticles processed via reversed-phase microemulsion using different amounts of starch, surfactant agent (Span 80), and oil/water (O/W) ratio for the preparation [96]. Their test indicated that the nanoparticles with the lower diameter (40 nm) were obtained using less amount of starch, O/W ratio, and high amount of surfactant agent (Figure 4.6e); while the nanoparticles with the highest diameter (400 nm) were obtained using less amount of surfactant agent (Figure 4.6d).

Previous studies reported that the addition of starch nanoparticles on a thermoplastic matrix increases the values of strength at break, elastic moduli (E), and glass transition temperature (T_g) of resulting nanocomposites [95–100]. However, changes in other properties are sometimes considered unfavorable, such as decomposition temperature (T_d), water uptake, and water vapor permeability [95,96].

The mechanisms that influence the property changes [7] are

- *Mechanical properties*: The increase in yield strength and Young´s modulus and a decrease in the elongation at break result from the reinforcing effect of the starch nanoparticles.
- *Glass transition*: The increase in glass transition temperature is due to the strengthened intermolecular interactions.
- *Moisture resistance*: The reduction is ascribed to the less hydrophilic nature of the starch nanoparticles.
- *Thermal stability*: The decrease is attributed to the sulfate groups on the acid-hydrolyzed starch nanoparticles.

For instance, Angellier et al. [101] prepared latex–starch nanocomposites using natural rubber as matrix and an aqueous suspension of waxy maize starch nanocrystals as the reinforcing phase. They obtained starch nanocrystals by the sulfuric acid hydrolysis of waxy maize starch granules. After mixing the latex and the starch nanocrystals, the resulting aqueous suspension was casted and evaporated. The solid nanocomposite films were characterized using scanning electron microscopy (SEM) and wide-angle x-ray diffraction analysis. They found that starch nanocomposites were evenly distributed in the rubber matrix and that the process did not affect the crystallinity of starch. They also investigated the barrier properties of the nanocomposites to water vapor and oxygen and found that the surface chemical modification of starch nanocrystals increased the swelling behavior and decreased the water uptake of the films.

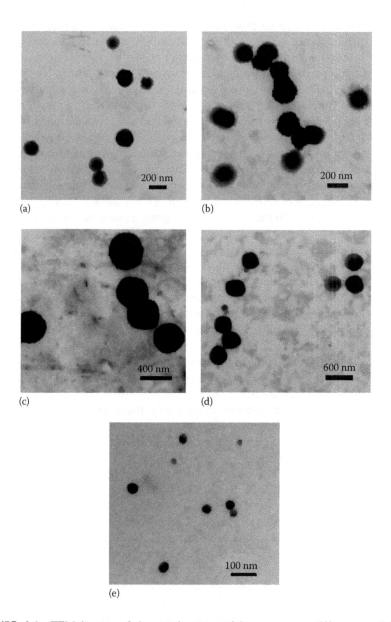

FIGURE 4.6 TEM images of the starch nanoparticles process at different conditions. The conditions used were: (a) 0.5 g Starch, 0.5 g Span 80 and 10:1 O/W; (b) 0.5g Starch, 0.5 g Span 80 and 15:1 O/W; (c) 1.0 g Starch, 0.5 g Span 80 and 10:1 O/W; (d) 0.5 g Starch, 0.2 g Span 80 and 10:1 O/W; and (e) 0.2 g Starch, 1.0 g Span 80 and 7:1 O/W. (Reproduced from García, N.L. et al., *Carbohydr. Polym.*, 84, 203, 2011. With permission.)

4.4 STARCH-BASED NANOCOMPOSITES FOR BIOMEDICAL APPLICATIONS

The characteristic properties of native starch such as good biocompatibility, bio-degradability, nontoxicity, proper mechanical properties, and degradability make this material suited to the development of biocomposites for biomedical applications [102–103]. The preparation of starch nanoparticles and nanocrystals has been widely studied, and several nanocomposites for the biomedical field have been reported. Due to its wide presence in food and its biodegradability, starch-based nanocomposites are considered *safe* materials. It is expected that potential allergic reactions will be experienced only in a restricted number of sensitive human recipients, as well as for other materials used for biomedical applications [104].

Starch-based nanocomposites have been widely used in several important biomedical applications [105– 116]. Some of them include the development of materials for bone regenerating treatments, tissue engineering, drug-delivery systems, hydrogels, and pharmaceutical products.

Fama et al. [107] developed starch-based nanocomposites containing very small quantities of multi walled carbon nanotubes (MWCNT), which can be used for the creation of tissue scaffolds or bone-regenerating treatments. The study of carbon nanotubes from a medical perspective has shown that besides use as reinforcement, they can stimulate bone formation [105]. Some researchers found that nanotubes work by severely damaging *Escherichia coli*'s cell walls, exhibiting powerful antimicrobial effects [106]. These materials exhibited highly improved tensile and impact properties as a consequence of wrapping MWCNTs with a starch–iodine complex composed by the same starch of the matrix. Even though these biodegradable composites are a very appealing alternative to traditional materials for different applications, there is little understanding of how they interact with humans and the environment.

In tissue engineering, fibrous structures that copy the morphology of natural extracellular matrices are considered promising scaffolds. For this reason, Martins et al. [57] developed a starch-based scaffold with the combination of SPCL micro-motifs and polycaprolactone nano-motifs produced by rapid prototyping and electrospinning techniques. They analyzed this material with SEM and microcomputed tomography showing the successful fabrication of a multilayered scaffold. The results also showed predominant cell attachment and spreading on the nanofiber meshes. These results supported the hypothesis that the integration of nanoscale fibers into 3D rapid prototyping scaffolds increases the biological performance in bone tissue engineering.

Drug-delivery systems have been improved over the last 20 years since the development of polymer based controlled drug delivery systems. Classical drug administration by injection causes plasma levels to rise and fall drastically when the drug is metabolized, leading to a cyclical pattern each time a dose is administered. In order to overcome this problem, a controlled drug-delivery mechanism is required close to the specific location where the drug is needed. Recently, attempts to use starch-based biodegradable plastics have resulted in enhanced drug delivery and eliminated the need for surgical retrieval of the polymeric material after drug administration [108]. The differential rates of drug release obtained by this method may be beneficial in cases where increased drug dosage is necessary at the beginning of therapy [109].

Simi and Abraham [79] produced a synthesis of modified hydrophobic starch nanoparticles using long-chain fatty acids. Based on this, they studied the drug loading and controlled release of the drug from the nanoparticles and found that this method can be used for drug-delivery applications.

Hydrogels are widely used in the biomedical field for tissue engineering due to their antimicrobial properties. Eid [110] synthesized a starch-based hydrogel by using a gamma radiation polymerization technique. He reported the formation of silver nanoparticles by the reduction of silver nitrate in the hydrogel. The development of a nanocomposite hydrogel prepared with silver nanoparticles, starch, and polyacrylamide was also reported by Abdel-Halim and Al-Deyab [111]. The nanosilver content and the antimicrobial activity were assessed. The results reported that a control sample without silver nanoparticles showed zero inhibition zones, while the samples containing silver nanoparticles showed different values of inhibition zones depending on the content of such nanoparticles. Silver nanoparticles were used to develop starch-based films with antibacterial properties for future biomedical applications [112]. Figure 4.7 shows the inhibitory zones of two sample films (a and b) against different bacterial strains (A: *E. coli*, B: *S. aureus*, and C: *B. cereus*).

Starch nanocomposites could offer a lot of benefits on eco-friendliness and compatibility for pharmaceutical and biomedical applications for large-scale production. Gao et al. [113] developed an eco-friendly method to synthesize silver nanoparticles by using biodegradable starch as a stabilizing agent. Core–shell Ag/starch nanoparticles were synthesized using biodegradable starch as a stabilizing agent via a green, quick, and simple method in the presence of glucose where the core Ag nanoparticles with starch layers were achieved. The nanoparticles produced were stable and uniform in size and shape and can be stored at room temperature for 3 months without any visible change. This method allows for the precise control of the diameter of nanoparticles and the thickness of layers by optimizing the reaction conditions.

Smitch et al. [114] prepared a fully biobased plastic material for biomedical applications. This material is a bionanocomposite based on halloysite (aluminosilicate clay mineral) nanotubes as nanofillers and plasticized starch as polymeric matrix prepared by melt-extrusion. The structural, morphological, thermal, and mechanical properties of plasticized starch/halloysite nanocomposites were investigated. It was found that the addition of halloysite nanotubes slightly enhanced the thermal stability of starch and significantly improved the tensile mechanical properties of starch without loss of ductility.

Silver nanowires were prepared on a waxy starch matrix by Valorkar et al. [115]. The nanocomposite exhibited bacterial effects and electrical conductivity. Also, Valorkar et al. [116] prepared water-soluble monodisperse copper nanoparticles using starch as green capping agent. The characterization of this nanocomposite showed excellent bactericidal action against Gram-negative and Gram-positive bacteria.

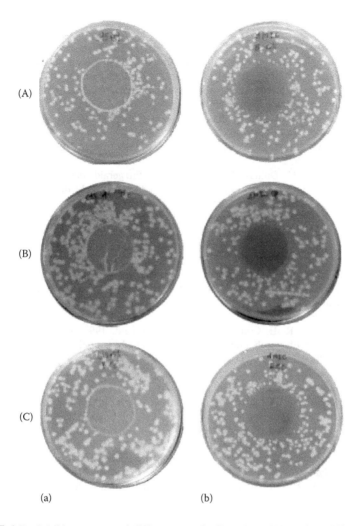

(A)

(B)

(C)

(a)   (b)

FIGURE 4.7 Inhibitory zones of different sample films (a and b) against different bacterial strains (A: *E. coli*, B: *S. aureus*, and C: *B. cereus*). (Reproduced from Yoksan, R. and Chirachanchai, S., *Mat. Sci. Eng. C*, 30, 891, 2010. With permission.)

4.5 CONCLUSIONS AND PERSPECTIVES

Starch is a natural polymer with outstanding biocompatible characteristics. This allows using it as a material for the development of new biocomposites. Starch can be used as both matrix and reinforcement. Starch particles and nanoparticles have been widely used for the creation of new biocomposites with different applications in the biomedical field. The applications of starch nanoparticles reported in the literature include tissue engineering, bone tissue engineering, and drug-delivery systems.

REFERENCES

1. Bogracheva, T. Y., C. Meares and C. L. Hedley. 2006. The effect of heating on the thermodynamic characteristics of potato starch. *Carbohydr. Polym.* 63:323–330.
2. Blennow, A., A. M. Bay-Smidt, P. Leonhardt, O. Bandsholm and M. H. Madsen. 2003. Starch paste stickiness is a relevant native starch selection criterion for wet-end paper manufacturing. *Starch/Starke* 55:381–389.
3. Pareta, R. and M. J. Edirisinghe. 2006. A novel method for the preparation of starch films and coatings. *Carbohydr. Polym.* 63:425–431.
4. Ramesh, M., J. R. Mitchell and S. E. Harding. 1999. Amylose content of rice starch. *Starch* 51:311–313.
5. Castro, J. V., C. Dumas, H. Chiou, M. A. Fitzgerald and R. G. Gilbert. 2005. Mechanistic information from analysis of molecular weight distributions of starch. *Biomacromolecules* 6:2248–2259.
6. Suortti, T., M. V. Gorenstein and P. Roger. 1998. Determination of the molecular mass of amylose. *J. Chromatogr. A* 828:515–521.
7. Xie, F., E. Pollet, P. J. Halley and L. Averous. 2013. Starch-based nano-biocomposites. *Progr. Polym. Sci.* 38:1590–1628.
8. Donald, A. M. 1994. Physics of foodstuffs. *Rep. Progr. Phys.* 57:1081–1135.
9. Torres, F. G., O. P. Troncoso, C. Torres, D. A. Díaz and E. Amaya. 2011. Biodegradability and mechanical properties of starch films from Andean crops. *Int. J. Biol. Macromol.* 48:603–606.
10. Jenkins, P. J., R. E. Cameron and A. M. Donald. 1993. A universal feature in the structure of starch granules from different botanical sources. *Starch/Starke* 45:417–420.
11. Perry, P. A. and A. M. Donald. 2000. The role of plasticization in starch granule assembly. *Biomacromolecules* 1:424–432.
12. Gidley, M. J. 2001. Starch: Advances. In: *Structure and Function, Royal Society of Chemistry*, eds. T. L. Barsby, A. M. Donald and P. J. Frazier, pp. 1–7. Food Chemistry Group, London, U.K.
13. Saibene, D., H. F. Zobel, D. B. Thompson and K. Seetharaman. 2008. Iodine-binding in granular starch: Different effects of moisture content for corn and potato. *Starch Starch–Stärke* 60:165–173.
14. Donovan, J. W. 1979. Phase transitions of the starch–water system. *Biopolymers* 18:263–275.
15. Jane, J., Y. Y. Chen, L. F. Lee et al. 1999. Effects of amylopectin branch chain length and amylose content on the gelatinization and pasting properties of starch. *Cereal Chem.* 76:629–637.
16. Biliaderis, C. G., C. M. Page, T. J. Maurice and B. O. Juliano. 1986. Thermal characterization of rice starches: A polymeric approach to phase transitions of granular starch. *J. Agric. Food Chem.* 34:6–14.
17. Jenkins, P. J. and A. M. Donald. 1995. The influence of amylose on starch granule structure. *Int. J. Biol. Macromol.* 17:315–321.
18. Srichuwong, S., T. C. Sunarti, T. Mishima, N. Isono and M. Hisamatsu. 2005. Starches from different botanical sources I: Contribution of amylopectin fine structure to thermal properties and enzyme digestibility. *Carbohydr. Polym.* 60:529–538.
19. Srichuwong, S., T. C. Sunarti, T. Mishima, N. Isono and M. Hisamatsu. 2005. Starches from different botanical sources II: Contribution of starch structure to swelling and pasting properties. *Carbohydr. Polym.* 62:25–34.
20. Hoover, R. 2001. Composition molecular structure and physicochemical properties of tuber and root starches. *Carbohydr. Polym.* 45:253–267.

21. Mweta, D. E., M. T. Labuschagne, S. Bonnet, J. Swarts and J. D. K. Saka. 2010. Isolation and physicochemical characterisation of starch from cocoyam (*Colocasia esculenta*) grown in Malawi. *J. Sci. Food Agric.* 90:1886–1896.

22. Torres, F. G., Troncoso, O. P., Díaz, D. A., Amaya, E. 2011. Morphological and thermal characterization of native starches from Adean crops. *Starch/Stärke* 63:381–389.

23. Karlsson, M. E. and Eliasson, A. 2003. Gelatinization and retrogradation of potato (*Solanum tuberosum*) starch in situ as assessed by differential scanning calorimetry (DSC). *Lebensm. Wiss. Technol.* 36:735–741.

24. Sandhu, K. S. and Singh, N. 2007. Some properties of corn starches II: Physicochemical, gelatinization, retrogradation, pasting and gel textural properties. *Food Chem.* 101:1499–1507.

25. Fleche, G. 1985. Chemical modification and degradation of starch. In: *Starch Conversion Technology*, eds. G. Van Beynum and J. A. Roels, pp. 73–100. Marcel Dekker, Inc., New York.

26. Agboola, S. O., J. O. Akingbala and G. B. Oguntimein. 1991. Physicochemical and functional properties of low DS cassava starch acetates and citrates. *Starch/Starke* 43:62–66.

27. Kaur, L., J. Singh and Q. Liu. 2007. Starch—A potential biomaterial for biomedical applications. In: *Nanomaterials and Nanosystems for Biomedical Applications*, ed. M. R. Mozafari, pp. 83–98. Springer, the Netherlands.

28. Shefer, A., S. Shefer, J. Kost and R. Langer. 1992. Structural characterization of starch networks in the solid state by cross-polarization magic-angle-spinning carbon-13 NMR spectroscopy and wide angle x-ray diffraction. *Macromolecules* 25:6756–6760.

29. Van Soest, J. J. G. and J. F.G, Vliegenthart. 1997. Crystallinity in starch plastics: consequences for material properties. *Trend Biotechnol.* 15:208–213.

30. Malafaya, P. B., F. Stappers and R. L. Reis. 2006. Starch-based microspheres produced by emulsion crosslinking with a potential media dependent responsive behavior to be used as drug delivery carriers. *J. Mater. Sci. Mater. Med.* 17:371–377.

31. Singh, J., Kaur, L. and McCarthy, O. J. 2007. Factors influencing the physico-chemical, morphological, thermal and rheological properties of some chemically modified starches for food applications—A review. *Food Hydrocoll.* 21:1–22.

32. Gustavsin, B. 1983. Cadexomer iodine: Introduction. In: *Cadexomer Iodine*, eds. J. A. Fox and H. Fischer. Schttauer, Stuttgart, New York.

33. Torres, F. G., S. Commeaux and O. P. Troncoso. 2013. Starch-based biomaterials for wound-dressing applications. *Starch/Starke* 65:543–551.

34. Sundberg, J. and R. Meller. 1993. A retrospective review of the use of cadexomer iodine in the treatment of chronic wounds. *Wounds: Compendium. Clin. Pract. Res.* 9:68–86.

35. Hillstrom, L. 1988. IODOSORB Compared to standard treatment in chronic venous leg ulcers—A multi centre study. *Acta Chir. Scand. Suppl.* 544:53–56.

36. Holloway, G. A., K. H. Johansen, R. W. Barnes and G. E. Pierce. 1989. Multicenter trial of cadexomer iodine to treat venous stasis ulcer. *West. J. Med.* 151:35–38.

37. Laudanska, H. and B. Gustavson. 1988. In-patients treatment of chronic varicose venous ulcers: A randomised trial of cadexomer-iodine versus standard dressing. *J. Int. Med. Res.* 16:428–435.

38. Moberg, S., L. Hoffman, M. L. Grennert and A. Holst. 1983. A randomized trial of cadexomer iodine in decubitus ulcers. *J. Am. Geriatr. Soc.* 31:462–465.

39. Ormiston, M. C., M. T. Seymour, G. E. Venn, R. I. Cohen and J. A. Fox. 1985. Controlled trial of IODOSORB in chronic venous ulcers. *Br. Med. J.* 291:308–310.

40. Skog, E., B. Arnesjo, T. Troeng, et al., 1983. A randomised trial comparing cadexomer iodine and standard treatment in the out-patient management of chronic venous ulcers. *Br. J. Dermatol.* 109:77–83.

41. Sangseethong, K., S. Lertphanich and K. Sriroth. 2009. Physicochemical properties of oxidized cassava starch prepared under various alkalinity levels. *Starch/Stärke* 61:92–100.

42. Lawal, O. S., K. O. Adebowale, B. M. Ogunsanwo, L. L Barba and N. S. Ilo. 2005. Oxidized and acid thinned starch derivatives of hybrid maize: Functional characteristics, wide-angle X-ray diffractometry and thermal properties. *Int. J Biol. Macromol* 35:71–79.

43. BeMiller, J. N. and R. L. Whistler. 1984. In: *Starch Chemistry and Technology*, 2nd edn., eds. R. L. Whustler, J. N. Bemiller and E. F. Paschall. Academic Press, New York.

44. Wang, H., Wang, W., Jiang, S., Jiang, S. et al. 2011. Poly(vinyl alcohol)/oxidized starch fibres via electrospinning technique: Fabrication and characterization. *Iran. Polym. J.* 20:551–558.

45. Kesler, C. C. and E. T. Hjermstad. 1950. Preparation of starch ethers in original granule form. U.S. Pat. 2,516,633.

46. Gallandat, R. C. G., A. W. Siemons, D. Baus, et al. 2000. A novel hydroxyethyl starch (HES 130/0.4) for effective perioperative plasma volume substitution in cardiac surgery. *Can. J. Anesth.* 47:1207–1215.

47. Marques A. P., R. L. Reis and J. A. Hunt. 2002. The biocompatibility of novel starch-based polymers and composites: In vitro studies. *Biomaterials* 23:1471–1478.

48. Mendes S. C., R. L. Reis, Y. P. Bovell, A. M. Cunha, C. A. van Blitterswijk and J. D. de Bruijn. 2001. Biocompatibility testing of novel starch-based materials with potential application in orthopaedic surgery: A preliminary study. *Biomaterials* 22:2057–2064.

49. Azevedo H. S., F. M. Gama and R. L. Reis. 2003. In vitro assessment of the enzymatic degradation of several starch-based biomaterials. *Biomacromolecules* 4:1703–1712.

50. Defaye J. and E. Wong. 1986. Structural studies of gum arabic, the exudate polysaccharide from acacia senegal. *Carbohydr. Res.* 150:221–231.

51. Reddy S. M., V. R. Sinha and D. S. Reddy. 1999. Novel oral colon-specific drug delivery systems for pharmacotherapy of peptides and nonpeptide drugs. *Drugs Today* 35:537–580.

52. Sinha V. R. and R. Kumria. 2001. Polysaccharides in colon-specific drug delivery. *Int. J. Pharm.* 224:19–38.

53. Williams, D. F. 1987. *Definitions in Biomaterials*. Elsevier, Amsterdam, the Netherlands.

54. Williams, D. F. 2008. On the mechanisms of biocompatibility. *Biomaterials* 29:2941–2953.

55. Marques, A. P., R. L. Reis and J. A. Hunt. 2005. An in vivo study of the host response to starch-based polymers and composites subcutaneously implanted in rats. *Macromol. Biosci.* 5:775–785.

56. Kozlowska, M., K. Fryder and B. Wolko. 2001. Peroxidase involvement in the defense response of red raspberry to *Didymella applanata. Acta Physiol. Plant.* 23:303–310.

57. Martins, A., S. Chung, A. J. Pedro, et al. 2009. Hierarchical starch-based fibrous scaffold for bone tissue engineering applications. *J. Tissue Eng. Regener. Med.* 3:37–42.

58. Azevedo, H. S. and R. L. Reis. 2009. Encapsulation of a-amylase into starch-based biomaterials: An enzymatic approach to tailor their degradation rate. *Acta Biomater.* 5:3021–3030.

59. Reddy, N. and Y. Yang. 2009. Preparation and properties of starch acetate fibers for potential tissue engineering applications. *Biotechnol. Bioeng.* 103:1016–1022.

60. Tuzlakoglu, K., I. Pashkuleva, M. T. Rodrigues, et al. 2010. A new route to produce starch-based fiber mesh scaffolds by wet spinning and subsequent surface modification as a way to improve cell attachment and proliferation. *J. Biomed. Mater. Res. Part A* 92:369–377.

61. Alves, N. M., I. B. Leonor, H. S. Azevedo, R. L. Reis and J. F. Mano. 2010. Designing biomaterials based on biomineralization of bone. *J. Mater. Chem.* 20:2911–2921.

62. Saikia, J. P., Banerjee, S., Konwar, B. K. and Kumar, A. 2010. Biocompatible novel starch/polyaniline composites: Characterization, anti-cytotoxicity and antioxidant activity. *Colloid Surf B: Biointerf.* 81:158–164.
63. Aswathy, R. G., Sivakumar, B., Brahatheeswaran, D., Yoshida, Y., Maekawa, T. and Kumar, D. S. Green synthesis, characterization and in vitro biocompatibility of starch capped PbSe nanoparticles. *Adv. Sci. Lett.* 16:69–75.
64. Lu, D. R., C. M. Xiao and S. J. Xu. 2009. Starch-based completely biodegradable polymer materials. *Express Polym. Lett.* 3:366–375.
65. Boesel, L. F., J. F. Mano and R. L. Reis. 2004. Optimization of the formulation and mechanical properties of starch-based partially degradable bone cements. *J. Mater. Sci. Mater. Med.* 15:73–83.
66. Gomes, M. E., V. I. Sikavitsas, E. Behravesh, R. L. Reis and A. G. Mikos. 2003. Effect of flow perfusion on the osteogenic differentiation of bone marrow stromal cells cultured on starch-based three-dimensional scaffolds. *J. Biomed. Mater. Res. Part A* 67:87–95.
67. Neves, N. M., A. Kouyumdzhiev and R. L. Reis. 2005. The morphology, mechanical properties and ageing behavior of porous injection molded starch-based blends for tissue engineering scaffolding. *Mater. Sci. Eng: C* 25:195–200.
68. Gomes, M. E., J. S. Godinho, D. Tchalamov, A. M. Cunha and R. L Reis. 2002. Alternative tissue engineering scaffolds based on starch: Processing methodologies, morphology, degradation and mechanical properties. *Mater. Sci. Eng. C.* 20:19–26.
69. Yang, J., Huang, Y., Gao, C., Liu, M., Zhang, X. 2014. Fabrication and evaluation of the novel reduction-sensitive starch nanoparticles for controlled drug release. *Coll. Surf. B. Biointerf.* 115:368–376.
70. Salgado, A. J., O. P. Coutinho, R. L. Reis and J. E. Davies. 2006. In vivo response to starch-based scaffolds designed for bone tissue engineering applications. *J. Biomed. Mater. Res. Part A* 80:983–989.
71. Darwish, L. R., M. Farag, M. T. El-Wakad and M. Emara. 2013. The use of starch matrix-banana fiber composites for biodegradable maxillofacial bone plates. In: *Proceedings of the 2013 International Conference on Biology, Medical Physics, Medical Chemistry, Biochemistry and Biomedical Engineering*, Innsbruck, Austria.
72. Gomes, M. E., H. S. Azevedo, A. R. Moreira, V. Ellä, M. Kellomäki and R. L. Reis. 2008. Starch–poly(ε-caprolactone) and starch–poly(lactic acid) fibre-mesh scaffolds for bone tissue engineering applications: Structure, mechanical properties and degradation behaviour. *J. Tissue Eng. Regenerative Med.* 2:243–252.
73. Santos, M. I., S. Fuchs, M. E. Gomes, R. E. Unger, R. L. Reis and C. J. Kirkpatrick. 2007. Response of micro- and macrovascular endothelial cells to starch-based fiber meshes for bone tissue engineering. *Biomaterials* 28:240–248.
74. Wang, Y., M. A. Rodriguez-Perez, R. L. Reis and J. F. Mano. 2005. Thermal and thermomechanical behaviour of polycaprolactone and starch/polycaprolactone blends for biomedical applications. *Macromol. Mater. Eng.* 290:792–801.
75. Chakraborty, S., B. Sahoo, I. Teraka, L. M. Miller and R. A. Gross. 2005. Enzyme-catalyzed regioselective modification of starch nanoparticles. *Macromolecules* 38:61–68.
76. Lenaerts, V., I. Moussa, Y. Dumoulin, et al. 1998. Cross-linked high amylose starch for controlled release of drugs: Recent advances. *J Controll. Rel.* 53:225–234.
77. Vandamme, Th. F., A. Lenourry, C. Charrueau and J. C. Chaumeil. 2002. The use of polysaccharides to target drugs to the colon. *Carbohydr. Polym.* 48:219–231.
78. Kost, J. and S. Shefer. 1990. Chemically-modified polysaccharides for enzymatically-controlled oral drug delivery. *Biomaterials* 11:695–698.
79. Simi, C. K. and E. T. Abraham. 2007. Hydrophobic grafted and cross-linked starch nanoparticles for drug delivery. *Bioprocess Biosyst. Eng.* 30:173–180.

80. Shaikh, M. M. and S. V. Lonikar. 2009. Starch–acrylics graft copolymers and blends: Synthesis, characterization, and applications as matrix for drug delivery. *J. Appl. Polym. Sci.* 114:2893–2900.
81. Balmayor, E. R., K. Tuzlakoglu, A. P. Marques, H. S. Azevedo and R. L. Reis. 2008. A novel enzymatically mediated drug delivery carrier for bone tissue engineering applications: Combining biodegradable starch based microparticles and differentiation agents. *J. Mater. Sci. Mater. Med.* 19:1617–1623.
82. Reis, A. V., M. R. Guilherme, T. A. Moia, L. H. C. Mattoso, E. C. Muniz and E. B. Tambourgi. 2008. Synthesis and characterization of a starch-modified hydrogel as potential carrier for drug delivery system. *J. Polym. Sci. Part A: Polym. Chem.* 46:2567–2574.
83. Peppas, N. A., P. Bures, W. Leobandung and H. Ichikawa. 2000. Hydrogels in pharmaceutical formulations. *Eur. J. Pharm. Biopharm.* 50:27–46.
84. Kordestani, S. S. 2014. Natural biopolymers: Wound care applications. In: *Encyclopedia of Biomedical Polymers and Polymeric Biomaterials*, ed. M. Mishra, CRC Press, U.K.
85. Pal, K., A. Banthia and D. Majumdar. 2009. Starch-based hydrogel with potential biomedical application as artificial skin. *ABNF J.* 9:23–29.
86. Shalviri, A., Q. Liu, M. J. Abdekhodaie and X. Y. Wu. 2010. Novel modified starch–xanthan gum hydrogels for controlled drug delivery: Synthesis and characterization. *Carbohydr. Polym.* 79:898–907.
87. Elvira, C., J. F. Mano, J. San Roman and R. L. Reis. 2002. Starch-based biodegradable hydrogels with potential biomedical applications as drug delivery systems. *Biomaterials* 23:1955–1966.
88. Wattanutchariya, W. and W. Changkowchai. 2012. Development of hemostatic agent from local material. In: *Proceedings of the Asia Pacific Industrial Engineering & Management Systems,* Phuket, Thailand.
89. Konwarh, R., N. Karak, C. E. Sawian, S. Baruah and M. Mandal. 2011. Effect of sonication and aging on the templating attribute of starch for "green" silver nanoparticles and their interactions at bio-interface. *Carbohydr. Polym.* 83:1245–1252.
90. Chang, P. R., R. Jian, J. Yu and X. Ma. 2010. Starch-based composites reinforced with novel chitin nanoparticles. *Carbohydr. Polym.* 80:420–425.
91. Chang, P. R., R. Jian, J. Yu and X. Ma. 2010. Fabrication and characterisation of chitosan nanoparticles/plasticised-starch composites. *Food Chem.* 120:736–740.
92. Vigneshwaran, N., Nachane, R. P., Balasubramanya, R. H. and Varadarajan, P. V. 2006. A novel one-pot 'green' synthesis of stable silver nanoparticles using soluble starch. *Carbohydr. Res.* 341:2012–2018.
93. Chung, Y., S. Ansari, L. Estevez, S. Hayrapetyan, E. P. Giannelis and H. Lai. 2010. Preparation and properties of biodegradable starch–clay nanocomposites. *Carbohydr. Polym.* 79:391–396.
94. Grande, C. J., Torres, F. G., Gomez, C. M., Troncoso, O. P., Canet-Ferrer, J., Martinez-Pastor, J. 2009. Development of self-assembled bacterial cellulose-starch nanocomposites. *Mat. Sci. Eng. C* 29:1098–1104.
95. Le Corre, D., J. Bras and A. Dufresne. 2010. Starch nanoparticles: A review. *Biomacromolecules* 11:1139–1153.
96. García, N. L., L. Ribba, A. Dufresne, M. I. Aranguren and S. Goyanes. 2011. Effect of glycerol on the morphology of nanocomposites made from thermoplastic starch and starch nanocrystals. *Carbohydr. Polym.* 84:203–210.
97. García, N. L., L. Ribba, A. Dufresne, M. I. Aranguren and S. Goyanes. 2009. Physicomechanical properties of biodegradable starch nanocomposites. *Macromol. Mater. Eng.* 294:169–177.
98. Viguié, J., S. Molina-Boisseau and A. Dufresne. 2007. Processing and characterization of waxy maize starch films plasticized by sorbitol and reinforced with starch nanocrystals. *Macromol. Biosci.* 7:1206–1216.

99. Ma, X., R. Jian, P. R. Chang and J. Yu. 2008. Fabrication and characterization of citric acid-modified starch nanoparticles/plasticized-starch composites. *Biomacromolecules* 9:3314–3320.

100. Angellier, H., S. Molina-Boisseau, P. Dole and A. Dufresne. 2006. Thermoplastic starch-waxy maize starch nanocrystals nanocomposites. *Biomacromolecules* 7:531–539.

101. Angellier, H., S. Molina-Boisseau, L. Lebrun and A. Dufresne. 2005. Processing and structural properties of Waxy maize starch nanocrystals reinforced natural rubber. *Macromolecules* 38:3783–3792.

102. Lane, M. E. 2011. Nanoparticles and the skin-applications and limitations. *J. Microencapsul.* 28:709–716.

103. Hakansson, L., A. Hakansson, O. Morales, L. Thorelius and T. Warfving. 1997. Spherex (degradable starch microspheres) chemo-occlusion—Enhancement of tumor drug concentration and therapeutic efficacy: An overview. *Semin. Oncol.* 24:100–109.

104. Gamucci, O., A. Bertero, M. Gagliardi and G. Bardi. 2014. Biomedical nanoparticles: Overview of their surface immune-compatibility. Coatings 4:139–159.

105. Harrison, B. S. and A. Atala. 2007. Carbon nanotube applications for tissue engineering. *Biomaterials* 28:344–353.

106. Valdés, M. G., A. C. V. González, J. A. G. Calzón and M. E. Díaz-García. 2009. Analytical nanotechnology for food analysis. *Microchim. Acta* 166:1–19.

107. Famá, L. M., V. Pettarin, S. N. Goyanes and C. R. Bernal. 2011. Starch/multi-walled carbon nanotubes composites with improved mechanical properties. *Carbohydr. Polym.* 83:1226–1231.

108. Mose, B. R. and S. M. Maranga. 2011. A review on starch-based nanocomposites for bioplastic materials. *J. Mater. Sci. Eng. B* 1:239–245.

109. Janssen, L. and L. Moscicki. 2009. *Thermoplastic Starch.* Willey-VCH Verlag GmbH & Co. KGaA, Weinheim, Germany.

110. Eid, M. 2011. Gamma radiation synthesis and characterization of starch-based polyelectrolyte hydrogels loaded silver nanoparticles. *J. Inorg. Organometal. Polym. Mater.* 21:297–305.

111. Abdel-Halim, E. S., S. S. Al-Deyab. 2014. Antimicrobial activity of silver/starch/poly-acrylamide nanocomposite. *Int. J. Biol. Macromol.* 68:33–38.

112. Yoksan, R. and Chirachanchai, S. 2010. Silver nanoparticle-loaded chitosan–starch-based films: Fabrication and evaluation of tensile, barrier and antimicrobial properties. *Mater. Sci. Eng: C* 30:891–897.

113. Gao, X., L. Wei, H. Yan and B. Xu. 2011. Green synthesis and characteristic of core-shell structure silver/starch nanoparticles. *Mater. Lett* 65:2963–2965.

114. Schmitt, H., K. Prashantha, J. Soulestin, M. F. Lacrampe and P. Krawczak. 2012. Preparation and properties of novel melt-blended halloysite nanotubes/wheat starch nanocomposites. *Carbohydr. Polym.* 89:920–927.

115. Valodkar, M., P. Sharma, D. K. Kanchan and S. Thakore. 2010. Conducting and antimicrobial properties of silver nanowire–waxy starch nanocomposites. *Int. J. Green Nanotechnol. Phys. Chem.* 2:10–19.

116. Valodkar, M., P. S. Rathore, R. N. Jadeja, M. Thounaojam, R. V. Devkar and S. Thakore. 2012. Cytotoxicity evaluation and antimicrobial studies of starch capped water soluble copper nanoparticles. *J. Hazard. Mater.* 201:244–249.

5 Polylactic Acid–Based Bionanocomposites

A State-of-the-Art Review Report

Inderdeep Singh and Kishore Debnath

CONTENTS

5.1 INTRODUCTION

The management of plastic products after the end of service has become one of the major environmental issues in the present scenario. Researchers worldwide are strategically focusing on the development of biopolymers because they can eliminate the disposal issue. Biopolymers may be broadly classified into four groups depending on the source from which they are derived, such as natural biopolymers (e.g., natural rubber, waxes, lipids, and lignin), biopolymers derived from renewable resources (e.g., polylactic acid [PLA], soy-based plastic, cellulosic plastic, and starch-based plastic), biopolymers synthesized from petrochemicals (e.g., polyesteramides, polycaprolactone, polyvinyl alcohol, and polyester amides), and microbial synthesized biopolymers (e.g., polyhydroxyalkanoates, polyhydroxybutyrate, and polyhydroxybutyrate-covalerate). Mostly biopolymers are used in packaging industries. It has been estimated that 41% of total production of plastic is used by packaging industries, where 47% of the plastic is used for packing of food items (Nishiyama and Kataoka 2006). Moreover, these materials are also widely used for the production of convenience products, such as disposable plates, cups, and cutlery.

95

Some specific applications of biopolymers are found in medical industries, where these materials are used in drug-delivery systems, surgical suture, and disposable gloves (McLauchlin and Thomas 2012). The major advantages associated with bio-polymers are they consume low energy during processing and are nontoxic to the environment (Bordes et al. 2009). Also, the limited petroleum resources can be preserved if biopolymers are used instead of petroleum-based synthetic polymers. Further, products based on biopolymers have no disposal issue after the end of ser-vice. But it is also true that biopolymers may not be used for manufacturing high-end sophisticated components. Low heat-distortion temperature, low melt viscosity, high gas permeability, and brittleness are a few properties that limit the biopolymers to expand their application spectrum (Sinha and Bousmina 2005). The cost of the bio-polymers is also substantially high as compared to the traditional petroleum-based polymers. The modification of the pristine biopolymer is mandatory in order to improve their performance. Hence, biopolymer-based bionanocomposites have been conceptualized and developed.

Nanocomposites are finding widespread acceptability due to their superior physi-cal and mechanical properties. Incorporation of a small amount (usually less than 10%) of nanoreinforcements into the polymer matrix results in improved physical and mechanical properties. According to the morphology, nanoreinforcements may be of three different types: acicular, spherical, and layered (Bordes et al. 2009). The size and shape of the nanoreinforcements significantly affect the mechanical behavior of the developed nanocomposites. A number of nanoreinforcement mate-rials have been developed, but the use of layered silicate clay mineral as nanore-inforcement has gained widespread attention among researchers for its low cost, easy availability, and environment friendly characteristics (Grim 1953; Lindblad et al. 2002). When nanoreinforcements are added to the biopolymer, the resultant material is called bionanocomposite. Three major processing techniques are com-monly used to prepare bionanocomposites: solution casting, in situ polymerization, and melt processing. The solution casting technique is a solvent system where both the nanoreinforcements and the polymer are dissolved in a predefined solvent. The in situ polymerization is a process where the nanoreinforcements are dispersed in the solution of monomer or in liquid monomer. The application of heat or radiation or suitable initiator results in the initiation of polymerization. The preparation of nanocomposites using the melt processing method involves two steps; in the first step, nanoreinforcements are mixed with polymer, and in second step, temperature (usually above the softening point of polymer) is applied to the mixture. The other processing methods such as processing at supercritical conditions and electrospin-ning have also gained widespread acceptance. The selection of processing technique mostly depends on the type of nanoreinforcements and biopolymer used for the development of bionanocomposites. The application spectrum of bionanocompos-ites is quite wide, which includes short-term application in agriculture, medical, and packaging sector. This chapter is designed to address the performance characteristics of various PLA-based bionanocomposites filled with different nanoreinforcements. A state-of-the-art literature review has been presented in the context of mechanical, electrical, thermal, rheological, and crystallization behavior of various PLA-based bionanocomposites.

5.2 POLYLACTIC ACID–BASED BIONANOCOMPOSITES: RESEARCH INITIATIVE

Polylactic acid has some unique characteristics, such as high strength, thermoplasticity, biocompatibility, and biodegradability. But the high degree of brittleness, high gas permeability, and slow crystallization rate of PLA limit its use in widespread applications. However, nanoreinforcements are extensively used to improve some of the properties of PLA. Nanoreinforcements such as silica, clays, graphene, hydroxyapatite (HAp), carbon nanotubes (CNTs), layered double hydroxide (LDH), and polyhedral oligomeric silsesquioxanes (POSS) are typically incorporated to improve certain properties of PLA (Ojijo and Sinha Ray 2013). The most widely used process for bionanocomposites is the solution casting method. Bionanocomposites based on graphene, silica, HAp, and POSS are prepared using the solution casting method. Further, these bionanocomposites may also be prepared by using the melt compounding technique. Among all the developed nanoreinforcements, clays and CNTs are mostly used for the development of bionanocomposites. In the following section, the properties of various PLA-based bionanocomposites have been discussed. The effects of various process parameters on the performance characteristics have also been highlighted in the context of PLA-based bionanocomposites.

5.2.1 Silica-Based Bionanocomposites

Bionanocomposites based on PLA and layered silicates, such as smectite, mica, and montmorillonite, have been developed in order to see the effect of layered silicates on the various properties of developed bionanocomposites (Krikorian and Pochan 2003; Lim et al. 2002; Maiti et al. 2002). A significant improvement in mechanical, gas barrier, fire retardancy, and other properties has been observed in the developed bionanocomposites as compared to the pristine polymer. For instance, poly(L-lactide) (PLLA)-based silica nanocomposites have been developed using sol-gel process to study the improvement in the properties (Yan et al. 2007). The investigation reveals that the tensile strength has been significantly improved even in the presence of a small amount of silica in PLLA. The thermal response has also been improved as the amount of silica content is increased from 0 to 12 wt.%. The infrared spectra measurement displays that the crystallization of PLLA is partially confined by silica network. Another investigation (Huang et al. 2009) has showed that the tensile, thermal, and hydrolysis behavior of PLA-based silica composites improves as the silica filler content is increased. It has also been noticed that the effect of nanosized silica particles on the mechanical and thermal stability is much better than the microscale silica particles. PLA-based SiO_2 bionanocomposites have been developed using melt mixing with the Haake mixing method (Zhu et al. 2010). For uniform dispersion of nanosized silica particles and attaining superior bonding between the PLA matrix and nanoreinforcements, the surface characteristics of the SiO_2 particles have been modified with oleic acid. The results show that the weight fraction of the modified SiO_2 particles has significant effect on the rheological properties of developed PLA bionanocomposites. The low weight percentage (less than 1%) of SiO_2 particles shows obvious plastication.

The authors finally conclude that the modified nanosilica particles improve the flexibility of PLA. The grafting of L-lactic oligomer with silica nanoreinforcements has been carried out (Yan et al. 2007). The results show that the dispersion of grafted SiO_2 (g-SiO_2) nanoreinforcements in PLA matrix is uniform as compared to unmodified SiO_2. However, at the 5% loading of g-SiO_2, the tensile strength and toughness of the materials are significantly improved. The rheological behavior during the in situ polymerization of L-lactide filled with silica particles has been studied (Prebe et al. 2010). The phase morphology, thermo-mechanical properties, and optical transparency of the PLA/silica nanocomposites have been investigated and compared with pristine PLA (Wen et al. 2009). The investigation reveals that the addition of silica particles results in significant improvement in crystallinity and crystallization speed as well. It has also been observed that both the tensile strength and modulus of the nanocomposites significantly improve. However, a slight improvement has been observed in impact strength and elongation at break (EB).

5.2.2 CLAY-BASED BIONANOCOMPOSITES

The understanding of the relationship between structure and property is an important aspect for designing bionanocomposites based on layered silicate with desired properties. In order to realize this, a number of bionanocomposites based on organically modified layered silicate and PLA have been developed using the melt extrusion process (Sinha Ray et al. 2003; Sinha Ray and Okamoto 2003). It has been observed that the heat-distortion temperature, biodegradability, oxygen gas permeability, and flexural properties of the developed bionanocomposites remarkably improve as compared to those of pristine PLA. PLA/layered silicate bionanocomposites have been developed by the melt extrusion of PLA and organically modified montmorillonite (C18-MMT) (Sinha Ray et al. 2002). It has been observed that the incorporation of a small amount of compatibilizer results in better parallel stacking of silicate layers and stronger flocculation as well. It has also been realized that the mechanical properties of the PLA/layered silicate bionanocomposites are much superior to those of the matrix without clay. Another study reveals that the mechanical properties obtained with PLA/clay bionanocomposites are much superior to those of the pristine PLA (Al-Mulla 2011). The decomposition temperature has also been found to be much higher than that of the pristine PLA. The PLLA-based modified clay has been blended using chloroform as cosolvent (Ogata et al. 1997). The analysis shows that dispersion of clay is not uniform, which means the clay existed in the form of tactoids. However, the influence of shearing force on the delamination of silicate layers has been found insignificant. Young's modulus of the blend is increased even with the addition of a small amount of clay. The tensile, antimicrobial, and water vapor barrier properties of the composite films based on PLA and different types of nanoclays (Cloisite 30B, Cloisite Na+, and Cloisite 20A) have been investigated (Rhim et al. 2009). A better intercalation and interaction have been observed between PLA and Cloisite 20A than between PLA and Cloisite 30B or Cloisite Na+. An extensive research work has been carried out focusing on the characterization of PLA-based clay bionanocomposites (Lin et al. 2007; McLauchlin and Thomas 2009; Wu and Wu 2006).

5.2.3 Graphene-Based Bionanocomposites

Due to the exceptional mechanical, thermal, and electrical properties, graphene has attracted many researchers and scientists in recent years (Compton and Nguyen 2010; Geim and Novoselov 2007; Zhu et al. 2010). Graphene is extensively used for the development of polymeric bionanocomposites. Graphene oxide (GO)-reinforced bio-degradable PLLA bionanocomposites have been developed at various loadings of GO ranging from 0.5 to 2 wt.% (Wang and Qiu 2012). It has been observed that the over-all isothermal melt crystallization rates are reduced as the crystallization temperature increases for both pristine PLLA and PLLA/GO bionanocomposites. The overall iso-thermal melt crystallization rates are substantially high for PLLA/GO as compared to the pristine PLLA. This may be ascribed to the fact that GO acts as a nucleating agent, which results in improved overall isothermal melt crystallization rates. It has also been observed that the overall isothermal melt crystallization rate and nonisothermal melt crystallization peak temperature of PLLA initially increase and thereafter decrease as the weight percentage of GO increases from 0.5 to 2 wt.%. Both the overall isother-mal melt crystallization rate and nonisothermal melt crystallization peak temperature have been found to be maximum at 1 wt.% GO loading. The crystallization behavior of PLLA/GO bionanocomposites at different loadings of GO has been studied (Wang and Qiu 2011). The findings show that with an increase in the content of GO, the maxi-mum crystallization temperature of PLLA shifts to low-temperature range. This means that the nonisothermal cold crystallization behavior of PLLA has been substantially improved with an increase in graphene loading. Further, it has been observed that the nonisothermal cold crystallization for both pristine PLLA and PLLA/GO bionano-composites accelerates as the heating rate increases. The feasibility of using conductive polymer composites (CPCs) as thermoelectric material has been studied (Antar et al. 2012). The major advantages of using CPCs over the conventional thermoelectric semi-conductor materials are ease of processing, environment friendliness, and low cost. Three different types of CPCs have been developed based on PLA matrix and reinforc-ing filler CNTs, expanded graphite (eGR), and CNT-eGR hybrid filler. The results show that the CNT-eGR hybrid filler significantly improves the electrical conductivity of the developed CPCs. It has also been observed that the eGR-based CPCs have the superior electrical conductivity than the CNT and CNT-eGR hybrid CPCs. The effect of eGR on the thermo-mechanical and fire-retardant properties of PLA has been evaluated (Murariu et al. 2010). The results show that the rigidity, tensile modulus, and storage modulus increase with eGR content. The thermal stability of the developed bionano-composites is also excellent. It has been recorded that the flame resistance capacity has improved. PLLA-based grafted graphite oxide bionanocomposites have been prepared by the in situ ring opening polymerization of L-lactide (Hua et al. 2010). It has been found that the electrical conductivity increases in the presence of graphite.

5.2.4 Hydroxyapatite-Based Bionanocomposites

One of the major mineral constituents of the vertebrate bones and teeth is HAp. It is a well-known fact that HAp can significantly improve the bioactivity and biocompat-ibility of developed biomaterials. Therefore, HAp is increasingly being in demand

and extensive efforts have been given to develop features based on HAp-based bion-anocomposites (Sadat-Shojai et al. 2013). HAp/PLLA bionanocomposites with fairly good mechanical properties have been fabricated using the modified in situ precipi-tation method. $Ca(OH)_2$ and H_3PO_4 have been used as precursors for the synthesis of HAp (Zhang et al. 2010). This modified in situ precipitation method has eluci-dated the aggregation of nanosized HAp particles into the PLLA matrix. The results show that both Young's modulus and compressive strength have been significantly improved when compared with the composites fabricated by the direct mixing of HAp and PLLA. This concludes the potential use of these composites in bone tissue engineering applications. The high molecular poly(D,L-lactide)-based Ca-deficient HAp nanocrystal (d-HAp) bionanocomposites have been developed using the solvent cast technique (Deng et al. 2001). The results show that the tensile modulus of the developed bionanocomposites increases as the content of Ca-deficient HAp nano-crystals is increased. Moreover, N,N-dimethylformamide has been found to be the best solvent among all PLA solvents used for the experimental work as the dispersion of Ca-deficient HAp nanocrystals is best in N,N-dimethylformamide. Another study reveals that the rate of mass loss increases with ageing time for HAp nanopowder (nHAp)-based medical-grade PLLA films (Delabarde et al. 2010). The rate of mass loss has also been found to be greater for amorphous PLLA films than for spherulitic films. However, the tensile strength and strain have been found to decrease with age-ing time, whereas the decrease in tensile properties is less for developed nHAp-based films as compared to the unmodified films as nHAp acts as an effective toughner. In order to obtain superior mechanical properties, nHAp has been surface grafted with PLLA (g-HAp) and further blended with PLLA to prepare PLLA/HAp bionano-composites (Hong et al. 2005). It has been found that the PLLA/g-HAp bionanocom-posites show higher impact energy and bending strength at approximately 4 wt.% of g-HAp, whereas at a higher g-HAp content, the modulus substantially increases. It indicates that PLLA can be strengthened and toughened if g-HAp nanoparticles are added to PLLA.

5.2.5 CARBON NANOTUBES–BASED BIONANOCOMPOSITES

Carbon nanotubes have some distinct properties such as high strength and stiffness and exceptional electrical and thermal properties. Because of these distinct proper-ties, CNTs are widely used for the development of bionanocomposites. The ther-mal, electrical, and mechanical properties of PLA/CNT bionanocomposites have been investigated (Moon et al. 2005). The study reveals that Young's modulus is slightly increased, whereas tensile strength and ultimate elongation decrease. The thermal stability of the developed bionanocomposites enhances in the presence of CNTs in PLLA. Another investigation shows that the DC conductivity increases as the multiwalled CNT (MWCNT) loading is increased in PLLA/MWCNT bionano-composites (Zhang et al. 2006). The effect of MWCNTs on the crystallization and melting behavior of PLLA has been studied (Shieh and Liu 2007). MWCNTs have been surface modified and grafted with PLLA to obtain PLLA-grafted MWCNTs. The results show that MWCNTs significantly improve the cold crystallization and nonisothermal melt crystallization rates of PLLA. In addition, the nucleation rate of

PLLA is enhanced by MWCNTs, which has been analyzed using polarized optical microscopy (POM). The effect of processing conditions during twin screw extrusion of PLA/MWCNTs has been experimentally investigated (Villmow et al. 2008). The effect of rotational speed on the dispersion of MWCNTs has been found maximum among all the input parameters such as MWCNT loading, temperature, screw profile, and rotation speed. As the rotation speed increases from 100 to 500 RPM, the number of agglomerates in PLA decreases. The electrical and mechanical properties of PLA/MWCNT-g-PLA bionanocomposites have been evaluated at 1 wt.% MWCNT content (Yoon et al. 2010). It has been observed that the morphological, electrical, and mechanical properties are strongly dependent on the length of the chain of PLA in the MWCNT-g-PLAs. The investigation reveals that the MWCNT-g-PLAs with longer PLA chain exhibit better dispersion of MWCNTs in the PLA matrix. The tensile properties of the developed bionanocomposites have also been improved as the length of PLA chain is increased. The electrical resistivity of the developed bionanocomposites has also been found to be increased, which may be attributed to the fact that the PLA-g-MWCNTs restrict the formation of the electrical conduction path of MWCNTs in the PLA matrix. The crystallization behavior of the PLA-based CNT nanocomposites has also been reported by many researchers (Barrau et al. 2011; Kuan et al. 2008; Wu et al. 2010).

5.2.6 LAYERED DOUBLE HYDROXIDE–BASED BIONANOCOMPOSITES

Layered double hydroxides are mineral and synthetic materials that possess positively charged brucite-type layers of mixed metal hydroxides (Nalawade et al. 2009). The development, processing, and characterization of LDH-based bionanocomposites are new areas of research in the field of materials science. PLA-based stearate-Mg_3Al LDH bionanocomposites have been developed using the solution casting method (Mahboobeh et al. 2010). It has been observed that the addition of 5 wt.% or less of stearate-Mg_3Al LDH produced exfoliated PLA bionanocomposites. The results show that the tensile strength and tensile modulus of the bionanocomposites do not change significantly in the presence of lower percentage (1 wt.%) of stearate-Mg_3Al LDH. Whereas the EB of the developed bionanocomposites is significantly enhanced to 650%. The EB of the bionanocomposites is about seven times higher than that of pristine PLA when stearate-Mg_3Al LDH content lies between 1 wt.% and 3 wt.%. The thermal degradation behavior of the PLLA/LDH bionanocomposites has been studied using thermogravimetric analysis (TGA) and pyrolysis-gas chromatography/mass spectroscopy (Py-GC/MS) in an inert atmosphere (Chiang et al. 2011). The bionanocomposites have been developed using organically modified magnesium/aluminum LDH (P-LDH) in tetrahydrofuran solution. Unfortunately, the TGA analysis reveals that the thermal stability of P-LDH is lower than that of pristine PLLA. The products of thermal degradation have been identified using Py-GC/MS, which shows that the incorporation of P-LDH into PLLA leads to a significant change in the thermal degradation process. The mechanical and thermophysical properties of the PLLA/LDH hybrids have been studied (Dagnon et al. 2009). The results show that some of the properties such as ultimate tensile strength, tensile modulus, and storage modulus have improved. It has also been observed that the thermal stability of the pristine PLLA is reduced. The cold crystallization has also been affected by LDH. The physical properties of the PLLA-based magnesium/aluminum LDH (MgAl-LDH) have been investigated (Chiang and Wu 2010). The surface of LDH has been modified by PLA with carboxyl end group (PLA-COOH) to improve the bonding between PLLA and LDH. It has been observed that the storage modulus has been significantly improved at 1.2 wt.% PLLA/P-LDH as compared to the pristine PLLA. PLLA-based organically modified LDH have been developed using the melt mixing process (Pan et al. 2008). The wide-angle x-ray diffraction results show that the layer distance of dodecyl sulfate-modified LDH (LDH-DS) is increased in the PLLA/LDH as compared to the organically modified LDH. Transmission electron microscopy analysis suggests that the dispersion of LDH-DS layers is homogenous in the PLLA matrix. It has also been observed that the effect of incorporating LDH-DS on the melting behavior and crystalline structure of PLLA is almost insignificant. However, the crystallization rate of PLLA increases with the addition of LDH-DS. POM observation indicates that the spherulite size of PLLA is reduced and nucleation density is increased in the presence of LDH-DS. The flame retarding behavior of PLA-based zinc-aluminum-LDH (Zn-Al-LDH) containing flame retardants such as pentaerythritol, ammonium polyphosphate, and melamine cyanurate nanocomposites has been studied (Wang et al. 2010). The results reveal that the incorporation of fire retardant and Zn-Al-LDH results in improved flame resistance properties of PLA-based bionanocomposites. In detail, total heat release, heat release rate, and heat release capacity of PLA bionanocomposites decrease as compared to those of pristine PLA, during combustion. The synthesis of PLA-LDHs bionanocomposites has been carried out by ROP (Katiyar et al. 2010). During in situ polymerization (in the presence of LDHs), the molecular weight of PLA is significantly reduced. This may be attributed to the chain termination via LDH surface hydroxyl groups and/or metal-catalyzed degradation. The effects of LDH carbonate (LDH-CO$_3$) and laurate-modified LDH (LDH-C$_{12}$) have also been studied. The investigation reveals that exfoliated bionanocomposites are obtained when using LDH-C$_{12}$, whereas using LDH-C$_{12}$ results in phase-separated morphology.

5.2.7 Polyhedral Oligomeric Silsesquioxanes–Based Bionanocomposites

Polyhedral oligomeric silsesquioxanes are an emerging nanostructured compounds that are mostly used to design novel hybrid bionanocomposites (Constable et al. 2004; Fu et al. 2004; Xu et al. 2002). POSS-reinforced PLLA bionanocomposites have been developed using the solution and coagulation method at various loading of POSS (Pan and Qiu 2010). The overall crystallization rate has improved for PLLA/POSS bionanocomposites as compared to that of pristine PLLA. Increasing POSS loading also results in improving the overall crystallization rate. However, the crystal structure and crystallization mechanism of PLLA remain unchanged in the presence of POSS. The storage modulus of PLLA/POSS bionancomposites is better than that of pristine PLA. It has also been observed that the hydrolytic degradation rates of the pristine PLLA have been enhanced with the addition of POSS. The crystallization behavior, crystal structure, spherulitic morphology, and thermal stability of the PLLA-based octavinyl-POSS (ovi-POSS) bionanocomposites have been investigated

(Yu and Qiu 2011). The experimental results reveal that both cold crystallization and nonisothermal melt response of the PLLA in the bionanocomposites have been enhanced in the presence of ovi-POSS, whereas the response is further improved as the weight percentage of ovi-POSS content is increased to 1 wt.%. The results also reveal that the overall crystallization rates are faster in PLLA/ovi-POSS as compared to those of pristine PLLA and further improved as the ovi-POSS loading is increased. It is also interesting to note that the crystal structure of PLLA remains unchanged in the developed bionanocomposites. However, the thermal stability of the PLLA is slightly reduced in the developed bionanocomposites as compared to that of pristine PLLA. The PLLA-based octa(3-chloropropylsilsesquioxane) (OCPS) films have been developed using the solution blending method (Zhang et al. 2011). It has been observed that when the content of OCPS is less than 3 wt.%, the dispersion of OCPS is good, but when the content of OCPS is increased to 5 wt.%, the OCPS begins to crystalize in the PLLA matrix. The study also reveals that the OCPS acts as a plasticizer to decrease both the glass transition temperature (T_g) and the melting temperature (T_m) of the PLLA matrix. The strain at break has also improved remarkably due to the plasticizer effect of OCPS. Further, the tensile test results indicate that the incorporation of OCPS into the PLLA results in a change in the tensile behavior, from brittle to ductile, of the developed hybrid films. The crystallization behavior of the PLA-based POSS-modified montmorillonite (POSS-MMT) bionanocomposites has been investigated (Lee and Jeong 2011). The PLA-based POSS-MMT (1–10 wt.%) bionanocomposites have been manufactured using the melt compounding technique. The results show that the overall melt crystallization is significantly improved by incorporating 3 wt.% POSS-MMT as compared to that of pristine PLA because POSS-MMT acts as an accelerating agent for the overall melt crystallization of PLA. The analysis also reveals that the nucleation density of PLA/POSS-NNT is higher than that of pristine PLA, whereas the spherulite growth rates in the PLA/POSS-NNT are comparable to those of pristine PLA. Poly(ε-caprolactone) and poly(L,L-lactide) covalently end-capped by POSS has led to the development of a new type of nanohybrid materials (Goffin et al. 2007). The nanohybrid materials have been developed by the coordination-insertion ROP of ε- caprolactone and L,L-lactide, respectively. Finally, the synthesis of a POSS-P(caprolactone-b-lactide) block copolymer has been carried out. PLAs/POSS have been developed by the ROP of L-lactide with 3-hydroxypropylheptaisobutyl POSS as an initiator in the presence of an Sn(Oct)$_2$ catalyst (Lee and Jeong 2010). Experimental investigation confirms that the hydroxyl-containing POSS molecules serve as an initiator for the polymerization of L-lactide. The thermal and thermo-oxidative degradation properties of the PLAs/POSS bionanocomposites improve at a lower POSS-PLA content (1%–20%) as compared to that of pristine PLA. The degradation properties of the bionanocomposites decrease at a higher content (30%) of POSS-PLA.

5.3　CONCLUDING REMARKS

Brittleness, high gas permeability, and slow crystallization rate are the properties that have restricted PLA in expanding its application spectrum. The modification of the pristine PLA is mandatory in order to improve the performance. It has been realized that incorporating nanoreinforcement into PLA improves various properties of PLA. When nanoreinforcements are added to the PLA, the resultant material is called bionanocomposite. The concept of bionanocomposites has been considered a novel route for the development of innovative materials with improved properties. A wide variety of nanoreinforcements such as silica, clays, graphene, HAp, CNTs, LDH, and POSS have been discovered in order to improve the performance characteristics of PLA. A significant improvement in mechanical, gas barrier, fire retardancy, and other properties has been observed in the bionanocomposites based on PLA and silica. Bionanocomposites based on clay and PLA have also shown remarkable improvement in HDT, biodegradability, oxygen gas permeability, and flexural properties. PLLA/GO bionanocomposites show better isothermal melt crystallization rates as compared to those of pristine PLLA, which may be due to the fact that GO acts as a nucleating agent. Bionanocomposites with fairly good mechanical properties can also be prepared using HAp and PLA, which can be used in bone tissue engineering applications. Due to some distinct properties such as high strength and stiffness and exceptional electrical and thermal properties, CNTs are also widely used for the development of bionanocomposites. Nanoreinforcements such as LDHs and POSS are also incorporated in PLA in order to improve properties such as tensile strength and modulus, storage modulus, EB, flame resistance, and the overall crystallization rate of the bionanocomposites.

REFERENCES

Al-Mulla, E.A.J. 2011. Preparation of new polymer nanocomposites based on poly (lactic acid)/fatty nitrogen compounds modified clay by a solution casting process. *Fibers and Polymers* 12: 444–450.

Antar, Z., Feller, J.F., Noël, H., Glouannec, P, and Elleuch, K. 2012. Thermoelectric behavior of melt processed carbon nanotube/graphite/poly(lactic acid) conductive biopolymer nanocomposites (CPC). *Materials Letters* 67: 210–214.

Barrau, S., Vanmansart, C., Moreau, M., Addad, A., Stoclet, G., Lefebvre, J.M., and Seguela, R. 2011. Crystallization behavior of carbon nanotube-polylactide nanocomposites. *Macromolecules* 44: 6496–6502.

Bordes, P., Pollet, E., and Avérous, L. 2009. Nano-biocomposites: Biodegradable polyester/ nanoclay systems. *Progress in Polymer Science* 34: 125–155.

Chiang, M.F., Chu, M.Z., and Wu, T.M. 2011. Effect of layered double hydroxides on the thermal degradation behavior of biodegradable poly (L-lactide) nanocomposites. Polymer Degradation and Stability 96: 60–66.

Chiang, M.F. and Wu, T.M. 2010. Synthesis and characterization of biodegradable poly (L-lactide)/layered double hydroxide nanocomposites. *Composites Science and Technology* 70: 110–115.

Compton, O.C. and Nguyen, S.T. 2010. Graphene oxide, highly reduced graphene oxide, and graphene: Versatile building blocks for carbon-based materials. *Small* 6: 711–723.

Constable, G.S., Lesser, A.J., and Coughlin, E.B. 2004. Morphological and mechanical evaluation of hybrid organic-inorganic thermoset copolymers of dicyclopentadiene and mono-or tris (norbornenyl)-substituted polyhedral oligomeric silsesquioxanes. *Macromolecules* 37: 1276–1282.

Dagnon, K.L., Ambadapadi, S., Shaito, A., Ogbomo, S.M., DeLeon, V., Golden, T.D., Rahimi, M, Nguyen, K, Braterman, P.S., and D'Souza, N.A. 2009. Poly (L-lactic acid) nanocomposites with layered double hydroxides functionalized with ibuprofen. *Journal of Applied Polymer Science* 113: 1905–1915.

Delabarde, C., Plummer, C.J.G., Bourban, P.E., and Månson, J.A.E. 2010. Accelerated ageing and degradation in poly-L-lactide/hydroxyapatite nanocomposites. *Polymer Degradation and Stability* 96: 595–607.

Deng, X., Hao, J., and Wang, C. 2001. Preparation and mechanical properties of nanocomposites of poly(D,L-lactide) with Ca-deficient hydroxyapatite nanocrystals. *Biomaterials* 22: 2867–2873.

Fu, B.X., Lee, A., and Haddad, T.S. 2004. Styrene-butadiene-styrene triblock copolymers modified with polyhedral oligomeric silsesquioxanes. *Macromolecules* 37: 5211–5218.

Geim, A.K. and Novoselov, K.S. 2007. The rise of graphene. *Nature Materials* 6: 183–191.

Goffin, A.L., Duquesne, E., Moins, S., Alexandre, M., and Dubois, P. 2007. New organic-inorganic nanohybrids via ring opening polymerization of (di)lactones initiated by functionalized polyhedral oligomeric silsesquioxane. *European Polymer Journal* 43: 4103–4113.

Grim, R.E. 1953. *Clay Mineralogy*. New York: McGraw-Hill.

Hong, Z., Zhang, P., He, C., Qiu, X., Liu, A., Chen, L., Chen, X., and Jing, X. 2005. Nano-composite of poly (L-lactide) and surface grafted hydroxyapatite: Mechanical properties and biocompatibility. *Biomaterials* 26: 6296–6304.

Hua, L., Kai, W., Yang, J., and Inoue, Y. 2010. A new poly (L-lactide)-grafted graphite oxide composite: Facile synthesis, electrical properties and crystallization behaviors. *Polymer Degradation and Stability* 95: 2619–2627.

Huang, J.W., Hung, Y.C., Wen, Y.L., Kang, C.C., and Yeh, M.Y. 2009. Polylactide/nano and microscale silica composite films. I. Preparation and characterization. *Journal of Applied Polymer Science* 112:1688–1694.

Katiyar, V., Gerds, N., Koch, C.B., Risbo, J., Hansen, H.C.B., and Plackett, D. 2010. Poly L-lactide-layered double hydroxide nanocomposites via in situ polymerization of L-lactide. *Polymer Degradation and Stability* 95: 2563–2573.

Krikorian, V. and Pochan, D.J. 2003. Poly (L-lactic acid)/layered silicate nanocomposite: Fabrication, characterization, and properties. *Chemistry of Materials* 15: 4317–4324.

Kuan, C.F., Chen, C.H., Kuan, H.C., Lin, K.C., Chiang, C.L., and Peng, H.C. 2008. Multiwalled carbon nanotube reinforced poly (L-lactic acid) nanocomposites enhanced by water-crosslinking reaction. *Journal of Physics and Chemistry of Solids* 69: 1399–1402.

Lee, J.H. and Jeong, Y.G. 2010. Preparation and characterization of nanocomposites based on polylactides tethered with polyhedral oligomeric silsesquioxane. *Journal of Applied Polymer Science* 115: 1039–1046.

Lee, J.H. and Jeong, Y.G. 2011. Preparation and crystallization behavior of polylactide nanocomposites reinforced with POSS-modified montmorillonite. *Fibers and Polymers* 12: 180–189.

Lim, S.T., Hyun, Y.H., Choi, H.J., and Jhon, M.S. 2002. Synthetic biodegradable aliphatic polyester/montmorillonite nanocomposites. *Chemistry of Materials* 14: 1839–1844.

Lin, L.H., Liu, H.J., and Yu, N.K. 2007. Morphology and thermal properties of poly (L-lactic acid)/organoclay nanocomposites. *Journal of Applied Polymer Science* 106: 260–266.

Lindblad, M.S., Liu, Y., Albertsson, A-C., Ranucci, E., and Karlsson, S. 2002. Polymer from renewable resources. *Advances in Polymer Science* 157: 139–61.

Mahboobeh, E., Yunus, W.M.Z.W., Hussein, Z., Ahmad, M., and Ibrahim, N.A. 2010. Flexibility improvement of poly (lactic acid) by stearate-modified layered double hydroxide. *Journal of Applied Polymer Science* 118: 1077–1083.

Maiti, P., Yamada, K., Okamoto, M., Ueda, K., and Okamoto, K. 2002. New polylactide/layered silicate nanocomposites: Role of organoclays. *Chemistry of Materials* 14: 4654–4661.

McLauchlin, A.R. and Thomas, N.L. 2009. Preparation and thermal characterisation of poly (lactic acid) nanocomposites prepared from organoclays based on an amphoteric surfactant. *Polymer Degradation and Stability* 94: 868–872.

McLauchlin, A.R. and Thomas, N.L. 2012. Biodegradable polymer nanocomposites. In *Advances in Polymer Nanocomposites: Types and Applications*, ed. F. Gao, pp. 398–430. Woodhead Publishing Limited, Cambridge, U.K.

Moon, S.I., Jin, F., Lee, C.J., Tsutsumi, S., and Hyon, S.H. 2005. Novel carbon nanotube/poly (L-lactic acid) nanocomposites; their modulus, thermal stability, and electrical conductivity. *Macromolecular Symposia* 224: 287–296.

Murariu, M., Dechief, A.L., Bonnaud, L., Paint, Y., Gallos, A., Fontaine, G., Bourbigot, S., and Dubois, P. 2010. The production and properties of polylactide composites filled with expanded graphite. *Polymer Degradation and Stability* 95: 889–900.

Nalawade, P., Aware, B., Kadam, V.J., and Hirlekar, R.S. 2009. Layered double hydroxides: A review. *Journal of Scientific and Industrial Research* 68: 267–272.

Nishiyama, N. and Kataoka, K. 2006. Current state, achievements, and future prospects of polymeric micelles as nanocarriers for drug and gene delivery. *Pharmacology & Therapeutics*, 112: 630–648.

Ogata, N., Jimenez, G., Kawai, H., and Ogihara, T. 1997. Structure and thermal/mechanical properties of poly (L-lactide)-clay blend. *Journal of Polymer Science Part B: Polymer Physics* 35: 389–396.

Ojijo, V. and Sinha Ray, S. 2013. Processing strategies in bionanocomposites. *Progress in Polymer Science* 38: 1543–1589.

Pan, H. and Qiu, Z. 2010. Biodegradable poly (L-lactide)/polyhedral oligomeric silsesquioxanes nanocomposites: Enhanced crystallization, mechanical properties, and hydrolytic degradation. *Macromolecules* 43: 1499–1506.

Pan, P., Zhu, B., Dong, T., and Inoue, Y. 2008. Poly (L-lactide)/layered double hydroxides nanocomposites: Preparation and crystallization behavior. *Journal of Polymer Science Part B: Polymer Physics* 46: 2222–2233.

Prebe, A., Alcouffe, P., Cassagnau, P., and Gérard, J.F. 2010. In situ polymerization of L-Lactide in the presence of fumed silica. *Materials Chemistry and Physics* 124: 399–405.

Rhim, J.W., Hong, S.I., and Ha, C.S. 2009. Tensile, water vapor barrier and antimicrobial properties of PLA/nanoclay composite films. *LWT—Food Science and Technology* 42: 612–617.

Sadat-Shojai, M., Khorasani, M.T., Dinpanah-Khoshdargi, E., and Jamshidi, A. 2013. Synthesis methods for nanosized hydroxyapatite with diverse structures. *Acta Biomaterialia* 9: 7591–7621.

Shieh, Y.T. and Liu, G.L. 2007. Effects of carbon nanotubes on crystallization and melting behavior of poly (L-lactide) via DSC and TMDSC studies. *Journal of Polymer Science Part B: Polymer Physics* 45: 1870–1881.

Sinha Ray, S. and Bousmina, M. 2005. Biodegradable polymers and their layered silicate nanocomposites: In greening the 21st century materials world. *Progress in Materials Science* 50(8): 962–1079.

Sinha Ray, S. and Okamoto, M. 2003. Biodegradable polylactide and its nanocomposites: Opening a new dimension for plastics and composites. *Macromolecular Rapid Communications* 24: 815–840.

Sinha Ray, S., Maiti, P., Okamoto, M., Yamada, K., and Ueda, K. 2002. New polylactide/layered silicate nanocomposites. 1. Preparation, characterization, and properties. *Macromolecules* 35: 3104–3110.

Sinha Ray, S., Yamada, K., Okamoto, M., Fujimoto, Y., Ogami, A., and Ueda, K. 2003. New polylactide/layered silicate nanocomposites. 5. Designing of materials with desired properties. *Polymer* 44: 6633–6646.

Sinha Ray, S., Yamada, K., Okamoto, M., and Ueda, K. 2003. Biodegradable polylactide/montmorillonite nanocomposites. *Journal of Nanoscience and Nanotechnology* 3: 503–510.

Villmow, T., Pötschke, P., Pegel, S., Häussler, L., and Kretzschmar, B. 2008. Influence of twin-screw extrusion conditions on the dispersion of multi-walled carbon nanotubes in a poly (lactic acid) matrix. *Polymer* 49: 3500–3509.

Wang, D.Y., Leuteritz, A., Wang, Y.Z., Wagenknecht, U., and Heinrich, G. 2010. Preparation and burning behaviors of flame retarding biodegradable poly (lactic acid) nanocomposite based on zinc aluminum layered double hydroxide. *Polymer Degradation and Stability* 95: 2474–2480.

Wang, H. and Qiu, Z. 2011. Crystallization behaviors of biodegradable poly(L-lactic acid)/graphene oxide nanocomposites from the amorphous state. *Thermochimica Acta* 526: 229–236.

Wang, H. and Qiu, Z. 2012. Crystallization kinetics and morphology of biodegradable poly (L-lactic acid)/graphene oxide nanocomposites: Influences of graphene oxide loading and crystallization temperature. *Thermochimica Acta* 527: 40–46.

Wen, X., Lin, Y., Han, C., Zhang, K., Ran, X., Li, Y., and Dong, L. 2009. Thermomechanical and optical properties of biodegradable poly (L-lactide)/silica nanocomposites by melt compounding. *Journal of Applied Polymer Science* 114: 3379–3388.

Wu, D., Wu, L., Zhou, W., Zhang, M., and Yang, T. 2010. Crystallization and biodegradation of polylactide/carbon nanotube composites. *Polymer Engineering & Science* 50: 1721–1733.

Wu, T.M. and Wu, C.Y. 2006. Biodegradable poly (lactic acid)/chitosan-modified montmorillonite nanocomposites: Preparation and characterization. *Polymer Degradation and Stability* 91: 2198–2204.

Xu, H., Kuo, S.W., Lee, J.S., and Chang, F.C. 2002. Preparations, thermal properties, and T_g increase mechanism of inorganic/organic hybrid polymers based on polyhedral oligomeric silsesquioxanes. *Macromolecules* 35: 8788–8793.

Yan, S., Yin, J., Yang, J., and Chen, X. 2007. Structural characteristics and thermal properties of plasticized poly (L-lactide)-silica nanocomposites synthesized by sol-gel method. *Materials Letters* 61: 2683–2686.

Yan, S., Yin, J., Yang, Y., Dai, Z., Ma, J., and Chen, X. 2007. Surface-grafted silica linked with L-lactic acid oligomer: A novel nanofiller to improve the performance of biodegradable poly (L-lactide). *Polymer* 48: 1688–1694.

Yoon, J.T., Lee, S.C., and Jeong, Y.G. 2010. Effects of grafted chain length on mechanical and electrical properties of nanocomposites containing polylactide-grafted carbon nanotubes. *Composites Science and Technology* 70: 776–782.

Yu, J. and Qiu, Z. 2011. Effect of low octavinyl-polyhedral oligomeric silsesquioxanes loadings on the melt crystallization and morphology of biodegradable poly (l-lactide). *Thermochimica Acta* 519: 90–95.

Zhang, C.Y., Lu, H., Zhuang, Z., Wang, X.P., and Fang, Q.F. 2010. Nano-hydroxyapatite/poly (L-lactic acid) composite synthesized by a modified in situ precipitation: Preparation and properties. *Journal of Materials Science: Materials in Medicine* 21: 3077–3083.

Zhang, D., Kandadai, M.A., Cech, J., Roth, S., and Curran, S.A. 2006. Poly (L-lactide) (PLLA)/multiwalled carbon nanotube (MWCNT) composite: Characterization and biocompatibility evaluation. *Journal of Physical Chemistry B* 110: 12910–12915.

Zhang, X., Sun, J., Fang, S., Han, X., Li, Y., and Zhang, C. 2011. Thermal, crystalline, and mechanical properties of octa(3-chloropropylsilsesquioxane)/poly(l-lactic acid) hybrid films. *Journal of Applied Polymer Science* 122: 296–303.

Zhu, A., Diao, H., Rong, Q., and Cai, A. 2010. Preparation and properties of polylactide-silica nanocomposites. *Journal of Applied Polymer Science* 116: 2866–2873.

Zhu, Y., Murali, S., Cai, W., Li, X., Suk, J.W., Potts, J.R., and Ruoff, R.S. 2010. Graphene and graphene oxide: Synthesis, properties, and applications. *Advanced Materials* 22: 3906–3924.

6 Tissue Engineering Researches on Biodegradable Polymer Nanocomposites
Designing Concepts, Properties, and Perspectives

Andreea Irina Barzic and Silvia Ioan

CONTENTS

6.1 INTRODUCTION

Progress in biomedicine is strongly related to the complexity and accuracy of diagnostic techniques, as well as to the development of biomaterials. During the past decades, research in this field has focused on biostable and biodegradable (hydrolytically and enzymatically degradable) compounds [1–6]. Among the available materials, polymers meet these criteria due to their functionality and ease of processing. Therefore, degradable polymeric biomaterials are often used in various biomedical fields, including pharmacology and tissue engineering. The latter represents a multidisciplinary domain involving application of knowledge in exact and life sciences in solving medical issues such as tissue loss and organ failure [7]. The main approach toward this direction consists in cell growth on bioactive degradable layers (scaffolds) that provide the physical and chemical indications to control their differentiation and assembly into 3D structures [8]. The success of tissue engineering lies in two main aspects: used biomaterials and fabrication technologies.

The bio-substrates should repair the failing organs/tissues or replace many of the permanent prosthetic devices used for temporary therapeutic applications with biodegradable devices that could help the body to regenerate the damaged tissues [9–11]. Therefore, biomaterials must be designed, on the one hand, to fulfill the requirements of specific cell response at the molecular level and, on the other, to exhibit the proper surface, physical, and mechanical properties [5]. Since conventional single-component polymer materials present insufficient stiffness and compressive strength, the proposed strategy is to prepare multicomponent polymer systems for upgrading the structural and functional properties. The introduction of nanofillers into biodegradable natural or synthetic polymers leads to nanocomposite materials with improved mechanical, morphological, and conductive properties [12,13]. The desired characteristics can be modified/enhanced depending on not only the nanoparticle type (organic or inorganic) and dispersion, but also on interactions occurring between the polymer chains and the nanoparticles and among the nanoparticles. Depending on the chosen system (polymer matrix and nanofiller), dense or porous scaffolds can be obtained, leading to a different response in cell seeding, migration, growth, mass transport, and tissue formation [14,15]. Besides the synthesis procedure, the fabrication and processing techniques play a key role in tissue engineering. The current design procedures include [16]:

- *Traditional methods*: Solvent casting and particulate leaching, gas foaming, phase separation, melt molding, freeze extraction
- *Advanced methods*: Electrospinning, rapid prototyping, microsphere sintering, shape deposition manufacturing, fused deposition modeling, nonfused liquid deposition modeling, 3D printing, selective laser sintering, transfer of liquid crystal texture

The preparation method generates specific architectural features, and consequently the interactions at the cell/substrate biointerface are different. The main challenges in scaffold manufacture lie in the production of customizable biodegradable constructs exhibiting properties that promote certain surface and bulk properties, which are compatible with the host tissue, with predictable degradation rate and biocompatibility [2,17].

This chapter presents the current researches on biodegradable polymer nano-composites for tissue engineering, highlighting the importance of the design concepts in the resulting physicochemical properties of the scaffold. The main results regarding the in vitro or in vivo cell culture analysis of the cell–scaffold interaction are also discussed for different types of biodegradable polymers nanocomposites. The combination of bioresorbable polymers and nanostructures opens new perspectives in the development of nanomaterials for tissue engineering applications with tunable mechanical, adhesion, and morphological properties.

6.2   DESIGNING CONCEPTS

It is widely known that in order to be used as scaffold, a biomaterial nanocomposite must satisfy the following requirements:

- Biodegradation to nonoxic products
- Processability into complicated shapes with appropriate porosity
- Ability to support cell growth and proliferation
- Suitable mechanical properties, as well as maintaining mechanical strength during most part of the tissue regeneration process

These demands can be accomplished depending on the used polymer matrix and nanofiller. The biodegradable polymers can be divided in two main categories [18–20]:

1. Natural-based materials, such as starch (alginate, chitin/chitosan, hyaluronic acid derivatives) or proteins (soy, collagen, fibrin gels, silk)
2. Synthetic materials, such as poly(lactic acid), poly(glycolic acid), poly(3-caprolactone) (PCL), poly(hydroxy butyrate)

Although these classes of biomaterials present many advantages, they also have some disadvantages, which can be overcome by introducing specific nanostructures. Regarding mechanical properties, it can be concluded that synthetic polymers are characterized by good mechanical strength and their degradation rate can be easily modified, while natural polymers have less mechanical resistance. When considering the polymer surface features, it can be noticed that synthetic polymers are hydrophobic and lack cell-recognition signals, whereas naturally derived compounds have the potential advantage of biological recognition that positively favor cell adhesion and function [5].

The current nanostructures inserted in biodegradable matrices are either organic or inorganic. Depending on the type of the inserted biocompatible particles, the main bionanocomposites for tissue engineering are categorized as follows:

- Ceramic: hydroxyapatite based [21–26]
- Metallic: gold, titanium, or silver based [27–29]
- Carbon: carbon nanotubes, graphene, or carbon nanofibers based [30–32]

The preparation of artificial supports with specific properties involves complex procedures to assembly the nanocomposites. The introduction of nanostructures into polymers can generally be done in different manners [33], as follows:

- *Solution method*: It involves dissolution of polymers in adequate solvent with nanoscale particles and evaporation of solvent or precipitation.
- *Melt mixing*: The polymer is directly melt mixed with nanoparticles.
- *In situ polymerization*: The nanoparticles are dispersed in liquid monomer or monomer solution; then polymerization occurs in the presence of nanoscale particles.
- *Template synthesis*: Using polymers as template, the nanoscale particles are synthesized from precursor solution.

Solvent casting, in situ polymerization, and template synthesis are processes that involve the utilization of a solvent in which the polymer is soluble. The effects of different solvents represent an essential factor in the film realization that must be elucidated. The solvent selection influences nanocomposite foil properties, heterogeneity of the surface, reorientation or mobility of the surface crystal segment, swelling, and deformation [34–36]. The solubility parameter of the polymer seems to be the factor that influences the surface structure. In nanocomposite preparation by the solvent casting process, the effects of solvents evaporation should be carefully examined. The dispersion of nanostructures in the solvent and consequently in the polymer matrix can be optimized by considering specific properties of solvent, such as electron-pair donicity, solvochromic parameter, hydrogen bond donation parameter, and dielectric constant.

The final architecture of the bionanocomposite scaffold can be

- Bidimensional (2D) dense films, where there is an effect of composition on the final properties
- Tridimensional (3D) porous architectures, where the morphology affects the nanocomposite properties

After the assembly of the nanocomposites, they are further processed through various methods in order to tailor their appearance as 2D or 3D structures. The most used fabrication procedures are further presented.

6.2.1 Solvent Casting and Particulate Leaching

Organic solvent casting and particulate leaching is one of the most popular methods used to fabricate biocomposite scaffolds [37,38]. The process is based on the dissolution of the polymer in an organic solvent, mixing with nanofillers and porogen particles, and casting the mixture into a predefined 3D mold. Subsequently, the solvent starts to evaporate, and the porogen particles are removed by leaching (Figure 6.1). However, residual solvents might cause toxicity effects in the scaffolds and thus become harmful to transplanted cells or host tissues. To avoid this problem, gas foaming can be used to prepare porous biopolymer nanocomposite foam.

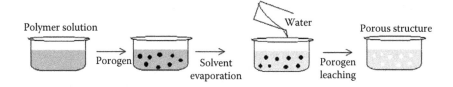

FIGURE 6.1 Schematic representation of the routes involved in solvent casting and particulate leaching process.

6.2.2 GAS FOAMING

Gas foaming involves saturation of biodegradable polymers subjected at high pressures with gas-foaming agents, such as carbon dioxide and nitrogen [39], water [40], or fluoroform [41]. Depending on the experimental conditions, the size of the gas bubbles can be controlled and thus pores with diameters ranging between 100 and 500 μm are formed in the polymer. The advantage of this method is that it does not require an organic solvent. The formation of a structure with largely unconnected pores and a nonporous external surface [42] limits the utilization of this technique (Figure 6.2).

6.2.3 PHASE SEPARATION

The nonsolvent-induced phase separation (NIPS) method consists of inducing a liquid–liquid phase separation of the polymer composite solution subjected to quenching. This results in the formation of two phases: a polymer-rich phase and a polymer-poor phase. When the latter is removed, the polymer-rich phase solidifies creating a highly porous polymer network [43] (Figure 6.3). The obtained scaffold exhibits a micro- and macrostructure that can be controlled by varying process parameters such as polymer concentration, quenching temperature, and quenching rate. Since the procedure is performed at low temperatures, it facilitates the incorporation of bioactive molecules in the structure.

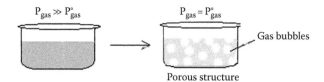

FIGURE 6.2 Schematic representation of the routes involved in gas foaming method.

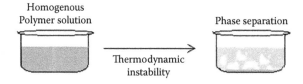

FIGURE 6.3 Schematic representation of the routes involved in phase separation process.

The thermally induced phase separation method produces scaffolds with very high porosities (~97%) and controlled microstructures for tissues such as nerve, muscle, tendon, intestine, bone, and teeth. The resulted cellular substrates are highly porous with anisotropic tubular morphology and extensive pore interconnectivity. The pore morphology, bioactivity, and degradation rates are strongly dependent on the polymer concentration in solution, volume fraction of secondary phase, quenching temperature, and the polymer and solvent characteristics. The utilization of the phase separation techniques allows the formation of a nanoscale fibrous structure that mimics natural extracellular matrix architecture and facilitates cell attachment and function [44].

6.2.4 MELT MOLDING

During the melt molding procedure, the solid polymer is mixed with a porogen and then introduced in a mold; it is subsequently heated above the glass-transition temperature of the polymer. The system is subjected to high pressure [45]. The raw materials bind together leading to a scaffold with designed-specified external shape. After removing the mold, the porogen is leached out and the porous layer is then dried (Figure 6.4). This is a nonsolvent fabrication method that assures independent control of morphology and shape. However, the presence of the residual porogen and high processing temperatures reduces the possibility of bioactive molecules incorporation.

6.2.5 FREEZE EXTRACTION

Freeze extraction is based on cooling down the polymer solution until the materials reach a frozen state and the solvent forms ice crystals, determining the polymer molecules to aggregate into the interstitial spaces. The application of a pressure lower than the equilibrium vapor pressure of the frozen solvent allows solvent removal. Once the solvent is sublimated, dry polymer scaffolds with an interconnected porous microstructure are formed [46,47] (Figure 6.5). The pore number can be controlled through the concentration of the polymer solution, whereas their size distribution is influenced by the freezing temperatures. This technique is also used to dry biological samples to protect their bioactivities [48].

6.2.6 ELECTROSPINNING

Electrospinning is a method that applies electrical charges to draw fine fibers from polymer solutions. The technique does not demand the use of coagulation chemistry or high temperatures to produce solid threads from solution. Also, it can be applied

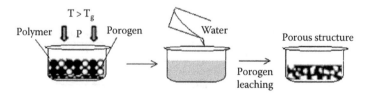

FIGURE 6.4 Schematic representation of the routes involved in melt molding procedure.

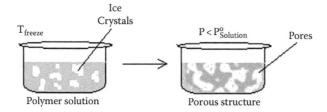

FIGURE 6.5   Schematic representation of the routes involved in freeze extraction procedure.

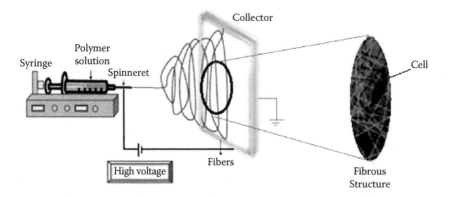

FIGURE 6.6   Schematic representation of the routes involved in electrospinning.

to molten samples, ensuring that no solvent can be carried over into the final product. The application of high voltage to the solution leads to electrostatic forces that counteract the surface tension (the droplet is stretched). If the molecular cohesion of the liquid is sufficiently high, stream breakup does not occur and a charged liquid jet is formed. During the jet drying in flight, the mode of current flow changes from ohmic to convective as the charge migrates to the surface of the fiber. The whipping process determines the elongation of the jet until it is deposited on the grounded collector (Figure 6.6).

Nanofibrous architectures favor more efficiently cell binding and spreading compared to micropore and microfibrous architectures since larger surface areas adsorb better proteins and present more binding sites to cell membrane receptors [49]. Cells growing in 3D nanofibrous structural environments easily exchange nutrients and utilize receptors throughout their surface, while those in flat culture are limited to nutrient exchange on only one side. Porous scaffolds with nanofibrous architectures can be produced with electrospinning, resulting in architectures that can mimic the structure and biological functions of the natural extracellular matrix [50]. The fiber diameters vary from 2 nm to several micrometers, using solutions of both natural and synthetic polymers, with small pore sizes and high surface-area-to-volume ratios. The experimental electrospinning setup is composed of three parts: a syringe pump containing the polymeric materials, a high-voltage source to generate high electric field for spinning, and a collector to collect the fibers [51]. The most important parameters that affect the fiber morphology are polymer solution parameters (viscosity, molecular weight of polymer, polymer conductivity, surface tension), processing parameters (applied voltage, distance between tip and collector, flow rate), and environment parameters (humidity, temperature). Nanofibers with high surface-area-to-volume ratios are optimal for tissue engineering purposes [52].

6.2.7 RAPID PROTOTYPING

An alternative method of scaffold preparation is rapid prototyping (RP). This approach is based on computer-assisted design (CAD) and manufacturing (CAM) techniques, offering better control of scaffold internal microstructure and external macroshape [53]. Based on the properties of different scaffold biomaterials, there are three basic RP system types: liquid-based, solid-based, and powder-based. The main advantage of the method is that it can build up a complex scaffold with an exactly predefined shape. Thus, a specific body shape can be obtained by the selective addition of material, layer by layer, guided by a computer program. The step-by-step procedure leads to an improved reproducibility, and thus morphological features of the scaffold such as porosity, interconnectivity, pore size, and geometric stability can be controlled more precisely [54]. Furthermore, cells can be printed on surfaces [55], thus favoring the insertion of living biological substances into the prefabricated layer before the final assembly [56] (Figure 6.7). However, the method resolution is influenced by the use of engineered precision machine tools, resulting scaffolds with resolutions in the range of 200–500 μm [57] depending on the used RP technology. The usage of a special RP fabrication technique demands specific material properties. Although many different applications to embody scaffolds under RP processing conditions are reported, the special requisitions of the polymer material limit the utilization of RP fabrication methods.

6.2.8 MICROSPHERE SINTERING

Microspheres are produced by different processes, such as spraying a polymer solution followed by NIPS [58]. The use of ultrasound [59] to emulsify water in a polymer solution is also reported. The water droplets from the water-in-oil-in-water emulsion may be loaded with a biological substance. Then, the emulsion of water-in-polymer solution is brought into an aqueous polymer solution to complete the NIPS by stirring for 3 h. Hot stirring of a paraffin/gelatin–water emulsion at 80°C is also described. The stirring is followed by an ice water quenching to obtain paraffin spheres for paraffin leaching [60]. The simplest way is to pour the organic polymer solution into the aqueous polymer solution. The system is stirred for a few hours, and

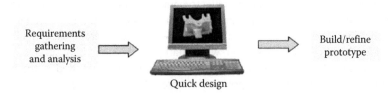

Requirements gathering and analysis ⟹ Quick design ⟹ Build/refine prototype

FIGURE 6.7 The main construction steps involved in rapid prototyping.

then microspheres that could be brought into a 3D shape are isolated and subjected to a sintering process to an in vivo characterized scaffold body [61,62]. This is a good method for obtaining composite structures from polymeric and inorganic substances for bone tissue engineering [63].

6.2.9   SHAPE DEPOSITION MANUFACTURING

Shape deposition manufacturing involves the fabrication of a layered scaffold in a tailor-made geometry by a computer-controlled cutting machine [56]. The biosubstrates are prepared incrementally from prefabricated cross-sectional layers of formed materials. Layers are assembled manually and joined to form 3D bodies using biodegradable or biostable fasteners. The concept of robotic microassembly is guided through the same principle [56]. In the first stage, differently designed block units are obtained [64], for example, by lithographic methods or other previously mentioned techniques. Second, the blocks are brought together with a precision robot with microgripping capabilities.

6.2.10   FUSED DEPOSITION MODELING

Porous scaffolds can be prepared using a 3D-fiber deposition technique of compressed polymer melts [65,66]. In this method, a polymer melt is processed into fibers with a temperature-controlled extruder. Its nozzle deposits the fiber or the filaments on a motor-driven x-y-z table. Initially, a layer of fibers with a well-defined distance is obtained. On the top, fiber layers are deposited, resulting in a 3D scaffold with an exact porous morphology and 100% interconnectivity. The positional control of the table is computer controlled and facilitates the construction of 3D structures (Figure 6.8). In the modification of the fused deposition modeling process, the filament preparation to feed the extrusion head as reported [56] is no longer required. The polymer material can be used as purchased: in the form of pellets and granules by precision extruding deposition.

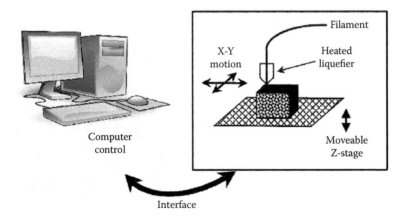

FIGURE 6.8   Schematic representation of the routes involved in fused deposition modeling.

A specific requirement is that the material must possess a suitable thermoplastic behavior. A disadvantage of biodegradability might be represented by the thickness of the pore walls stemming from the fiber diameters [67,68], and the dimensions of the scaffolds are often rectangular [69,70].

6.2.11 NONFUSED LIQUID DEPOSITION MODELING

The deposition of extruded strands or the plotting of dots in 3D is not always correlated with high temperatures and polymer melts. A good alternative is the usage of pastes or slurries, solutions and dispersions of polymers or reactive oligomers [71]. Special experimental setup, with adapted processing options, is mandatory for transforming these materials into 3D scaffolds. The multiphase jet solidification process for biomaterials [72] generally implies utilization of a dispersion of different phases, for instance, solid ceramic particles and a binder solution [73] in RP. The bioplotter [74,75] or reactive plotter [76] dispenses pastes or dispersions into a matching plotting liquid with the right density. After leaving the nozzle and contacting the previous layer of the body that is being constructed, the plotting medium gets solid. No supports are required since the plotting liquid medium compensates the gravity.

6.2.12 3D PRINTING

In the 3D printing procedure (3D-P), the shaped bodies are achieved by a layering printing process with adhesive bonding, using powder as a base material [76]. In the first stage, over a building platform, a layer of powder is spread and then covered with a binder solution through an ink-jet print head. The aim is to join single powder particles and to obtain a 2D layer profile [77]. Another layer of powder is laid down and the process is repeated. The binder is dried, and the nonjoined powder is removed by an air jet flow. The resolution of 3D-P is determined by the particle size of the powder, the nozzle dimension, and the degree of control over the position controller that defines print-head movement (Figure 6.9).

The appropriate particle size for biomedical applications usually ranges between 80 and 250 μm, and thus the powder of materials demands certain pretreatments [78].

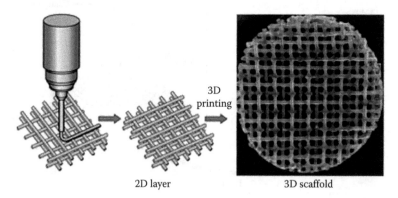

3D printing

2D layer   3D scaffold

FIGURE 6.9 Schematic representation of the routes involved in 3D printing process.

The powder particles must flow well with a defined size range resulting a good interaction with the liquid binder in an amount of at least 500 mL granulate [78,79]. The success of this process also lies in the adaptation of an appropriate binder for different base materials. A preferred solvent with regard to biocompatibility is water, suitable for natural biopolymers. Organic solvents as binders (chloroform or methylene chloride) lead to harmful reactions in the human body and are difficult to remove completely [80,81].

6.2.13 SELECTIVE LASER SINTERING

Selective laser sintering involves utilization of deflected laser beams (infrared laser, CO_2 laser) to sinter thin layers [82] of powdered polymeric materials to produce solid 3D scaffolds (Figure 6.10). The laser beam selectively scans over the powder surface. The interaction of the laser beam with the powder increases the powder temperature in the range between the glass-transition temperature and the melting point of the used material. The powder particles that are in contact start to deform and to fuse together. The layers of powder are deposited by a roller, forming a novel sintered layer on top of the previous one. The laser-beam diameter (of about 400 µm) or the powder particle size restricts the dimension of the created scaffold structures. Considering the Gaussian distribution of the laser energy and the principle of powder

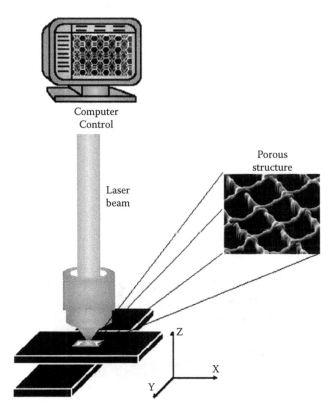

FIGURE 6.10 Schematic representation of scaffold preparation by selective laser sintering.

bonding (different powder particle forms), it is difficult to prepare special shaped scaffolds with sharp corners or clear boundaries. Still, some problems related to laser spot size, powder size, and trapped loose powder from scaffolds have to be solved [83]. The used materials must be achieved under the form of powder that must demonstrate a suitable melting and welding behavior.

6.2.14 STEREOLITHOGRAPHY

Stereolithography relies on the initiation of a chemical reaction (photopolymerization [84] or crosslinking [85]) in certain polymer liquids by electromagnetic radiation. Light from a laser beam is focused onto selected regions of a layer of liquid polymer causing solidification in the irradiated areas. Another layer of polymer solution can be laser exposed for the initiation of the chain reaction by lowering of the nascent-shaped body, which is placed in a polymer liquid bath. The working principle is repeated creating 3D scaffolds (Figure 6.11).

Many attempts were made to improve hydrogel stability (usage of polymer mixtures) [84] in order to incorporate living cells during the formation process (optimizing of processing conditions to prevent toxic free radicals) [86,87].

Other research directions are concerned with the improvement in the acuteness of the prepared structures—more precise laser beam moves connected with the expansion of the material base or using photolithographic techniques with x-rays and electron or ion beams [88]. The stereolithographic technique requires materials that are able to react to light, activating a chemical reaction.

6.2.15 TRANSFER OF LIQUID CRYSTAL TEXTURE

Literature reports few investigations on patterned polymer films that can induce a guided cell growth [89]. The main interest is to control cell morphology (which is

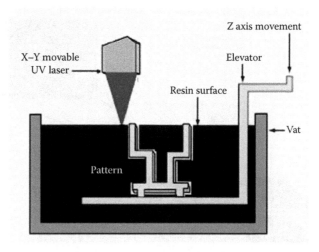

FIGURE 6.11 Schematic representation of the routes involved in stereolithography procedure.

closely related to cell functions) through the polymer surface topography. When cells are brought in contact with a randomly oriented polymer surface, they adopt a bidimensional monolayer culture of cells, whereas when they are casted on an anisotropic morphology, the cells develop tridimensional biological structures. Tissue engineering is focused on obtaining 3D cell spheroids, which are spherical mass composed of many cells and extracellular matrices, because they appear to mimic not only the morphology but also the physiological functions of cells in living tissues and organs. These tridimensional biological units sustain viability for extended culture periods and maintain high levels of cell functions when compared with those of cells as monolayers. However, it is not easy to prepare multicellular spheroids from cells that do not easily aggregate and, in addition, to obtain numerous spheroids from the cell culture.

In this context, many methods for patterning polymer film surface were reported. Recently, a new method of patterning isotropic polymer films was developed based on the banded texture of a sheared liquid crystal polymer (LCP) solution [90–92]. Polymers with semi-rigid chains, like cellulose derivatives, develop after the cessation of shearing a special morphology in organic solvents at a certain concentration. Due to the longer relaxation time of LCPs, the resulted texture can be maintained until solidification and transferred to other biocompatible polymers, such as poly(amic acid)s (PAAs). Hydroxypropyl cellulose (HPC) solutions can be used as LC matrix since high shearing conditions change their cholesteric texture into a banded one (Figure 6.12). This type of structural organization can be obtained in special conditions depending on the solvent, concentration, shear rate, and time of shearing [93]. Atomic force microscopy studies reveal that HPC

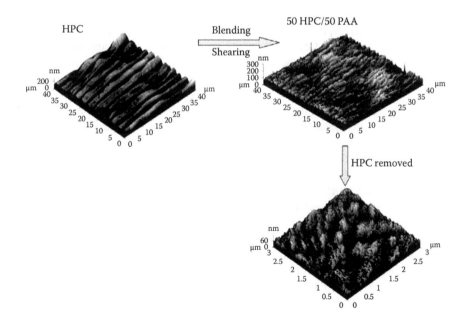

FIGURE 6.12   Schematic representation of LCP texture transfer to PAA.

films prepared from sheared concentrated solutions exhibit anisotropic surface characterized by two periodicities. The main pattern is slightly tilted from the shear direction and is observed as fine, long, parallel, equidistant lines running perpendicular to the deformation. These bands appear as a result of the sinusoidal variation in the fibrilar (oriented HPC molecules) trajectory. The secondary bands (also named *torsads*) are formed parallel to the shear direction, and they are the result of some competitive processes, such as orthogonal deformation to bulk orientation and hydrodynamics of the solvent evaporation. When mixing HPC with PAA, the regular morphology is maintained, whatever its content in the system. The bands are still discernible after removal of the matrix with a selective solvent. This type of surface pattern is useful in obtaining biosubstrates that are able to produce tridimensional cell steroids.

6.3   PROPERTIES OF IMPORTANCE IN TISSUE ENGINEERING

Naturally produced ceramic organic composites can combine good mechanical properties with an open porosity. Among the ceramic bionanocomposites, those that are based on hydroxyapatite (HA) have gained great importance since it is a major mineral component of the human body. The HA-derived materials are expected to have excellent biocompatibility with bones, teeth, skin, and muscles. Due to the similarity with the bone mineral [94], natural or synthetic HA is employed in the fabrication of scaffolds for bone regeneration in orthopedic surgery and dentistry [95]. The combination of the tough polymer phase with the compressive strength of the inorganic one leads to the improvement in the mechanical properties and degradation profiles of the bioactive materials.

In the past years, it was shown that the osteoconductive properties of HA composites can be controlled by changing their composition, size, and morphology. When the Ca/P ratio ranges between 1.50 and 1.67, a better promotion of bone regeneration is obtained. In addition, a nanosized inorganic component tends to be more bioactive than a microsized one because the specific surface area is enhanced considerably, thus favoring protein adsorption and osteoblast adhesion [96]. Also, microparticles induce some undesired effects since in most cases they are embedded in the pore wall and are piled together between or within the pores. Thus, it has been demonstrated that microparticles may lead to inflammatory reactions.

The nanometer surface topography of HA particles determines the conformation of adsorbed vitronectin, which is a linear protein, 15 nm in length, that mediates osteoblast adhesion. This aspect brings new information on understanding the mechanisms of enhanced osteoblast functions. Moreover, increased initial calcium adsorption to nanoceramic surfaces increased the binding of vitronectin, which subsequently facilitated osteoblast adhesion [97]. Regarding the shape of HA ceramics, it was reported that precipitation method allows to obtain needle-like particles (10–30 nm in width and 50–100 nm in length) [98] or rod-like by the wet chemical method (37–65 nm in width and 100–400 nm in length) [99]. The latter method allows to obtain spherical HA nanoparticles [100]. It has been revealed that needle-shaped particles cause inflammatory reaction (especially when they are microsized), comparatively with the spherical ones, which present an inhibition rate that increases with time and concentration. In vitro study of cell response to spherical nanocrystalline HA particles indicates that they can function as an effective biomaterial for bone tumorectomy repair, while having little adverse effect [101]. However, HAs are generally brittle, and thus their utilization (as scaffolds) is sometimes compromised.

Introduction of these ceramic nanoparticles in biodegradable polymers opened new perspective in tissue engineering. Besides their good osteoconductivity, osteoinductivity, and biodegradability, these reinforced materials exhibit considerably improved physical properties even at a very low filler concentration. Literature reports various nanocomposites based on HA and different biodegradable matrices, such as poly(ε-caprolactone), poly(L-lactic acid) (PLLA), poly(3-hydroxybutyrate-co-3-hydroxyval) (PHBHV) [102], chitosan [103], and poly(hydroxy butyrate) [104]. Besides the HA amount and shape, the type of the polymer matrix is an essential factor influencing the mechanical and morphological properties. Figure 6.13 shows the variation of the compressive modulus and porosity for some of the most representative biodegradable polymers containing 15% HA.

The intrinsic mechanical characteristics of the bionanocomposites used for scaffolding or their postprocessing properties should match those of the host tissue. Recent mechanobiology investigations revealed that when exerting traction forces on a scaffold, many mature cell types (such as epithelial cells, fibroblasts, muscle cells, and neurons) sense the stiffness of the substrate and show dissimilar morphology and adhesive characteristics. This mechanosensitivity has also been

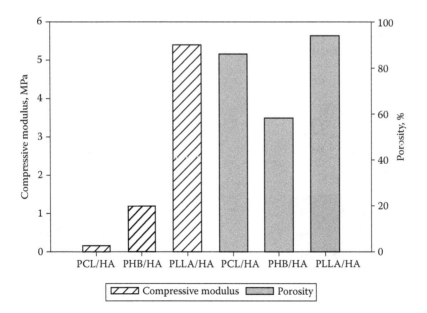

FIGURE 6.13 Compressive modulus and porosity for some biodegradable polymers containing 15% HA nanoparticles.

observed for naive mesenchymal stem cells [105], for which the tendency to differentiate is controlled by the stiffness of the matrix. Soft matrices that imitate brain are neurogenic, whereas stiffer matrices that mimic muscle are myogenic, and comparatively rigid matrices that reproduce collagenous bone features prove to be osteogenic. After several weeks in culture, the cells commit to the lineage specified by matrix elasticity, consistent with the elasticity-insensitive commitment of differentiated cell types.

On the other hand, the internal architectures of porous implants affect the mechanical properties of the implants and the degree of tissue regeneration [5]. Structural heterogeneity of the porous scaffold with designed micro-architecture is one of the main goals in tissue engineering applications. For instance, the success of a bone scaffold depends on the pore size and porosity, which can be tailored by the variation in both the size and the content of the porogen particles. However, the lack of interaction between the polymer and the HA nanoparticles can lead to deleterious effects on the mechanical properties, when added at high loadings. In order to enhance the matrix/nanofiller interactions and to avoid and HA aggregation, coupling agents are used. The traditional problem of HA clustering can be overcome by precipitation of the apatite crystals within the polymer solution. The porous scaffolds obtained through this method present well-developed structural features and pore configuration to induce cell growth. For example, grafting HA nanoparticles (g-HA) can enhance their interfacial interactions with the PLLA matrix as reflected in the enhancement of the mechanical properties and cell compatibility [106]. The chemical binding of PLLA on HA surface and subsequently blending with PLLA lead to more uniform distribution of the g-HA nanoparticles on the film surface and increased interactions of the human chondracytes cells with the bioactive material surface. As shown in Figure 6.14, the presence of bioactive g-HA/PLLA may have positive biological effects because the loss of the g-HAP particles that takes place in contact with the culture medium results in a coarse surface for cell adhesion and

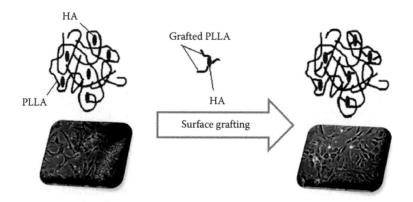

FIGURE 6.14 Scanning electron microscopy (SEM) images of cell culture on PLLA/HA and PLLA/g-HA nanocomposites.

proliferation. Moreover, the g-HAP particles disengaged from matrix and exposed to body fluid might generate a microenvironment change, positively influencing the cell metabolism. These nanocomposites containing grafted fillers are of interest to tissue engineering field because they have a structure that induces and promotes new bone formation at the required site.

Another type of ceramic-based scaffold contains coral mineral (aragonite or calcite forms of calcium carbonate). The main advantages of this material are given by its porous structure (150–500 µm), which is similar to that of cancellous bone and its ability to form chemical bonds with bone and soft tissues in vivo. The ingrowth of fibrovascular tissue or bone from the host is facilitated by a favorable pore size and microstructural composition. Pore interconnection sizes are of utmost importance when hard and soft tissue ingrowth is involved. The best ingrowth is observed for implants with average pore sizes of around 260 µm when compared to no implants [107]. Coral-based scaffolds were used in clinical settings for osseous regeneration of the distal phalanx of a thumb in an avulsion injury [108]. The high dissolution rate as well as poor longevity and stability makes coralline calcium carbonate unsuitable for some types of implants.

Metal-based nanocomposites represent another category of biocompatible materials used as scaffolds. Nanoparticles of noble metals have significantly distinct physical, chemical, and biological properties comparatively with the ceramic ones. It has been shown that the electromagnetic, optical, and catalytic properties of noble-metal nanoparticles such as gold, silver, titanium, and platinum are affected by shape and size. The size-dependent characteristics of small metal particles yield special optical, electrochemical, and electronic properties [5]. Many efforts have been focused on the synthesis routes that allow better control of shape and size.

Biomedical applications of metal nanoparticles have been dominated by the use of nanobioconjugates that are used as probes for electron microscopy to visualize cellular components, drug delivery (vehicle for delivering proteins, peptides, plasmids), detection, diagnosis, and therapy (targeted and nontargeted) [5]. Considerable research activities are being done regarding the introduction of metal and semiconductor clusters in plastics [109]. The main interest is to achieve small particle sizes, narrow size distributions, and well-stabilized metal particles. Because of surface effects and the dramatic changes in properties occurring when the critical length is reached, metal clusters exhibit unique properties, such as plasmon absorption, near-IR photoluminescence, or superparamagnetism. The simplest way to protect clusters and keep the advantage of their physical characteristics is to insert the nanoscopic metal structures into polymeric matrices. Traumatic injuries can disrupt muscle contraction by damaging the skeletal muscle and/or the peripheral nerves. The healing process results in scar tissue formation that obstructs muscle function. Polymer fibers embedded metal nanoparticles can create a scaffold that will trigger muscle cell elongation, orientation, fusion, and striation.

Gold–PLLA scaffolds nanocomposites have been prepared by electrospinning as fiber scaffolds for rat primary muscle cells [110]. Fluorescent images of each type of scaffold reveal that cells are shown to have elongated and grown together to form

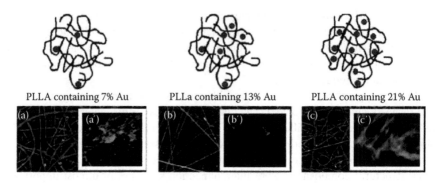

FIGURE 6.15 SEM images (a–c) of PLLA/gold electrospun nanocomposites and fluorescent images (a′–c′) of the cell culture deposited on these scaffolds.

multinucleated constructs. The cellular growth on the PLLA scaffolds was significantly lower than on the PLLA containing 7%, 13%, and 21% gold nanoparticles (Figure 6.15). These electrospun gold-based scaffolds can be utilized to create a biodegradable, biocompatible, and conductive substrate for skeletal muscle repair. Gold/chitosan films can be used in skin tissue engineering since it increases the attachment of keratinocytes and promote their growth [111].

Given the disinfecting effect of silver, its corresponding polymer composites have found applications in traditional medicines. According to electron microscopy investigations, the antimicrobial properties are dependent on the silver nanoparticles' size, which generate different interactions with bacteria [112]. Silver nanoparticles have the capability to release silver ions in a controlled manner, generating a powerful antibacterial activity against a large number of microorganisms [113–115]. The nanostructured silver materials present a high surface contact area and thus inhibitory capacity is enhanced [116]. The aggregation problem of the silver nanoparticles (favored by its high surface free energy) is solved by embedding them into biodegradable polymer matrices [116]. Low amounts of silver nanoparticles produce surface morphological changes in the polymer matrix and affect surface nanocomposite wettability and roughness. These aspects can influence the bacterial adhesion process on the nanocomposite surface. Moreover, silver/collagen composites are used in neural tissue engineering. This type of scaffold presents superior functionality in the adsorption to laminin and subsequent regeneration of damaged peripheral nerves [117].

Other metal-based nanocomposites for tissue engineering are those prepared from titanium (Ti) or aluminum (Al). Titanium-derived materials have found applications as vascular stents since they enhance endothelial and vascular smooth muscle cell functions [118]. Also, Ti nanoparticles improve compressive strength and osteoconductivity of poly(methyl methacrylate) composite [119], while poly(lactic-co-glycolic acid)/Ti scaffolds present increased osteogenic functions [120]. Aluminum composites present higher flexural and compressive strength, and additionally aluminum's good thermal conductivity enhances the degradation rate of the scaffold [121].

Carbon-based nanocomposites represent one of the most investigated categories of biomaterials. There are many types of carbon nanofillers—fullerenes, carbon nanotubes (CNTs), carbon nanofibers (CNFs), graphene, nanodiamonds (NDs)—and a wide variety of carbon-related forms [122]. The physical and biological properties of scaffolds are dependent on the shape and size of the carbon particles. Besides the good mechanical properties, the electrical conductivity of the polymer containing carbon nanostructures is a useful tool to direct cell growth because they can conduct an electrical stimulus in the tissue healing process.

A fullerene is a molecule made entirely of carbon, in the form of a hollow sphere, ellipsoid, and many other shapes. Photoluminescent fullerene nanoparticles/PLLA nanofibers biocomposites were fabricated by electrospinning method and subsequently they were characterized to check their potential utilization in bioimaging. The fullerene nanoparticles were introduced in the PLLA uniform nanofibers (with diameters ranging from 300 to 600 nm), forming a core–shell structure. The fibrous scaffolds presented excellent hydrophilic surface due to the addition of water-soluble fullerene nanoparticles. The suitability of these composite substrates for bioimaging was evaluated with human liver carcinoma HepG2 cells. The fullerene nanoparticles signal is almost displayed in every cell, implying that the potential of fluorescent fullerene nanoparticles/PLLA nanofibers can be used for the pursued application [123].

Carbon nanotubes have the potential in providing the needed structural reinforcement for biomedical scaffold. To enhance their dispersion in polymer matrix and their compatibility in biological fluids, sidewall functionalization has been performed [124]. Nanotubes sustained osteoblast matrix deposition and allowed mineralization, cell differentiation, and bone-like tissue forming functions. Neurons grown on CNTs coated with bioactive molecules elaborate multiple neurites and present extensive branching, making such nanocomposites utilizable as substrates for nerve cell growth and as probes of neuronal function at the nanometer scale. Considering the fact that CNTs are similar in shape and size to nerve cells, they could assist to structurally and functionally reconnect injured neurons. Hippocampal neurons grown on nanotubes display a sixfold increase in the frequency of spontaneous postsynaptic currents, reflecting the functional synapse formation [125]. Therefore, CNTs are considered support devices for bridging and integrating functional neuronal networks. Honeycomb-like matrices of multiwall CNTs (MWCNTs) or vertically aligned CNT functionalized with carboxylic acid groups were obtained as potential scaffolds for tissue engineering [126]. Mouse fibroblast cells were cultured on the CNT networks, forming a confluent layer with no cytotoxicity effects. In vitro cytotoxicity of single-walled CNT (SWNT)/poly(propylene fumarate) (PPF) nanocomposites was tested [127]. The results show that almost 100% cell viability was observed on the nanocomposites and good cell attachment on their surfaces. The nature of the functional group at the CNT surface represents an essential factor for improving the dispersion of CNTs in polymer matrix and in the mechanism of interaction with cells. The sidewall carboxylic functionalized SWNTs exhibited a nucleation surface, which is able to produce a biomimetic apatite coating. PLLA/MWCNT nanocomposites were subjected to alternating current stimulation and the osteoblast proliferation on such substrates was analyzed [128]. An increase in osteoblast proliferation and extracellular calcium deposition on the nanocomposites was noticed comparatively with the control samples.

Carbon nanofibers are cylindrical or conical structures having diameters that range from a few to hundreds nanometers and lengths varying from less than a micron to a few millimeters. Scaffolds based on chitosan/CNF composites were prepared by precipitation, resulting highly porous materials [129]. The elastic modulus of the biomaterials is of 28.1 ± 3.3 kPa, being similar to that measured for rat myocardium. The scaffolds were seeded with neonatal rat heart cells, without electrical stimulation. After 14 days of culture, the scaffold pores throughout the construct volume were filled with cells. The metabolic activity of cells in chitosan/carbon constructs was significantly high. The presence of CNFs also led to increased expression of cardiac-specific genes involved in muscle contraction and electrical coupling. The obtained biosubstrates improved the properties of cardiac tissue constructs, presumably through enhanced transmission of electrical signals between the cells [129].

Incorporation of NDs into polymer matrices increases the strength, toughness, and thermal stability of the corresponding nanocomposites [130]. The purified NDs are constituted of particles with 5 nm average diameter, composed from an inert diamond core surrounded by functional groups, such as COOH, OH, and NH_2 [130]. Multifunctional bone scaffold materials were prepared from PLLA and octadecylamine-functionalized ND (ND-ODA) via solution casting, followed by compression molding [131]. Addition of 10 wt.% of ND-ODA resulted in a 280% increase in the strain to failure and a 310% increase in fracture energy comparatively to the pure PLLA. The biomineralization of the nanocomposite scaffolds was evaluated using simulated body fluid (SBF) [132]. The apatite nucleation and growth occurred faster on the reinforced PLLA than on neat matrix, recommending these materials for bone surgical fixation devices and regenerative medicine.

Graphene is a single-layer 2D material consisting of carbon atoms forming six-membered rings. The utilization of graphene sheets as nanofillers for composites leads to many unique properties [133]. Thermoplastic polyurethane/graphene oxide (GO) composite scaffolds were obtained using the thermally induced phase separation technique. Cell viability on the porous scaffolds was tested via live/dead fluorescent staining and scanning electron microscopy (SEM) observation. SEM images revealed that the average pore diameter of the composite scaffolds decreased as the amount of GO increased. Additionally, the surface of the biocomposites became rougher due to the embedded GO. The compressive modulus of scaffolds was increased by almost 200% and 300% with the addition of 5% and 10% GO, respectively, comparatively with the pure matrix. The fibroblast culture tests showed no apparent cytotoxicity at low amounts of GO, whereas at high loading of GO, cell proliferation on the specimens is delayed [134].

6.4   FUTURE PERSPECTIVES

The future of bionanocomposite scaffolds can be developed in several directions, including the synthesis, processing, mechanical properties, biodegradability, bioactivity, and sterilization. The utilization of polymer nanocomposites in tissue engineering enables mimicking of the complex architecture of some tissues. Synthetic or natural polymer matrices provide a wide range of mechanical properties and present different biodegradation characteristics, whereas the embedded nanoparticles provide the indispensable bioactivity. Also, new synthetic biodegradable polymer matrices should be developed, which can be produced in large scale under controlled conditions and with predictable and reproducible mechanical properties, degradation rate, and microstructure. It must be noted that the literature lacks in investigations on multiphase nanocomposite scaffolds. This could be a good solution to improve current biomaterials and to develop advanced nanocomposite scaffolds that imitate the structural and morphological organization of some tissues at the deepest levels. An important aspect that should be addressed in more detail in the design and fabrication of composite scaffolds is the interfacial properties between the filler and the matrix phases. It seems that this issue has been less analyzed in the context of bone engineering, although great efforts were made in the enhancement of the interfacial adhesion in conventional polymer matrix composites. Therefore, the development of coupling methodologies that enhance the adhesion of the nanoparticles (particularly the ceramic ones) toward the polymer should be explored.

The complex interactions between nanocomposites and bone tissue are still to be fully elucidated. From the point of view of their biocompatibility and physical properties, there are some disadvantages of polymer nanocomposites, including uncertain biocompatibility, component stability, and structural integrity in long-term service, and the related mechanical strength, especially the fatigue limit under periodic external stress. Consequently, the design of bionanocomposites for applications in bone tissue regeneration must take in consideration the optimization of the balance between good mechanical properties, biocompatibility, and controlled resorbability. Furthermore, these properties should be maintained during long-term service and the evaluation of their time dependence is mandatory. More importantly, more effort should be dedicated to apply biodegradable polymer nanocomposites in clinical and surgical settings. This could lead to a better understanding of the mechanism of nanocomposite–bone tissue interactions and to optimize the composition, structure, and properties of different polymer nanocomposites, in order to finally obtain the entire potential of these scaffolds in bone tissue regeneration. Also, the investigations should be extended to other tissues than bone, cartilage, ligament, skin, vascular tissues, neural tissues, and skeletal muscle.

Building upon a firm background of in vitro and preliminary in vivo studies, significant progress will be made over the next decade in applying some less studied biodegradable nanostructures, such as bacterial cellulose (BC) nanoparticles or cellulose nanowhiskers (CNWs) to tissue engineering. The combination of high stiffness and tensile strength with the highly hydrated (perhaps hydrogel-like) nature of BC will garner future interest. Thus, engineering of tensile load-bearing tissues, such as skeletal muscle, ligaments, tendons, and indeed blood vessels, could advance beyond preliminary in vitro studies. Other fields such as bone and neural tissue engineering may perhaps not progress to the same extent and probably not as far as the clinic. It must be noted that there are potential issues in the utilization of BC and cellulose more generally in tissue engineering. The most obvious are in fact two aspects of the same problem: the inherent nonanimal origin of cellulose and the lack of true biodegradation in vivo. Many attempts focused on controlling and/or facilitating biodegradation in vivo are likely to emerge in the future years and serious long-term in vivo investigations on BC and CNWs will be essential for the development of therapeutic applications.

The future development of CNWs in bioapplications is hard to predict, given the small number of studies already published. In terms of tissue engineering, however, it is possible that the high aspect ratio of CNWs will be used to obtain structurally oriented tissues, such as skeletal muscle, tendons, ligaments, and nerves. In order to prepare 3D scaffolds that contain CNWs, however, composite materials must be developed. In the shorter term, future studies will be focused on cell targeting and delivery of molecules such as drugs and probes using CNWs. For instance, the potential functionalization of CNWs with peptide/glycan motifs to elicit specific targeting and signaling has not yet been reported. Also, it is likely that CNWs having the ability to cross the cell plasma membrane delivering genetic material for transfection would be explored. Such applications are to be expected in the coming years.

REFERENCES

1. Gunatillake, P. A. and Adhikari, R. 2003. Biodegradable synthetic polymers for tissue engineering. *Eur. Cells Mater.* 5:1–16.
2. Okamoto, M. and John, B. 2013. Synthetic biopolymer nanocomposites for tissue engineering scaffolds. *Progr. Polym. Sci.* 38:1487–1503.
3. Allo, B. A., Costa, D. O., Dixon, S. J., Mequanint, K., and Rizkalla, A. S. 2012. Bioactive and biodegradable nanocomposites and hybrid biomaterials for bone regeneration. *J. Funct. Biomater.* 3:432–463.
4. Naira, L. S. and Laurencin, C. T. 2007. Biodegradable polymers as biomaterials. *Prog. Polym. Sci.* 32:762–798.
5. Armentano, I., Dottori, M., Fortunati, E., Mattioli, S., and Kenny, J. M. 2010. Biodegradable polymer matrix nanocomposites for tissue engineering: A review. *Polym. Degrad. Stab.* 95:2126–2146.
6. Platt, D. K. 2006. *Biodegradable Polymers, Market Report.* London, U.K.: Rapra Technology Ltd.
7. Langer, R. and Vacanti, J. P. 1993. Tissue engineering. *Science* 260:920–926.
8. Seunarine, K., Gadegaard, N., Tormen, M., Meredith, D. O., Riehle, M. O., and Wilkinson, C. D. 2006. 3D polymer scaffolds for tissue engineering. *Nanomedicine* 1:281–296.
9. Zhang, R. and Ma, P. X. 2001. Processing of polymer scaffolds: Phase separation. In *Methods of Tissue Engineering*, eds. Atala A., and Lanza R., p. 715. San Diego, CA: Academic Press.
10. Shalak, R. and Fox, C. F. 1988. Preface. In: *Tissue Engineering*, eds. Shalak R. and Fox C. F., pp. 26–29. New York: Alan R. Liss.
11. Nagura, I., Fujioka, H., Kokubu, T., Makino, T., Sumi Y., and Kurosaka, M. 2007. Repair of osteochondral defects with a new porous synthetic polymer scaffold. *J. Bone Joint Surg.* 89:258–264.
12. Schmitt, H., Creton, N., Prashantha, K., Soulestin, J., Lacrampe, M. F, and Krawczak, P. 2014. Preparation and characterization of plasticized starch/halloysite porous nanocomposites possibly suitable for biomedical applications. *J. Appl. Polym. Sci.* DOI: 10.1002/app.41341.
13. Vishnoi, T. and Kumar, A. 2013. Conducting cryogel scaffold as a potential biomaterial for cell stimulation and proliferation. *J. Mater. Sci. Mater. Med.* 24:447–459.
14. Gay, S., Arostegui, S., and Lemaitre, J. 2009. Preparation and characterization of dense nanohydroxyapatite/PLLA composites. *Mater. Sci. Eng. C* 29:172–177.

15. Ma, P. X. 2004. Scaffolds for tissue fabrication. *Mater. Today* 7:30–40.
16. Zhu, N. and Chen, X. 2013. Biofabrication of tissue scaffolds. In *Advances in Biomaterials Science and Biomedical Applications*, ed. Pignatello R., pp. 315–328. Croatia: InTech.
17. Mohanty, A. K., Misra, M., and Hinrichsen, G. 2000. Biofibers. Biodegradable polymers and biocomposites: An overview. *Macromol. Mater. Eng.* 276:1–24.
18. Shin, H., Jo, S., and Mikos, A. G. 2003. Biomimetic materials for tissue engineering. *Biomaterials* 24:4353–4364.
19. Wen, X. and Tresco, P. A. 2006. Fabrication and characterization of permeable degradable poly(DL-lactide-co-glycolide) (PLGA) hollow fiber phase inversion membranes for use as nerve tract guidance channels. *Biomaterials* 27:3800–3809.
20. Koegler, W. S. and Griffith, L. G. 2004. Osteoblast response to PLGA tissue engineering scaffolds with PEO modified surface chemistries and demonstration of patterned cell response. *Biomaterials* 25:2819–2830.
21. Curtin, C. M., Cunniffe, G. M., Lyons, F. G., Bessho, K., Dickson, G. R., Duffy, G. P., and O'Brien, F. J. 2012. Innovative collagen nano-hydroxyapatite scaffolds offer a highly efficient non-viral gene delivery platform for stem cell-mediated bone formation. *Adv. Mater.* 24:749–754.
22. Dey, S. and Pal, S. 2009. Evaluation of collagen-hydroxyapatite scaffold for bone tissue engineering. In *13th International Conference on Biomedical Engineering IFMBE Proceedings*, Singapore, 23:1267–1270.
23. Li, X., Feng, Q., and Cui, F. 2006. In vitro degradation of porous nano-hydroxyapatite/collagen/PLLA scaffold reinforced by chitin fibres. *Mater. Sci. Eng. C* 26:716–720.
24. Zhou, C, Ye, X., Fan, Y., Ma, L., Tan, Y., Qing, F., and Zhang, X. 2014. Biomimetic fabrication of a three-level hierarchical calcium phosphate/collagen/ hydroxyapatite scaffold for bone tissue engineering. *Biofabrication* 6:035013.
25. Campos D. M., Anselme K., and Dulce de Almeida Soares G. 2011. In vitro biological evaluation of 3-D hydroxyapatite/collagen (50/50 wt. (%)) scaffolds. *Mat. Res.* 15 (1): 1–8. http://www.scielo.br/pdf/mr/v15n1/aop1000.pdf (accessed August 4, 2014).
26. Huang Z., Tian J., Yu B., Xu Y., and Feng Q. 2009. A bone-like nano-hydroxyapatite/collagen loaded injectable scaffold. *Biomed. Mater.* 4:055005.
27. Luderer F., Begerow I., Schmidt W., Martin H., Grabow N., Bünger C.M., Schareck W., Schmitz K.P., and Sternberg K. 2013. Enhanced visualization of biodegradable polymeric vascular scaffolds by incorporation of gold, silver and magnetite nanoparticles. *J. Biomater. Appl.* 28:219–231.
28. Tencomnao, T., Apijaraskul, A., Rakkhithawatthan, V., Chaleawlert-umpon, S., Pimpa, N., Sajomsang, W., and Saengkrit, N. 2011. Gold/cationic polymer nanoscaffolds mediated transfection for non-viral gene delivery system. *Carbohyd. Polym.*184:216–222.
29. Kundu, S., Huitink, D., Wang, K., and Liang, H. 2010. Photochemical formation of electrically conductive silver nanowires on polymer scaffolds. *J. Colloid Interf. Sci.* 344:334–342.
30. Zhou, K., Thouas, G. A., Bernard, C. C., Nisbet, D. R., Finkelstein, D. I., Li, D., and Forsythe, J. S. 2012. Method to impart electro- and biofunctionality to neural scaffolds using graphene-polyelectrolyte multilayers. *ACS Appl. Mater. Interf.* 4:4524–4531.
31. Vasita, R. and Katti, D. S. 2006. Nanofibers and their applications in tissue engineering. *Int. J. Nanomed.* 1:15–30.
32. Liu, S. F., Petty, A. R., Sazama, G. T., and Swager, T. M. 2015. Single-walled carbon nanotube/metalloporphyrin composites for the chemiresistive detection of amines and meat spoilage. *Angew. Chem. Int. Ed. Engl.* 54:6554–6557.

33. Dai, P. and Chen, J. 2011. Research progress on the preparation methods of single polymer composites. In *IEEE 2011 International Conference on Remote Sensing, Environment and Transportation Engineering,* Nanjing, China, (June): 6277–6282. http://ieeexplore. ieee.org/xpl/login.jsp?tp=&arnumber=5965792&url=http%3A%2F%2Fieeexplore.ieee. org%2Fxpls%2Fabs_all.jsp%3Farnumber%3D5965792 (accessed August 4, 2014).

34. Xiao, G. 1995. Solvent-induced changes on corona-discharge-treated polyolefin surfaces probed by contact angle measurement. *J. Colloid Interf. Sci.* 171:200–204.

35. Otsuka, H., Nagasaki, Y., and Kataoka, K. 2000. Dynamic wettability study on the functionalized PEGylated layer on a polylactide surface constructed by coating of aldehyde-ended poly(ethylene glycol) (PEG)/polylactide (PLA) block copolymer. *Sci. Technol. Adv. Mater.* 1:21–29.

36. Tang, Z. G., Black, R. A., Curran J. M., Hunt, J. A., Rhodes, N. P., and Williams, D. F. 2004. Surface properties and biocompatibility of solvent-cast poly[3-caprolactone] films. *Biomaterials* 25:4741–4748.

37. Mikos, A. G., Thorsen, A. J., Czerwonka, L. A., Bao, Y., Langer, R., and Winslow, D. N. 1994. Preparation and characterization of poly(L-lactic acid) foams. *Polymer* 35:1068–1077.

38. Mikos, A. G., Sarakinos, G., Vacanti, J. P., Langer, R., and Cima, L.G. 1996. Biocompatible polymer membranes and methods of preparation of three dimensional membrane structures. United States Patent No. 5514378.

39. Di Maio, E., Mensitieri, G., Iannace, S., Nicolais, L., Li, W., and Flumerfelt, R. W. 2005. Structure optimization of polycaprolactone foams by using mixtures of CO_2 and N_2 as blowing agents. *Polym. Eng. Sci.* 45:432–441.

40. Haugen, H., Ried, V., Brunner, M., Will, J., and Wintermantel, E. 2004. Water as foaming agent for open cell polyurethane structures. *J. Mater. Sci. Mater. Med.* 15:343–346.

41. Parks, K. L. and Beckman, E. J. 1996. Generation of microcellular polyurethane foams via polymerization in carbon dioxide. 2. Foam formation and characterization. *Polym. Eng. Sci.* 36:2417–2431.

42. Quirk, R. A., France, R. M., Shakesheff, K. M., and Howdle, S. M. 2004. Supercritical fluid technologies and tissue engineering scaffolds. *Curr. Opin. Solid State Mater. Sci.* 8:313–321.

43. Lee, K. W. D., Chan, P. K., and Feng, X. S. 2004. Morphology development and characterization of the phase-separated structure resulting from the thermal-induced phase separation phenomenon in polymer solutions under a temperature gradient. *Chem. Eng. Sci.* 59:1491–1504.

44. Ma, P. X. and Zhang, R. Y. 1999. Synthetic nano-scale fibrous extracellular matrix. *J. Biomed. Mater. Res.* 46:60–72.

45. Thomson, R. C., Wake, M. C., Yaszemski, M. J., and Mikos, A. G. 1995. Biodegradable polymer scaffolds to regenerate organs. *Adv. Polym. Sci.* 122:245–274.

46. Pikal, M. J., Shah, S., Roy, M. L., and Putman, R. 1990. The secondary drying stage of freeze-drying kinetics as a function of temperature and chamber pressure. *Int. J. Pharm.* 60:203–217.

47. Liapis, A. I. and Bruttini, R. 1994. A theory for the primary and secondary drying stages of the freeze-drying of pharmaceutical crystalline and amorphous solutes - comparison between experimental—data and theory. *Separat. Technol.* 4:144–155.

48. Bischof, J. C. and He, X. M. 2005. Thermal stability of proteins. *Ann. NY. Acad. Sci.* 1066:12–33.

49. Stevens, M. M. and George J. H. 2005. Exploring and engineering the cell surface interface. *Science* 310:1135–1138.

50. Huang, Z. M., Zhang, Y. Z., Kotaki, M., and Ramakrishna, S. 2003. A review on polymer nanofibers by electrospinning and their applications in nanocomposites. *Compos. Sci. Technol.* 63:2223–2253.

51. Pham, Q. P., Sharma, U., and Mikos, A. G. 2006. Electrospinning of polymeric nanofibers for tissue engineering applications: A review. *Tissue Eng.* 12:1197–1211.
52. Jain, K. K. 2006. Role of nanotechnology in developing new therapies for diseases of the nervous system. *Nanomedicine* 1:9–12.
53. Yeong, W. Y., Chua, C. K., Leong, K. F., and Chandrasekaran, M. 2004. Rapid prototyping in tissue engineering: Challenges and potential. *Trends Biotechnol.* 22:643–652.
54. Chua, C. K., Leong, K. F., Cheah, C. M., and Chua, S. W. 2003. Development of a tissue engineering scaffold structure library for rapid prototyping. Part 1: Investigation and Classification. *J. Adv. Manufac. Technol.* 21:291–301.
55. Mironov, V., Boland, T., Trusk, T., Forgacs, G., and Markwald, R. R. 2003. Organ printing: Computer aided jet-based 3D tissue engineering. *Trends Biotechnol.* 21:157–161.
56. Hutmacher, D. W., Sittinger, M., and Risbud, M. V. 2004. Scaffold-based tissue engineering: Rationale for computer-aided design and solid freeform fabrication systems. *Trends Biotechnol.* 22:354–362.
57. Song, B. R., Yang, S. S., Jin, H., Lee, S. H., Park, D. Y., Lee, J. H., Park, S. R., Park, S. H., and Min, B. H. 2015. Three dimensional plotted extracellular matrix scaffolds using a rapid prototyping for tissue engineering application. *Tissue Eng. Regen. Med.* 12:172–180.
58. Albrecht, W., Luetzow, K., Weigel, T., Groth, T., Schossig, M., and Lendlein, A. 2006. Development of highly porous microparticles from poly(ether imide) prepared by a spraying/coagulation process. *J. Membr. Sci.* 273:106–115.
59. Newman, K. D. and McBurney, M. W. 2004. Poly(D,L lactic-co-glycolic acid) microspheres as biodegradable microcarriers for pluripotent stem cells. *Biomaterials* 25: 5763–5771.
60. Zhang, J., Zhang, H., Wu, L., and Ding, J. 2006. Fabrication of three dimensional polymeric scaffolds with spherical pores. *J. Mater. Sci.* 41:1725–1731.
61. Borden, M., Attawia, M., Khan, Y., El-Amin, S. F., and Laurencin, C. T. 2004. Tissue engineered bone formation in vivo using a novel sintered polymeric microsphere matrix. *J. Bone Joint Surg. Br.* 86:1200–1208.
62. Borden, M., Attawia, M., and Laurencin, C. T. 2002. The sintered microsphere matrix for bone tissue engineering: In vitro osteoconductivity studies. *J. Biomed. Mater. Res.* 61:421–429.
63. Khan, Y. M., Katti, D. S., and Laurencin C. T. 2004. Novel polymer-synthesized ceramic composite based system for bone repair: An in vitro evaluation. *J. Biomed. Mater. Res. Part A* 69A:728–737.
64. Dollar, A. M. and Howe, R. D. 2006. A robust compliant grasper via shape deposition manufacturing. *IEEE ASME Trans. Mechatron.* 11:154–161.
65. Malda, J., Woodfieldm T. B. F., and van der Vloodt F. 2005. The effect of PEGT/PBT scaffold architecture on the composition of tissue engineered cartilage. *Biomaterials* 26:63–72.
66. Woodfield, T. B. F., Malda, J., de Wijn J., Peters, F., Riesle, J., and van Blitterswijk, C. A. 2004. Design of porous scaffolds for cartilage tissue engineering using a three-dimensional fiber-deposition technique. *Biomaterials* 25:4149–4161.
67. Zein, I., Hutmacher, D. W., Tan, K. C., and Teoh, S. H. 2001. Fused deposition modeling of novel scaffold architectures for tissue engineering applications. *Biomaterials* 23:1169–1185.
68. Chen, Z., Li, D., Lu, B., Tang, Y., Sun, M., and Xu, S. 2004. Fabrication of osteo-structure analogous scaffolds via fused deposition modeling. *Scr. Mater.* 52:157–161.
69. Hutmacher, D. W., Schantz, T., Zein, I., Ng, K. W., Teoh, S. H., and Tan, K. C. 2001. Mechanical properties and cell cultural response of polycaprolactone scaffolds designed and fabricated via fused deposition modeling. *J. Biomed. Mater. Res.* 55:203–216.
70. Schantz, J. T., Ng, M. M. L., and Netto, P. 2002. Application of an X-ray microscopy technique to evaluate tissue-engineered bone-scaffold constructs. *Mater. Sci. Eng. C* C20:9–17.

71. Landers, R. and Mulhaupt, R. 2000. Desktop manufacturing of complex objects, prototypes and biomedical scaffolds by means of computer-assisted design combined with computer-guided 3D plotting of polymers and reactive oligomers. *Macromol. Mater. Eng.* 282:17–21.
72. Koch, K. U., Biesinger, B., Arnholz, C., and Jansson, V. 1998. Creating of biocompatible, high stress resistant and resorbable implants using multiphase jet solidification technology. http://publica.fraunhofer.de/dokumente/PX-8787.html (accessed August 4, 2014).
73. Ruecker, M., Laschke, M. W., and Junker, D. 2006. Angiogenic and inflammatory response to biodegradable scaffolds in dorsal skinfold chambers of mice. *Biomaterials* 27:5027–5038.
74. Sachlos, E. and Czernuszka, J. T. 2003. Making tissue engineering scaffolds work. Review on the application of solid freeform fabrication technology to the production of tissue engineering scaffolds. *Euro. Cells Mater.* 5:29–40.
75. Landers, R., Pfister, A., Huebner, U., John, H., Schmelzeisen, R., and Muelhaupt, R. 2002. Fabrication of soft tissue engineering scaffolds by means of rapid prototyping techniques. *J. Mater. Sci.* 37:3107–3116.
76. Sachs, E. M., Haggerty, J. S., Cima, M. J., and Williams, P. A. 1989. Three-dimensional printing techniques. United States Patent No. 5204055.
77. Leukers, B., Guelkan, H., and Irsen, S. H. 2005. Hydroxyapatite scaffolds for bone tissue engineering made by 3D printing. *J. Mater. Sci. Mater. Med.* 16:1121–1124.
78. Curodeau, A., Sachs, E., and Caldarise, S. 2000. Design and fabrication of cast orthopedic implants with freeform surface textures from 3-D printed ceramic shell. *J. Biomed. Mater. Res.* 53:525–535.
79. Irsen, S. H., Leukers, B., Hoeckling, C., Tille, C., and Seitz, H. 2006. Bioceramic granulates for use in 3D printing: Process engineering aspects. *Materialwissenschaft und Werkstofftechnik* 37:533–537.
80. Lam, C. X. F., Mo, X. M., Teoh, S. H., and Hutmacher, D. W. 2002. Scaffold development using 3D printing with a starch-based polymer. *Mater. Sci. Eng. C* C20:49–56.
81. Giordano, R. A., Wu, B. M., Borland, S. W., Cima, L. G., Sachs, E. M., and Cima, M. J. 1996. Mechanical properties of dense polylactic acid structures fabricated by three dimensional printing. *J. Biomater. Sci. Polym. Ed.* 8:63–75.
82. Tan, K. H., Chua, C. K., and Leong, K. F. 2005. Selective laser sintering of biocompatible polymers for applications in tissue engineering. *Bio-Med. Mater. Eng.* 15:113–124.
83. Tan, K. H., Chua, C. K., and Leong, K. F. 2003. Scaffold development using selective laser sintering of polyetheretherketone-hydroxyapatite biocomposite blends. *Biomaterials* 24:3115–3123.
84. Dhariwala, B., Hunt, E., and Boland, T. 2004. Rapid prototyping of tissue-engineering constructs, using photopolymerizable hydrogels and stereolithography. *Tissue Eng.* 10:1316–1322.
85. Cooke, M. N., Fisher, J. P., Dean, D., Rimnac, C., and Mikos, A. G. 2003. Use of stereolithography to manufacture critical-sized 3D biodegradable scaffolds for bone ingrowth. *J. Biomed. Mater. Res. Part B.* 64B:65–69.
86. Matsuyama, H., Yuasa, M., Kitamura, Y., Teramoto, M., and Lloyd, D. R. 2000. Structure control of anisotropic and asymmetric polypropylene membrane prepared by thermally induced phase separation. *J. Membr. Sci.* 179:91–100.
87. Chen, J., Cui, L., Liu, W., and Cao, Y. 2003. Development on solvent casting/particulate leaching. *Zhongguo Shengwu Gongcheng Zazhi* 23:32–35.
88. Lawes, R. A. 2000. Future trends in high-resolution lithography. *App. Surf. Sci.* 154–155:519–526.
89. Matsumoto, N., Hiruma, H., Nagaoka, S., Fujiyama, K., Kaneko, A., and Kawakami, H. 2008. Cell processing on polyimide surface patterned by rubbing. *Polym. Adv. Technol.* 19:1002–1008.

90. Cosutchi, A. I., Hulubei, C., Stoica, I., and Ioan, S. 2011. A new approach for patterning epiclon-based polyimide precursor films using a lyotropic liquid crystal template. *J. Polym. Res.* 18:2389–2402.
91. Cosutchi, A. I., Hulubei, C., Stoica, I., and Ioan, S. 2010. Morphological and structural-rheological relationship in epiclon-based polyimide/hydroxypropyl cellulose blend systems. *J. Polym. Res.* 17:541–550.
92. Cosutchi, A. I. 2009. Thermodynamics and morphology of complex polymer structures, PhD Thesis, Petru Poni Institute of Macromolecular Chemistry of Iasi, Romania.
93. Navard, P. 1986. Formation of band textures in hydroxypropyl cellulose liquid crystals. *J. Polym. Sci. B* 24:435–442.
94. Freed, L. E., Novakovic, G. V., Biron, R. J., Eagles, D. B., Lesnoy, D. C., and Barlow, S. K. 1994. Biodegradable polymer scaffolds for tissue engineering. *Biotechnology* 12:689–693.
95. Rezwan, K., Chen, Q. Z., Blaker, J. J., and Boccaccini, A. R. 2006. Biodegradable and bioactive porous polymer/inorganic composite scaffolds for bone tissue engineering. *Biomaterials* 27:3413–3431.
96. Webster, T. J., Ergun, C., Doremus, R. H., Siegel, R. W., and Bizios, R. 2000. Enhanced functions of osteoblasts on nanophase ceramics. *Biomaterials* 2:1803–1810.
97. Webster, T. J., Schadler, L. S., Siegel, R. W., and Bizios, R. 2001. Mechanisms of enhanced osteoblast adhesion on nanophase alumina involve vitronectin. *Tissue Eng.* 7:291–301.
98. Nishiguchi, H., Kato, H., Fujita, H., Kim, H. M., Miyaji, F., and Kokubo, T. 1999. Enhancement of bone-bonding strength of titanium alloy implants by alkali and heat treatments. *J. Biomed. Mater. Res. B* 48:689–696.
99. Nejati, E., Mirzadeh, H., and Zandi, M. 2008. Synthesis and characterization of nano-hydroxyapatite rods/poly(l-lactide acid) composite scaffolds for bone tissue engineering. *Compos. Part A* 39:1589–1596.
100. Fu, Q., Zhou, N., Huang, W., Wang, D., Zhang, L., and Li, H. 2004. Preparation and characterization of a novel bioactive bone cement: Glass based nanoscale hydroxyapatite bone cement. *J. Mater. Sci. Mater. Med.* 15:1333–1338.
101. Fu, Q. Rahaman, M. N., Zhou, N., Huang, W., Wang, D., Zhang, L., and Li, H. 2008. In vitro study on different cell response to spherical hydroxyapatite nanoparticles. *J. Biomater. Appl.* 23:37–50.
102. Baei, S. M. and Rezvani A. 2011. Nanocomposite (PHBHV/HA) fabrication from biodegradable polymer. *Middle-East J. Sci. Res.* 7: 46–50.
103. Hu, Q. L., Li, B. Q., Wang, M., and Shen, J. C. 2004. Preparation and characterization of biodegradable chitosan/hydroxyapatite nanocomposite rods via in situ hybridization: A potential material as internal fixation of bone fracture. *Biomaterials* 25:779–785.
104. Porter, M. M., Lee, S., Tanadchangsaeng, N., Jaremko, M. J., Yu, J., Meyers, M., and McKittrick, J. 2013. Porous Hydroxyapatite-polyhydroxybutyrate composites fabricated by a novel method via centrifugation. *Mech. Biol. Syst. Mater.* 5:63–71.
105. Engler, A. J., Sen, S., Sweeney, H. L., and Discher, D. E. 2006. Matrix elasticity directs stem cell lineage specification. *Cell.* 126:677–689.
106. Hong, Z., Zhang, P., He, C., Qiu, X., Liu, A., Chen, L., Chen, X., and Jing, X. 2005. Nano-composite of poly(l-lactide) and surface grafted hydroxyapatite: Mechanical properties and biocompatibility. *Biomaterials* 26:6296–6304.
107. Kuhne, J. H., Bartl, R., and Frisch, B. 1994. Bone formation in coralline hydroxyapatite. Effects of pore size studied in rabbits. *Acta Orthop. Scand.* 65: 246–252.
108. Carinci, F., Santarelli, A., Laino, L., Pezzetti, F., De Lillo, A., Parisi, D., Bambini, F., Procaccini, M., Testa, N. F., Cocchi, R., and Lo Muzio, L. 2014. Pre-clinical evaluation of a new coral-based bone scaffold. *Int. J. Immunopathol. Pharmacol.* 27:221–234.

109. Mangeney, C., Ferrage, F., Aujard, I., Marchi-Artzner, V., Jullien, L., and Ouari, O. 2002. Synthesis and properties of water-soluble gold colloids covalently derivatized with neutral polymer monolayers. *J. Am. Chem. Soc.* 124:5811–5821.

110. McKeon-Fischer, K. D. and Freeman, J. W. 2011. Characterization of electrospun poly(L-lactide) and gold nanoparticle composite scaffolds for skeletal muscle tissue engineering. *J. Tissue. Eng. Regen. Med.* 5:560–568.

111. Zhang, Y., He, H., Gao, W. J., Lu, S. Y., Liu, Y., and Gu, H. Y. 2009. Rapid adhesion and proliferation of keratinocytes on the gold colloid/chitosan film scaffolds. *Mater. Sci. Eng. C* 29:908–912.

112. Morones, J. R., Elechiguerra, J. L., Camacho, A., Holt, K., Kouri J. B., and Ramirez, J. T. 2005. The bactericidal effect of silver nanoparticles. *Nanotechnology* 16:2346–2353.

113. Falletta, E., Bonini, M., Fratini, E., Lo Nostro, A., Pesavento, G., and Becheri, A. 2008. Clusters of poly(acrylates) and silver nanoparticles: Structure and applications for anti-microbial fabrics. *J. Phys. Chem. C* 112:11758–11766.

114. Evanoff Jr., D. D. and Chumanov, G. 2005. Synthesis and optical properties of silver nanoparticles and arrays. *Chem. Phys. Chem.* 6:1221–1231.

115. Dobos-Necula, A. M. and Ioan, S. 2012. Silver nanoparticles in cellulose derivative matrix. In *Nanotechnology in Polymers*, eds. V. K. Thakur, A. S. Singha, pp. 191–248. Houston, TX: Studium Press LLC.

116. Necula, A. M., Stoica, I., Olaru, N., Doroftei, F., and Ioan, S. 2011. Silver nanoparticles in cellulose acetate polymers. Rheological and morphological properties. *J. Macromol. Sci. B* 50:639–651.

117. Ding, T., Luo, Z. J., Zheng, Y., Hu, X. Y., and Ye, Z. X. 2010. Rapid repair and regeneration of damaged rabbit sciatic nerves by tissue engineered scaffold made from nanosilver and collagen type I. *Injury* 41:522–527.

118. Choudhary, S., Haberstrih, K. M., and Webster, T. J. 2007. Enhanced functions of vascular cells on nanostructured Ti for improved stent applications. *Tissue Eng.* 13:1421–1430.

119. Goto, K., Tamura, J., Shinzato, S., Fujibayashi, S., Hashimoto, M., Kawashita, M., Kokubo, T., and Nakamura, T. 2005. Bioactive bone cements containing nano-sized titania particles for use as bone substituents. *Biomaterials* 26:6496–6505.

120. Liu, H., Slamovich, E. B., and Webster, T. J. 2006. Increased osteoblast functions among nanophase titania/poly(lactide-co-glycolide) composites of the highest nanometer surface roughness. *J. Biomed. Mater. Res. A* 78A:798–807.

121. Horch, R. A., Shahid, N., Mistrry, A. S., Timmer, M. D., Mikos, A. G., and Rarron A. R., 2004. Nanoreinforcement of poly(propylene fumarate)-based networks with surface modified alumoxane nanoparticles for bone tissue engineering. *Biomacromolecules* 5:1990–1998.

122. Dresselhaus, M. S., Dresselhaus, G., and Eklund, P. C. 2001. *Science of Fullerenes and Carbon Nanotubes*. San Diego, CA: Academic Press.

123. Liu, W., Wei, J., Chen, Y., Huo, P., and Wei, Y. 2013. Electrospinning of poly(L-lactide) nanofibers encapsulated with water-soluble fullerenes for bioimaging application. *ACS Appl. Mater. Interf.* 5:680–685.

124. Shi, X., Hudson, J. L., Spicer, P. P., Tour, J. M., Krishnamoorti, R., and Mikos, A. G. 2006. Injectable nanocomposites of single-walled carbon nanotubes and biodegradable polymers for bone tissue engineering. *Biomacromolecules* 7:2237–2242.

125. Lovat, V., Pantarotto, D., Lagostena, L., Cacciari, B., Grolfo, M., and Righi, M. 2005. Nanotube substrates boost neuronal electrical signaling. *Nano. Lett.* 5:1107–1110.

126. Mwenifumbo, S., Shaffer, M. S., and Stevens, M. M. 2007. Exploring cellular behaviour with multi-walled carbon nanotube constructs. *J. Mater. Chem.* 17:1894–1902.

127. Shi, X., Hudson, J. L., Spicer, P. P., Tour, J. M., Krishnamoorti, R., and Mikos, A. G. 2005. Rheological behaviour and mechanical characterization of injectable poly(propylene fumarate)/single-walled carbon nanotube composites for bone tissue engineering. *Nanotechnology* 16:S531–S538.

128. Supronowicz, P. R., Ajayan, P. M., Ullmann, K. R., Arulanandam, B. P., Metzger, D. W., and Bizios, R. 2002. Novel current-conducting composite substrates for exposing osteoblasts alternating current stimulation. *J. Biomed. Mater. Res.* 59:49–506.
129. Martins, A. M., Eng, G., Caridade, S. G., Mano, J. F., Reis, R. L., and Vunjak-Novakovic, G. 2014. Electrically conductive chitosan/carbon scaffolds for cardiac tissue engineering. *Biomacromolecules* 15:635–643.
130. Mochalin, V. N., Shenderova, O., Ho, D., and Gogotsi, Y. 2012. The properties and applications of nanodiamonds. *Nat. Nanotechnol.* 7:11–23.
131. Zhang, Q., Mochalin, V. N., Neitzel, I., Hazeli, K., Niu, J., Kontsos, A., Zhou, J. G., Lelkes, P. I., and Gogotsi Y. 2012. Mechanical properties and biomineralization of multifunctional nanodiamond-PLLA composites for bone tissue engineering. *Biomaterials* 33:5067–5075
132. Kokubo, T. and Takadama, H. 2006. How useful is SBF in predicting in vivo bone bioactivity?. *Biomaterials* 27:2907–2915.
133. Kim, H. and Macosko, C. W. 2009. Processing-property relationships of polycarbonate/graphene composites. *Polymer* 50:3797–3809.
134. Jing, X., Mi, H. Y., Salick, M. R., Peng, X. F., and Turng, L. S. 2014. Preparation of thermoplastic polyurethane/graphene oxide composite scaffolds by thermally induced phase separation. *Polym. Compos.* 35:1408–1417.

7 Biocomposites and Hybrid Biomaterials of Calcium Orthophosphates with Polymers

Sergey V. Dorozhkin

CONTENTS

ABBREVIATIONS

BMP	Bone morphogenetic protein
BSA	Bovine serum albumin
EVOH	Copolymer of ethylene and vinyl alcohol
HDPE	High-density polyethylene
HIPS	High impact polystyrene
HPMC	Hydroxypropylmethylcellulose
PBT	Polybutyleneterephthalate

PCL	Poly(ε-caprolactone)
PDLLA	Poly(D,L-lactic acid)
PE	Polyethylene
PEEK	Polyetheretherketone
PEG	Polyethylene glycol
PGA	Polyglycolic acid
PHB	Polyhydroxybutyrate
PHBHV	Poly(hydroxybutyrate-*co*-hydroxyvalerate)
PLA	Polylactic acid
PLGA	Poly(lactic-*co*-glycolic) acid
PLLA	Poly(L-lactic acid)
PMMA	Polymethylmethacrylate
PP	Polypropylene
PPF	Poly(propylene-*co*-fumarate)
PS	Polysulfone
PTFE	Polytetrafluoroethylene
PVA	Polyvinyl alcohol
SEVA-C	Blend of EVOH with starch
UHMWPE	Ultrahigh molecular weight polyethylene

7.1   INTRODUCTION

The fracture of bones due to various traumas or natural aging is a typical type of tissue failure. An operative treatment frequently requires implantation of a temporary or a permanent prosthesis, which still is a challenge for orthopedic surgeons, especially in the cases of large bone defects. Fast aging of the population and serious drawbacks of natural bone grafts make the situation even worse; therefore, there is a high clinical demand for bone substitutes. Unfortunately, a medical application of xenografts (e.g., bovine bone) is generally associated with potential viral infections. In addition, xenografts have a low osteogenicity and an increased immunogenicity, and they usually resorb more rapidly than autogenous bone. Similar limitations are also valid for human allografts (i.e., tissue transplantation between individuals of the same species but of nonidentical genetic composition), where the concerns about potential risks of transmitting tumor cells, a variety of bacterial and viral infections, as well as immunological and blood group incompatibility are even stronger [1,2]. Moreover, harvesting and conserving allografts (exogenous bones) are additional limiting factors. Autografts (endogenous bones) are still the *golden standard* among any substitution materials because they are osteogenic, osteoinductive, osteoconductive, completely biocompatible, nontoxic, and do not cause any immunological problems (nonallergic). They contain viable osteogenic cells and bone matrix proteins as well as support bone growth. Usually, autografts are well accepted by the body and are rapidly integrated into the surrounding bone tissues. Due to these reasons, they are used routinely for a long period with good clinical results [2–4]; however, it is fair to say on complication cases, those frequently happened in the past [5]. Unfortunately, a limited number of donor sites restrict the quantity of autografts harvested from the iliac crest or other locations of the patient's own body. In addition, their medical application is always associated with additional traumas and scars resulting from the extraction of a donor tissue during a superfluous surgical operation, which requires further healing at the donation site and can involve long-term postoperative pain. Thus, any types of biologically derived transplants appear to be imperfect solutions, mainly due to a restricted quantity of donor tissues, donor-site morbidity, as well as potential risks of an immunological incompatibility and disease transfer [6–8]. In this light, man-made materials (alloplastic or synthetic bone grafts) stand out as a reasonable option because they are easily available and might be processed and modified to suit the specific needs of a given application. What is more is that there are no concerns about potential infections, immunological incompatibility, sterility, and donor-site morbidity. Therefore, investigations on artificial materials for bone tissue repair appear to be one of the key subjects in the field of biomaterials research for clinical applications [9,10].

Currently, several classes of synthetic bone-grafting biomaterials are available for in vivo applications. The examples include natural coral, coral-derived materials, bovine porous demineralized bone, human demineralized bone matrix, bioactive glasses, glass-ceramics, and $CaPO_4$ [11,12]. Among them, porous bioceramics made of $CaPO_4$ appear to be very prominent due to both excellent biocompatibility and bonding ability to living bone in the body. This is directly related to the fact that the inorganic material of mammalian calcified tissues, that is, of bone and teeth, consists of $CaPO_4$ [13–15]. Due to this reason, other artificial materials are normally encapsulated by fibrous tissue, when implanted in body defects, while $CaPO_4$ are not. Many types of $CaPO_4$-based bioceramics with different chemical composition are already on the market. Unfortunately, as for any ceramic material, $CaPO_4$ bioceramics alone lack the mechanical and elastic properties of the calcified tissues. Scaffolds made of $CaPO_4$ suffer only from low elasticity, high brittleness, poor tensile strength, low mechanical reliability and fracture toughness, which leads to various concerns about their mechanical performance after implantation [16,17]. Besides, in many cases, it is difficult to form $CaPO_4$ bioceramics into the desired shapes.

The superior strength and partial elasticity of biological calcified tissues (e.g., bones) are due to the presence of bioorganic polymers (mainly, collagen type I fibers) rather than to a natural ceramic [mainly, a poorly crystalline ion-substituted calcium-deficient hydroxyapatite (CDHA), often referred to as *biological apatite*] phase [18–21]. The elastic collagen fibers are aligned in bone along the main stress directions. The biochemical composition of bones is given in Table 7.1 [22].

A decalcified bone is very flexible and can be easily twisted, whereas a bone without collagen is very brittle; thus, the inorganic nanosized crystals of biological apatite provide hardness and stiffness, while the bioorganic fibers are responsible for elasticity and toughness. In bones, both types of materials integrate each other into a nanometric scale in such a way that the crystallite size, fibers orientation, short-range order between the components, etc., determine their nanostructure and, therefore, the function and mechanical properties of the entire composite. From the mechanical point of view, bone is a tough material at low strain rates but fractures more like a brittle material at high strain rates; generally, it is rather weak in tension and shear, particularly along the longitudinal plane. Besides, bone is an anisotropic material because its properties are directionally dependent [18–21].

TABLE 7.1
Biochemical Composition[a] of Bones

Inorganic Phases	wt.%	Bioorganic Phases	wt.%
CaPO$_4$ (biological apatite)	~60	Collagen type I	~20
Water	~9	Non-collagenous proteins: osteocalcin, osteonectin, osteopontin, thrombospondin, morphogenetic proteins, sialoprotein, serum proteins	~3
Carbonates	~4	Other traces: polysaccharides, lipids, cytokines	Balance
Citrates	~0.9	Primary bone cells: osteoblasts, osteocytes, osteoclasts	Balance
Sodium	~0.7		
Magnesium	~0.5		
Other traces: Cl$^-$, F$^-$, K$^+$ Sr^{2+}, Pb^{2+}, Zn^{2+}, Cu^{2+}, Fe^{2+}	Balance		

Source: Murugan, R. and Ramakrishna, S., *Compos. Sci. Technol.*, 65, 2005, 2385.

[a] The composition is varied from species to species and from bone to bone.

It remains a great challenge to design the ideal bone graft that emulates nature's own structures or functions. Certainly, the successful design requires an appreciation of the bones' structure. According to expectations, the ideal bone graft should be benign; available in a variety of forms and sizes, all with sufficient mechanical properties for use in load-bearing sites; form a chemical bond at the bone–implant interface; as well as be osteogenic, osteoinductive, osteoconductive, biocompatible, completely biodegradable at the expense of bone growth, and moldable to fill and restore bone defects [16,23,24]. Further, it should resemble the chemical composition of bones (thus, the presence of CaPO$_4$ is mandatory), exhibit contiguous porosity to encourage invasion by the live host tissue, as well as possess both viscoelastic and semi-brittle behavior, as bones do [25–27]. Moreover, the degradation kinetics of the ideal implant should be adjusted to the healing rate of the human tissue with absence of any chemical or biological irritation and/or toxicity caused by substances, which are released due to corrosion or degradation. Ideally, the combined mechanical strength of the implant and the ingrowing bone should remain constant throughout the regenerative process. Furthermore, the substitution implant material should not disturb significantly the stress environment of the surrounding living tissue [28]. Finally, there is an opinion that, in the case of a serious trauma, bone should fracture rather than the implant [16]. Good sterilizability, storability, and processability, as well as a relatively low cost, are also of great importance to permit a clinical application. Unfortunately, no artificial biomaterial is yet available, which embodies all these requirements and unlikely it will appear in the nearest future. To date, most of the available biomaterials appear to be either predominantly osteogenic or osteoinductive or else purely osteoconductive [1].

Careful consideration of the bone type and mechanical properties are needed to design bone substitutes. Indeed, in high load-bearing bones such as femur, the stiffness of the implant needs to be adequate—not too stiff to result in strain shielding, but rigid enough to present stability. However, in relatively low load-bearing applications such as cranial bone repairs, it is more important to have stability and the correct 3D shapes for aesthetic reasons. One of the most promising alternatives is to apply materials with similar composition and nanostructure to that of bone tissue. Mimicking the structure of calcified tissues and addressing the limitations of the individual materials, development of organic–inorganic hybrid biomaterials provides excellent possibilities for improving the conventional bone implants. In this sense, suitable biocomposites of tailored physical, biological, and mechanical properties with the predictable degradation behavior can be prepared combining biologically relevant $CaPO_4$ with bioresorbable polymers [29]. As a rule, the general behavior of such biocomposites is dependent on nature, structure, and relative contents of the constitutive components, although other parameters such as the preparation conditions also determine the properties of the final materials. Currently, $CaPO_4$ is incorporated as either a filler or a coating (or both), either into or onto a biodegradable polymer matrix, in the form of particles or fibers, are increasingly considered for using as bone tissue engineering scaffolds due to their improved physical, biologic, and mechanical properties [30–34]. Thus, through the successful combinations of ductile polymer matrices with hard and bioactive particulate bioceramic fillers, optimal materials can be designed and, ideally, this approach could lead to a superior construction to be used as either implants or posterior dental restorative material [29,35,36].

A lint-reinforced plaster was the first composite used in clinical orthopedics as an external immobilizer (bandage) in the treatment of bone fracture by Mathijsen in 1852 [37], followed by Dreesman in 1892 [38]. Great progress in the clinical application of various types of composite materials has been achieved since then. Based on both experience and the newly gained knowledge, various composite materials with tailored mechanical and biological performance can be manufactured and used to meet various clinical requirements [39]. However, this chapter presents only a brief history and advances in the field of $CaPO_4$/polymer biocomposites and hybrid biomaterials suitable for biomedical application.

7.2 GENERAL INFORMATION ON COMPOSITES AND BIOCOMPOSITES

A composite material (also called a composition material or shortened to composite) is a material made from two or more constituent materials with significantly different physical or chemical properties that, when combined, produce a material with characteristics different from the individual components. The individual components remain separate and distinct within the finished structure [40]. Thus, composites are always heterogeneous. Furthermore, the phases of any composite retain their identities and properties, and are bonded, which is why an interface is maintained between them. This provides improved specific or synergistic characteristics that are not obtainable by any of the original phases alone [41]. Following the point of view of some predecessors, we also consider that "for the purpose of this review, composites are defined as those having a distinct phase distributed through their bulk, as opposed to modular or coated components" [42, p. 1329]. For this reason, with a few important exceptions, the structures obtained by soaking of various materials in supersaturated solutions containing ions of calcium and orthophosphate (e.g., Refs. [43–46]), those obtained by coating of various materials by $CaPO_4$ (reviewed in Refs. [47–49]), as well as $CaPO_4$ coated by other compounds [50–54] have not been considered; however, composite coatings have been considered. Occasionally, porous $CaPO_4$ scaffolds filled by cells inside the pores [55–58], as well as $CaPO_4$ impregnated by biologically active substances [59,60], are also defined as composites and/or hybrids; nevertheless, such structures have not been considered either.

Any composite has two major categories of constituent materials: a matrix (or a continuous phase) and a dispersed phase (or phases). To create a composite, at least one portion of each type is required. General information on the major fabrication and processing techniques might be found elsewhere [42,61]. The continuous phase is responsible for filling the volume, as well as it surrounds and supports the dispersed material(s) by maintaining their relative positions. The dispersed phase(s) is(are) usually responsible for enhancing one or more properties of the matrix. Most of the composites target an enhancement of mechanical properties of the matrix, such as stiffness and strength; however, other properties, such as erosion stability, transport properties (electrical or thermal), radiopacity, density, or biocompatibility might also be of great interest. This synergism produces the properties that are unavailable from the individual constituent materials [61,62]. What is more is that by controlling the volume fractions and local and global arrangement of the dispersed phase, the properties and design of composites can be varied and tailored to suit the necessary conditions. For example, in the case of ceramics, the dispersed phase serves to impede crack growth. In this case, it acts as reinforcement. A number of methods, including deflecting crack tips, forming bridges across crack faces, absorbing energy during pullout, and causing a redistribution of stresses in regions adjacent to crack tips, can be used to accomplish this [63]. Other factors to be considered in composites are the volume fraction and orientation of the dispersed phase(s) and homogeneity of the overall composite. For example, higher volume fractions of reinforcement phases tend to improve the mechanical properties of the composites, while continuous and aligned fibers best prevent crack propagation with the added property of anisotropic behavior. From a structural point of view, composites are anisotropic in nature: their mechanical properties are different in different directions. Furthermore, the uniform distribution of the dispersed phase is also desirable as it imparts consistent properties to the composite [40,61,62].

In most cases, three interdependent factors must be considered in designing any composite: (1) selection of a suitable matrix and dispersed materials, (2) choice of appropriate fabrication and processing methods, and (3) both internal and external design of the device itself [42]. Furthermore, any composite must be formed to shape. To do this, the matrix material can be added before or after the dispersed material has been placed into a mold cavity or onto the mold surface. The matrix material experiences a melding event that, depending on the nature of the matrix material, can occur in various ways such as chemical polymerization, setting, curing, or solidification from a melted state. Due to general inhomogeneity, the physical properties of many composite materials are not isotropic but rather orthotropic (i.e., there are different properties or strengths in different orthogonal directions) [40,61,62].

In order to prepare any type of composite, at least two different materials must be mixed. Thus, the phase miscibility phenomenon appears to be of paramount

TABLE 7.2

General Respective Properties from the Bioorganic and Inorganic Domains, to Be Combined in Various Composites and Hybrid Materials

Inorganic	Bioorganic
Hardness, brittleness	Elasticity, plasticity
High density	Low density
Thermal stability	Permeability
Hydrophilicity	Hydrophobicity
High refractive index	Selective complexation
Mixed valence slate (red-ox)	Chemical reactivity
Strength	Bioactivity

Source: Vallet-Regi, M. and Arcos, D., *Curr. Nanosci.*, 2, 2006, 179.

importance [64,65]. Furthermore, the interfacial strength among the phases is a very important factor because lack of adhesion among the phases will result in an early failure at the interface and thus in a decrease in mechanical properties, especially tensile strength. From the chemical point of view, we can distinguish several types of the interactions among composite components: materials with strong (covalent, coordination, ionic) interactions; those with weak interactions (van der Waals forces, hydrogen bonds, hydrophilic–hydrophobic balance), or without chemical interactions among the components [66]. Wetting is also important in bonding or adherence of the materials. It depends on the hydrophilicity or polarity of the filler(s) and the available polar groups of the matrix.

Biocomposites are defined as nontoxic composites able to interact well with the human body in vivo and, ideally, contain one or more component(s) that stimulate(s) the healing process and uptake of the implant [67]. Thus, for biocomposites the biological compatibility appears to be more important than any other type of compatibility [39,68–70]. Interestingly, according to the databases, the first paper with the term *biocomposite* in the title was published in 1987 [71] and the one containing a combination of terms *biocomposite* and HA in the title was published in 1991 [72]. Thus, this subject appears to be quite new. The most common properties from the bioorganic and inorganic domains to be combined in biocomposites have been summarized in Table 7.2 [23]. For general advantages of the modern $CaPO_4$/polymer biocomposites over $CaPO_4$ bioceramics and bioresorbable polymers individually, interested readers are advised to get through the "Composite Materials Strategy" section of Ref. [29].

7.3 MAJOR CONSTITUENTS

7.3.1 Calcium Orthophosphates

The main driving force behind the use of $CaPO_4$ as bone substitute materials is their chemical similarity to the mineral component of mammalian bones and teeth [13–15]. As a result, in addition to being nontoxic, they are biocompatible, not recognized as foreign materials in the body and, most importantly, both exhibit bioactive behavior and integrate into living tissue by the same processes active in remodeling healthy bone. This leads to an intimate physicochemical bond between the implants and bone, termed osteointegration. More to the point, $CaPO_4$ is also known to support osteoblast adhesion and proliferation. Even so, the major limitations of using $CaPO_4$ as load-bearing biomaterials are their mechanical properties: they are brittle with poor fatigue resistance [16,17]. The poor mechanical behavior is even more evident for highly porous ceramics and scaffolds because porosity greater than 100 µm is considered the requirement for proper vascularization and bone cell colonization [73,74]. That is why in biomedical applications, $CaPO_4$ is used primarily as fillers and coatings [15].

The complete list of known $CaPO_4$, including their standard abbreviations and major properties, is given in Table 7.3, while the detailed information on $CaPO_4$ might be found in special books and monographs [15,75–78].

7.3.2 POLYMERS

Polymers are a class of materials consisting of large molecules, often containing many thousands of small units, or monomers, joined together chemically to form one giant chain, thus creating very ductile materials. In this respect, polymers are comparable with major functional components of the biological environment: lipids, proteins, and polysaccharides. They differ from each other in chemical composition, molecular weight, polydispersity, crystallinity, hydrophobicity, solubility, and thermal transitions. Besides, their properties can be fine-tuned over a wide range by varying the type of polymer, chain length, as well as by copolymerization or blending of two or more polymers [79,80]. Opposite to ceramics, polymers exhibit substantial viscoelastic properties and easily can be fabricated into complex structures, such as sponge-like sheets, gels, or complex structures with intricate porous networks and channels [81]. Being x-ray transparent and nonmagnetic, polymeric materials are fully compatible with the modern diagnostic methods such as computed tomography and magnetic resonance imaging. Unfortunately, most of them are unable to meet the strict demands of the in vivo physiological environment. The main requirements to polymers suitable for biomedical applications are that they must be biocompatible, not eliciting an excessive or chronic inflammatory response upon implantation, and for those that degrade, they breakdown into nontoxic products only. Unfortunately, polymers, for the most part, lack rigidity, ductility, and ultimate mechanical properties required in load-bearing applications. Thus, despite their good biocompatibility, many of the polymeric materials are mainly used for soft tissue replacements (such as skin, blood vessel, cartilage, ligament replacement, etc.). Moreover, the sterilization processes (autoclave, ethylene oxide, and ^{60}Co irradiation) may affect the polymer properties [82].

A variety of biocompatible polymers are suitable for biomedical applications [83,84]. For example, polyacrylates, poly(acrylonitrile-co-vinylchloride), and polylysine have been investigated for cell encapsulation and immunoisolation [85–87]. Polyorthoesters and poly(ε-caprolactone)(PCL) have been investigated as

TABLE 7.3

Existing Calcium Orthophosphates and Their Major Properties

Ca/P Molar Ratio	Compound	Formula	Solubility at 25°C, $-\log(K_s)$	Solubility at 25°C, g/L	pH Stability Range in Aqueous Solutions at 25°C
0.5	Monocalcium phosphate monohydrate (MCPM)	$Ca(H_2PO_4)_2 \cdot H_2O$	1.14	~18	0.0–2.0
0.5	Monocalcium phosphate anhydrous (MCPA or MCP)	$Ca(H_2PO_4)_2$	1.14	~17	c
1.0	Dicalcium phosphate dihydrate (DCPD), mineral brushite	$CaHPO_4 \cdot 2H_2O$	6.59	~0.088	2.0–6.0
1.0	Dicalcium phosphate anhydrous (DCPA or DCP), mineral monetite	$CaHPO_4$	6.90	~0.048	c
1.33	Octacalcium phosphate (OCP)	$Ca_8(HPO_4)_2(PO_4)_4 \cdot 5H_2O$	96.6	~0.0081	5.5–7.0
1.5	α-Tricalcium phosphate (α-TCP)	$\alpha\text{-}Ca_3(PO_4)_2$	25.5	~0.0025	a
1.5	β-Tricalcium phosphate (β-TCP)	$\beta\text{-}Ca_3(PO_4)_2$	28.9	~0.0005	a
1.2–2.2	Amorphous calcium phosphates (ACP)	$Ca_xH_y(PO_4)_z \cdot nH_2O$, $n = 3\text{–}4.5$; 15%–20% H_2O	b	b	~5–12 d
1.5–1.67	Calcium-deficient hydroxyapatite (CDHA or Ca-def HA)[e]	$Ca_{10-x}(HPO_4)_x(PO_4)_{6-x}(OH)_{2-x}$ (0<x<1)	~85	~0.0094	6.5–9.5
1.67	Hydroxyapatite (HA, HAp, or OHAp)	$Ca_{10}(PO_4)_6(OH)_2$	116.8	~0.0003	9.5–12
1.67	Fluorapatite (FA or FAp)	$Ca_{10}(PO_4)_6F_2$	120.0	~0.0002	7–12
1.67	Oxyapatite (OA, OAp, or OXA),[f] mineral voelckerite	$Ca_{10}(PO_4)_6O$	~69	~0.087	a
2.0	Tetracalcium phosphate (TTCP or TetCP), mineral hilgenstockite	$Ca_4(PO_4)_2O$	38–44	~0.0007	a

Source: Dorozhkin, S.V., *Calcium Orthophosphates: Applications in Nature, Biology, and Medicine,* Pan Stanford, Singapore, 2012.

[a] These compounds cannot be precipitated from aqueous solutions.

[b] Cannot be measured precisely. However, the following values were found: 25.7 ± 0.1 (pH = 7.40), 29.9 ± 0.1 (pH = 6.00), 32.7 ± 0.1 (pH = 5.28). The comparative extent of dissolution in acidic buffer is ACP ≫ α-TCP ≫ β-TCP > CDHA ≫ HA > FA.

[c] Stable at temperatures above 100°C.

[d] Always metastable.

[e] Occasionally, it is called "precipitated HA (PHA)."

[f] Existence of OA remains questionable.

drug-delivery devices, the latter for long-term sustained release because of their slow degradation rates [88]. PCL is a hydrolytic polyester having appropriate resorption period and releases nontoxic byproducts upon degradation [89,90]. Polyurethanes are in use in the engineering of both hard and soft tissues, as well as in nanomedicine [91]. Polymers considered for orthopedic purposes include polyanhydrides, which have also been investigated as delivery devices (due to their rapid and well-defined surface erosion) for bone augmentation or replacement since they can be photopolymerized in situ [88,92,93]. To overcome their poor mechanical properties, they have been copolymerized with imides or formulated to be crosslinkable in situ [93]. Other polymers, such as polyphosphazenes, can have their properties (e.g., degradation rate) easily modified by varying the nature of their side groups and have been shown to support osteoblast adhesion, which makes them candidates for skeletal tissue regeneration [93]. PPF has emerged as a good bone replacement material, exhibiting good mechanical properties (comparable to trabecular bone), possessing the capability to crosslink in vivo through the C=C bond, and being hydrolytically degradable. It has also been examined as a material for drug-delivery devices [88,92–95]. Polycarbonates have been suggested as suitable materials to make scaffolds for bone replacement and have been modified with tyrosine-derived amino acids to render them biodegradable [88,96]. Polydioxanone has also been tested for biomedical applications [97]. PMMA is widely used in orthopedics, as a bone cement for implant fixation, as well as to repair certain fractures and bone defects, for example, osteoporotic vertebral bodies [98,99]. However, PMMA sets by a polymerization of toxic monomers, which also evolves significant amounts of heat that damages tissues. Moreover, it is neither degradable nor bioactive, does not bond chemically to bones, and might generate particulate debris leading to an inflammatory foreign body response [92,100]. A number of other nondegradable polymers applied in orthopedic surgery include PE in its different modifications such as low-density PE, HDPE, and UHMWPE (used as the articular surface of total hip replacement implants [101,102]), polyethylene terephthalate, PP, and PTFE, which are applied to repair knee ligaments [103]. Polyactive™, a block copolymer of PEG and PBT, was also considered for biomedical application [104–106]. Cellulose [107,108] and its esters [109,110] are also popular. Finally yet importantly, polyethylene oxide, PHB, and blends thereof have also been tested for biomedical applications [29].

Nonetheless, the most popular synthetic polymers used in medicine are the linear aliphatic poly(α-hydroxyesters) such as PLA, PGA, and their copolymers—PLGA (Table 7.4). These materials have been extensively studied; they appear to be the only synthetic and biodegradable polymers with an extensive FDA approval history [29,93,111]. They are biocompatible, mostly noninflammatory, as well as degrade in vivo through hydrolysis and possible enzymatic action into products that are removed from the body by regular metabolic pathways [88,93,112–116]. Besides, they might be used for drug-delivery purposes [117]. Poly(α-hydroxyesters) have been investigated as scaffolds for the replacement and regeneration of a variety of tissues, cell carriers, controlled delivery devices for drugs or proteins (e.g., growth

TABLE 7.4

Major Properties of Several FDA-Approved Biodegradable Polymers

Polymer	Thermal Properties,[a] °C	Tensile Modulus, GPa	Degradation Time, Months
Polyglycolic acid (PGA)	$t_g = 35$–40 $t_m = 225$–230	7.0	6–12 (strength loss within 3 weeks)
L-polylactic acid (LPLA)	$t_g = 60$–65 $t_m = 173$–178	2.7	>24
D,L-polylactic acid (DLPLA)	$t_g = 55$–60 Amorphous	1.9	12–16
85/15 D,L-polylactic-co-glycolic acid (85/15 DLPLGA)	$t_g = 50$–55 Amorphous	2.0	5–6
75/25 D,L-polylactic-co-glycolic acid (75/25 DLPLGA)	$t_g = 50$–55 Amorphous	2.0	4–5
65/35 D,L-polylactic-co-glycolic acid (65/35 DLPLGA)	$t_g = 45$–50 Amorphous	2.0	3–4
50/50 D,L-polylactic-co-glycolic acid (50/50 DLPLGA)	$t_g = 45$–50 Amorphous	2.0	1–2
poly(ε-caprolactone) (PCL)	$t_g = (-60) - (-65)$ $t_m = 58$–63	0.4	>24

Source: Thomas, V. et al., *Curr. Nanosci.*, 2, 2006, 155.

[a] t_g, glass transition temperature; t_m, melting point.

factors), membranes or films, screws, pins, and plates for orthopedic applications [88,93,118,119]. Additionally, the degradation rate of PLGA can be adjusted by varying the amounts of the two component monomers (Table 7.4), which in orthopedic applications can be exploited to create materials that degrade in concert with bone ingrowth [115,120]. Furthermore, PLGA is known to support osteoblast migration and proliferation [36,93,112,121], which is a necessity for bone tissue regeneration. Unfortunately, such polymers on their own, though they reduce the effect of stress-shielding, are too weak to be used in load-bearing situations and are only recommended in certain clinical indications, such as ankle and elbow fractures [161]. In addition, they exhibit bulk degradation, leading to both loss in mechanical properties and lowering of the local solution pH that accelerates further degradation in an autocatalytic manner. As the body is unable to cope with the vast amounts of implant degradation products, this might lead to an inflammatory foreign body response. Finally, poly(α-hydroxyesters) do not possess bioactive and osteoconductive properties [93,122]. Further details on polymers suitable for biomedical applications are available in literature [82,119,123–129], which the interested readers can check. Good reviews on the synthesis of different biodegradable polymers [130], as well as on the experimental trends in polymer composites [131], are available elsewhere.

7.4 BIOCOMPOSITES AND HYBRID BIOMATERIALS BASED ON CALCIUM ORTHOPHOSPHATES

7.4.1 BIOCOMPOSITES WITH POLYMERS

Typically, the polymeric components of biocomposites and hybrid biomaterials comprise polymers that have shown good biocompatibility and are routinely used in surgical applications. In general, since polymers have low modulus (2–7 GPa, as the maximum) as compared to that of bone (3–30 GPa), $CaPO_4$ bioceramics need to be loaded at a high weight percent ratio. Besides, general knowledge on composite mechanics suggests that any high aspect ratio particles, such as whiskers or fibers, significantly improve the modulus at a lower loading. Thus, some attempts have already been performed to prepare biocomposites containing whisker-like [132–136] or needle-like [137–139] $CaPO_4$, as well as $CaPO_4$ fibers [140].

The history of implantable $CaPO_4$/polymer formulations started in 1981 (however, a more general topic, "ceramic-plastic material as a bone substitute," is at least 18 years older [141]) from the pioneering study by Prof. William Bonfield and colleagues at Queen Mary College, University of London, performed on HA/PE blends [142,143]. That initial study introduced a bone-analogue concept, when proposed biocomposites comprised a polymer ductile matrix of PE and a ceramic stiff phase of HA, and was substantially extended and developed in further investigations by that research group [69,144–154]. More recent studies included investigations on the influence of surface topography of HA/PE composites on cell proliferation and attachment [155–158]. The material is composed of a particular combination of HA particles at a volume loading of ~40% uniformly dispensed in an HDPE matrix. The idea was to mimic bones by using a polymeric matrix that can develop a considerable anisotropic character through adequate orientation techniques reinforced with a bone-like bioceramics that assures both mechanical reinforcement and bioactive character of the composite. Following FDA approval in 1994, this material became commercially available in 1995 under the trade name HAPEX™ (Smith and Nephew, Richards, Tennessee, USA), and to date it has been implanted in more than 300,000 patients with successful results. It remains the only clinically successful bioactive composite, which was a major step in the implant field [17,159]. The major production stages of HAPEX™ include blending, compounding, and centrifugal milling. A bulk material or device is then created from this powder by compression and injection molding [39]. Besides, HA/HDPE biocomposites might be prepared by a hot-rolling technique that facilitated uniform dispersion and blending of the reinforcements in the matrix [160]. In addition, PP might be used instead of PE [161–163].

A mechanical interlock between both phases of HAPEX™ is formed by the shrinkage of HDPE onto the HA particles during cooling [69,70,164]. Both HA particle size and their distribution in the HDPE matrix were recognized as important parameters affecting the mechanical behavior of HAPEX™. Smaller HA particles were found to lead to stiffer composites due to general increasing of interfaces between the polymer and the ceramics; furthermore, rigidity of HAPEX™ was found to be proportional to HA volume fraction [149]. Furthermore, coupling agents, for example, 3-trimethoxysiyl propylmethacrylate for HA and acrylic acid for HDPE, might be used to improve bonding (by both chemical adhesion and mechanical coupling) between HA and HDPE [165,166]. Obviously, other $CaPO_4$ might be used instead of HA in biocomposites with PE [167].

Various studies revealed that HAPEX™ attached directly to bones by chemical bonding (a bioactive fixation), rather than forming fibrous encapsulation (a morphological fixation). Initial clinical applications of HAPEX™ came in orbital reconstruction [168], but since 1995, the main uses of this composite have been in the shafts of middle ear implants for the treatment of conductive hearing loss [169,170]. In both applications, HAPEX™ offers the advantage of in situ shaping, so a surgeon can make final alterations to optimize the fit of the prosthesis to the bone of a patient, and subsequent activity requires only limited mechanical loading with virtually no risk of failure from insufficient tensile strength [69,70]. As compared to cortical bones, HA/PE composites have a superior fracture toughness for HA concentrations below ~40% and similar fracture toughness in the 45%–50% range. Their Young's modulus is in the range of 1–8 GPa, which is quite close to that of bone. Examination of the fracture surfaces has revealed that only mechanical bond occurs between HA and PE. Unfortunately, the HA/PE composites are not biodegradable, the available surface area of HA is low, and the presence of bioinert PE decreases the ability to bond to bones. Furthermore, HAPEX™ has been designed with a maximized density to increase its strength, but the resulting lack of porosity limits the ingrowth of osteoblasts when the implant is placed into the body [16]. Further details on HAPEX™ are available elsewhere [69,70]. Except HAPEX™, other types of HA/PE biocomposites are also known [171–177].

Both linear and branched PE was used as a matrix, and the biocomposites with the former were found to give a higher modulus [172]. The reinforcing mechanisms in $CaPO_4$/polymer formulations have yet to be convincingly disclosed. Generally, if a poor filler choice is made, the polymeric matrix might be affected by the filler through reduction in molecular weight during composite processing, formation of an immobilized shell of polymer around the particles (transcrystallization, surface-induced crystallization, or epitaxial growth) and changes in conformation of the polymer due to particle surfaces and interparticle spacing [69,70]. On the other hand, the reinforcing effect of $CaPO_4$ particles might depend on the molding technique employed: a higher orientation of the polymeric matrix was found to result in a higher mechanical performance of the composite [177,178].

Many other blends of $CaPO_4$ with various polymers are possible, including rather unusual formulations with dendrimers [179]. Even light-curable $CaPO_4$/polymer formulations are known [180]. The list of appropriate $CaPO_4$ is shown in Table 7.3 (except MCPM and MCPA—both are too acidic and, therefore, are not biocompatible [15]; nevertheless, to overcome this drawback, they might be mixed with basic compounds, such as HA, TTCP, $CaCO_3$, CaO, etc.) and many biomedically suitable polymers have been listed earlier. The combination of $CaPO_4$ and polymers into biocomposites has a twofold purpose. The desirable mechanical properties of polymers compensate for a poor mechanical behavior of $CaPO_4$ bioceramics, while in turn the desirable bioactive properties of $CaPO_4$ improve those of polymers, expanding the possible uses of each material within the body [113–115,181–185]. Polymers have been added to $CaPO_4$ in order to improve their mechanical strength [113,181], while $CaPO_4$ fillers have been blended with polymers to improve their compressive strength and modulus, in addition to increasing their osteoconductive properties [115,122,186–189]. In the 1990s, it was established that with an increase in the $CaPO_4$ content, both Young's modulus and bioactivity of the biocomposites generally increased, while ductility decreased [16]. However, later investigations revealed that the mechanical properties of $CaPO_4$/polymer biocomposites were not so straightforward: the strength was found to decrease with increasing $CaPO_4$ content in such biocomposites [190]. Nevertheless, biocompatibility of such biocomposites is enhanced because $CaPO_4$ fillers induce an increased initial flash spread of serum proteins compared to the more hydrophobic polymer surfaces [191]. What is more is that experimental results of these biocomposites indicated favorable cell–material interactions with increased cell activities as compared to each polymer alone [183]. Furthermore, such formulations can provide a sustained release of calcium and orthophosphate ions into the milieus, which is important for mineralized tissue regeneration [182]. Indeed, a combination of two different materials draws on the advantages of each one to create a superior biocomposite with respect to the materials on their own.

It is logical to assume that a proper biocomposite of $CaPO_4$ (for instance, CDHA) with a bioorganic polymer (for instance, collagen) would yield physical, chemical, and mechanical properties similar to those of human bones. Different ways have already been realized to bring these two components together into biocomposites, like mechanical blending, compounding, ball milling, dispersion of ceramic fillers into a polymer–solvent solution, melt extrusion of a ceramic/polymer powder mixture, co-precipitation, and electrochemical co-deposition [22,39,192–194]. Three methods for preparing a homogeneous blend of HA with PLLA were compared [192]. A dry process consisting in mixing ceramic powder and polymer pellets before a compression-molding step was used. The second technique was based on the dispersion of ceramic fillers into a polymer–solvent solution. The third method was the melt extrusion of a ceramic/polymer powder mixture. Mixing dry powders led to a ceramic particle network around the polymer pellets, whereas the solvent and melt methods also produced a homogeneous dispersion of HA in the matrix. The main drawback of the solvent casting method is the risk of potentially toxic organic solvent residues. The melt extrusion method was shown to be a good way to prepare homogeneous ceramic/polymer blends [192].

Besides, there is an in situ formation involving either synthesizing the reinforcement inside a preformed matrix material or synthesizing the matrix material around the reinforcement [39,195,196]. This is one of the most attractive routes since it avoids extensive particle agglomeration. For example, several papers have reported the in situ formation technique to produce various composites of apatites with carbon nanotubes [197–200]. Other examples comprise using amino-acid-capped gold nanosized particles as scaffolds to grow CDHA [201] and preparation of nanosized HA/polyamide biocomposites [202,203]. In certain cases, a mechano-chemical route [204], emulsions [205–208], freeze-drying [209], and freeze-thawing techniques [210] or gel-templated mineralization [211] might be applied to produce $CaPO_4$/polymer biocomposites. Various fabrication procedures are well described elsewhere [22,39,192], where the interested readers are referred to.

The interfacial bonding between $CaPO_4$ and a polymer is an important issue of any biocomposite. Four types of mutual arrangements of nanodimensional particles to polymer chains have been classified by Kickelbick (Figure 7.1): (1) inorganic particles embedded in inorganic polymer, (2) incorporation of particles by bonding to the polymer backbone, (3) an interpenetrating network with chemical bonds, and (4) an inorganic–organic hybrid polymer [212].

If adhesion among the phases is poor, the mechanical properties of a biocomposite suffer. To solve the problem, various approaches have been already introduced. For example, a diisocyanate coupling agent was used to bind PEG/PBT (Polyactive™) block copolymers to HA filler particles. Using surface-modified HA particles as a filler in a PEG/PBT matrix significantly improved the elastic modulus and strength of the polymer as compared to the polymers filled with ungrafted HA [187,213]. Another group used processing conditions to achieve a better adhesion of the filler to the matrix by pressing blends of varying PLLA and HA content at different temperatures and pressures [113,114,214,215]. The researchers found that maximum compressive strength was achieved at ~15 wt.% of PLLA. By using blends with 20 wt.% of PLLA, the authors also established that increasing the pressing temperature and pressure improved the mechanical properties. The former was explained by the decrease in the viscosity of the PLLA associated with a temperature increase, hence leading to improved wettability of HA particles. The latter was explained by increased compaction and penetration of pores at higher pressure, in conjunction with a greater fluidity of the polymer at higher temperatures. The combination of high pressures and temperatures was found to decrease porosity and guarantee a close apposition of a polymer to the particles, thereby improving the compressive strength [181] and fracture energy [285] of the biocomposites. The PLLA/HA biocomposites scaffolds were found to improve cell survival over plain PLLA scaffolds [216].

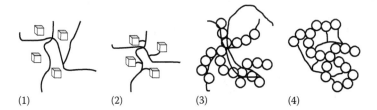

(1)   (2)   (3)   (4)

FIGURE 7.1 Four types of mutual arrangements of nanosized particles to a polymer chain: (1) inorganic particles embedded in an inorganic polymer, (2) incorporation of particles by bonding to the polymer backbone, (3) interpenetrating network with chemical bonds, and (4) inorganic–organic hybrid polymer. (Reprinted from Kickelbick, G., *Prog. Polym. Sci.*, 28, 83, 2003. With permission.)

It is also possible to introduce porosity into $CaPO_4$/polymer biocomposites, which is advantageous for most applications as bone substitution material. The porosity facilitates migration of osteoblasts from surrounding bones to the implant site [115,217,218]. Various material processing strategies to prepare composite scaffolds with interconnected porosity comprise thermally induced phase separation, solvent casting and particle leaching, solid freeform fabrication techniques, microsphere sintering and coating [123,219–222]. A supercritical gas foaming technique might be used as well [192,223,224].

7.4.1.1 Apatite-Based Formulations

A biological apatite is known to be the major inorganic phase of mammalian calcified tissues [13,14]. Consequently, CDHA, HA, carbonateapatite (both with and without dopants), and, occasionally, FA have been applied to prepare biocomposites with other compounds, usually with the aim to improve bioactivity. For example, PS composed with HA can be used as a starting material for long-term implants [225–227]. Retrieved in vivo, HA/PS biocomposite-coated samples from rabbit distal femurs demonstrated direct bone apposition to the coatings, as compared to the fibrous encapsulation that occurred when uncoated samples were used [225]. The resorption time of such biocomposites is a very important factor, which depends on polymer's microstructure and the presence of modifying phases [226].

Various apatite-containing biocomposites with PVA [210,228–233] and several other polymeric components [234–245] have been already developed. PVA/CDHA biocomposite blocks were prepared by the precipitation of CDHA in aqueous solutions of PVA [210]. An artificial cornea consisted of a porous nanosized HA/PVA hydrogel skirt and a transparent center of PVA hydrogel has been prepared as well. The results displayed good biocompatibility and interlocking between artificial cornea and host tissues [229,230]. Greish and Brown developed HA/Ca poly(vinyl phosphonate) biocomposites [237–239].

PEEK [132,134,246–253] and HIPS [252] were also applied to create biocomposites with HA having a potential for clinical use in load-bearing applications. The study on reinforcing PEEK with thermally sprayed HA particles revealed that the mechanical properties increased monotonically with the reinforcement concentration, with a maximum value in the study of ~40% volume fraction of HA particles [247–249]. The reported ranges of stiffness within 2.8–16.0 GPa and strength within 45.5–69 MPa exceeded the lower values for human bone (7–30 GPa and 50–150 MPa, respectively) [248]. Modeling of the mechanical behavior of HA/PEEK biocomposites is available elsewhere [250].

Biodegradable poly(α-hydroxyesters) are well established in clinical medicine. Currently, they provide with a good choice when a suitable polymeric filler material is sought. For example, HA/PLGA composites were developed, which appeared to possess a cellular compatibility suitable for bone tissue regeneration [254–263]. Zhang and Ma seeded highly porous PLLA foams with HA particles in order to improve the osteoconductivity of polymer scaffolds for bone tissue engineering [186]. They pointed out that hydration of the foams prior to incubation in simulated body fluid increased the amount of carbonated CDHA material due to an increase in COOH and OH groups on the polymer surface, which apparently acted as nucleation sites for apatite. The mechanical properties of PLA/CaPO$_4$ biocomposites fabricated using different technique, as well as the results of in vitro and in vivo experiments with them, are available in literature [262].

On their own, PGA and PLA are known to degrade to acidic products (glycolic and lactic acids, respectively) that both catalyze polymer degradation and cause inflammatory reactions of the surrounding tissues [264]. Thus, in biocomposites of poly(α-hydroxyesters) with CaPO$_4$, the presence of slightly basic compounds (HA, TTCP) to some extent neutralizes the acid molecules, provides with a weak pH-buffering effect at the polymer surface, and, therefore, more or less compensates these drawbacks [122,262,265–267]. However, additives of even more basic chemicals (e.g., CaO, CaCO$_3$) might be necessary [123,266,268,269]. Extensive cell culture experiments on pH-stabilized composites of PGA and carbonateapatite were reported, which were afterward supported by extensive in vitro pHstudies [270]. A consequent development of this approach has led to the designing of functionally graded composite skull implants consisting of polylactides, carbonateapatite, and CaCO$_3$ [271,272]. Besides the pH-buffering effect, inclusion of CaPO$_4$ was found to modify both surface and bulk properties of the biodegradable poly(α-hydroxyesters) by increasing the hydrophilicity and water absorption of the polymer matrix, thus altering the scaffold degradation kinetics. For example, polymer biocomposites filled with HA particles were found to hydrolyze homogeneously due to water penetrating into interfacial regions [273].

Biocomposites of poly(α-hydroxyesters) with CaPO$_4$ are prepared mainly by incorporating the inorganic phase into a polymeric solution, followed by drying under vacuum. The resulting solid biocomposites might be shaped using different processing techniques. One can also prepare these biocomposites by mixing HA particles with L-lactide prior the polymerization [265] or by a combination of slip-casting technique and hot pressing [274]; however, other production techniques are known [262]. Addition of a surfactant (surface-active agent) might be useful to keep the suspension homogeneity [275]. Furthermore, HA/PLA [206,207] and HA/PLGA [208] microspheres might be prepared by a microemulsion technique. More complex carbonated-FA/PLA [276] and PLGA/carbon nanotubes/HA [277] porous biocomposite scaffolds are also known. An interesting list of references, assigned to the different ways of preparing HA/poly(α-hydroxyesters) biodegradable composites, might be found in publications by Durucan and Brown [30,278,279]. The authors prepared CDHA/PLA and CDHA/PLGA biocomposites by the solvent casting technique with a subsequent hydrolysis of α-TCP to CDHA in aqueous solutions. The presence of both polymers was found to inhibit α-TCP hydrolysis, if compared with that of single-phase α-TCP; what is more, the inhibiting effect of PLA exceeded that of PLGA [30,278,279]. The physical interactions between CaPO$_4$ and poly(α-hydroxyesters) might be easily seen in Figure 7.2 [30]. Another set of good pictures might be found in Ref. [54]. Nevertheless, it should not be forgotten that typically non-melt-based routes lead to the development of composites with lower mechanical performance and many times require the use of toxic solvents and intensive hand labor [125].

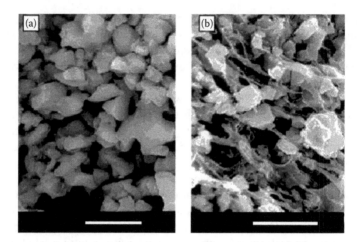

FIGURE 7.2   SEM micrographs of (a) α-TCP compact and (b) α-TCP/PLGA biocomposite (bars = 5 μm). (Reprinted from Durucan C. and Brown P.W., *Adv. Eng. Mater.*, 3, 227, 2001. With permission.)

The mechanical properties of poly(α-hydroxyesters) could be substantially improved by the addition of $CaPO_4$ [280,281]. CDHA/PLLA biocomposites of very high mechanical properties were developed [122] and mini-screws and mini-plates made of these composites were manufactured and tested. These fixation tools revealed easy handling and shaping according to the implant site geometry, total resorbability, good ability to bond directly to the bone tissue without interposed fibrous tissue, osteoconductivity, biocompatibility, and high stiffness retainable for the period necessary to achieve bone union [273]. The initial bending strength of ~280 MPa exceeded that of cortical bone (120–210 MPa), while the modulus was as high as 12 GPa [122]. The strength could be maintained above 200 MPa up to 25 weeks in phosphate-buffered saline solution. Such biocomposites were obtained from the precipitation of a PLLA/dichloromethane solution, where small granules of uniformly distributed CDHA microparticles (average size of 3 μm) could be prepared [121]. Porous scaffolds of PDLLA and HA have been manufactured as well [224,282,283]. Upon implantation into rabbit femora, a newly formed bone was observed and biodegradation was significantly enhanced if compared to single-phase HA bioceramics. This might be due to the local release of lactic acid, which in turn dissolves HA. In other studies, PLA and PGA fibers were combined with porous HA scaffolds. Such reinforcement did not hinder bone ingrowth into the implants, which supported further development of such biocomposites as bone graft substitutes [29,30,262,263].

Blends (named SEVA-C) of EVOH with starch filled with 10–30 wt.% HA have been fabricated to yield biocomposites with modulus up to ~7 GPa with a 30% HA loading [284–288]. The incorporation of bioactive fillers such as HA into SEVA-C aimed to assure the bioactive behavior of the composite and to provide the necessary stiffness within the typical range of human cortical bone properties. These biocomposites exhibited a strong in vitro bioactivity that was supported by the polymer's water-uptake capability [289]. However, the reinforcement of SEVA-C by HA particles was found to affect the rheological behavior of the blend. A degradation model of these biocomposites has been developed [290].

Higher homologues poly(3-hydroxybutyrate), 3-PHB, and poly(3-hydroxyvalerate) show almost no biodegradation. Nevertheless, biocomposites of these polymers with $CaPO_4$ showed good biocompatibility both in vitro and in vivo [291–296]. Both bioactivity and mechanical properties of these biocomposites can be tailored by varying the volume percentage of $CaPO_4$. Similarly, biocomposites of PHBHV with both HA and amorphous carbonated apatite [almost amorphous calcium phosphate (ACP)] appeared to have a promising potential for repair and replacement of damaged bones [297–300].

Along this line, PCL is used as a slowly biodegradable but well-biocompatible polymer. PCL/HA and PCL/CDHA biocomposites have been already discussed as suitable materials for substitution, regeneration, and repair of bone tissues [219,301–313]. For example, biocomposites were obtained by the infiltration of ε-caprolactone monomer into porous apatite blocks and in situ polymerization [304]. The composites were found to be biodegradable and might be applied as cancellous or trabecular bone replacement material or for cartilage regeneration. Both mechanical performance and biocompatibility in osteoblast cell culture of PCL were shown to be strongly increased when HA was added [314]. Several preparation techniques of PCL/HA biocomposites are known. For example, to make biocomposite fibers of PCL with nanodimensional HA, the desired amount of nanodimensional HA powder was dispersed in a solvent using magnetic stirrer followed by ultrasonication for 30 min. Then, PCL was dissolved in this suspension, followed by the solvent evaporation [315]. The opposite preparation order is also possible: PCL was initially dissolved in chloroform at room temperature (7%–10% weight/volume); then HA (~10 μm particle size) was suspended in the solution, sonicated for 60 s, followed by solvent evaporation [115] or salt-leaching [316]. The mechanical properties obtained by this technique were about one-third that of trabecular bone. In a comparative study, PCL and biological apatite were mixed in the ratio 19:1 in an extruder [317]. At the end of the preparation, the mixture was cooled in an atmosphere of nitrogen. The authors observed that the presence of biological apatite improved the modulus while concurrently increasing the hydrophilicity of the polymeric substrate. Besides, an increase in apatite concentration was found to increase both the modulus and yield stress of the composite, which indicated to good interfacial interactions between the biological apatite and PCL. It was also observed that the presence of biological apatite stimulated osteoblasts attachment to the biomaterial and cell proliferation [317]. In another study, a PCL/HA biocomposite was prepared by blending in melt form at 120°C until the torque reached equilibrium in the rheometer attached to the blender [318]. Then, the sample was compression molded and cut into specimens of appropriate size for testing. It was observed that the composite containing 20 wt.% HA had the highest strength [318]. However, a direct grafting of PCL on the surface of HA particles seems to be the most interesting preparation technique [301]. In another study, HA porous scaffolds were coated by a PCL/HA composite coating [31]. In this system, PCL, as a coating component, was able to improve the brittleness and low strength of the HA scaffolds, while the particles in the coating were to improve the osteo-conductivity and bioactivity of the coating layer. More complex formulations, such as PDLLA/PCL/HA [319], PLLA/PCL/HA [320], and supramolecular PCL/func-tionalized HA [321] biocomposites, have been prepared as well. Further details on both the PCL/HA biocomposites and the processing methodologies thereof might be found elsewhere [219].

The spread of attached human osteoblasts onto PLA and PCL films reinforced with CDHA and sintered HA was shown to be higher than that for the polymers alone [130]. Moreover, biochemical assays relating cell activity to DNA content allowed concluding that cell activity was more intense for the composite films [130]. Kim et al. coated porous HA blocks with PCL from dichloromethane solu-tion and performed drug release studies. The antibiotic tetracycline hydrochloride was added into this layer, yielding a bioactive implant with drug release for longer than a week [31].

Yoon et al. investigated the highest mechanical and chemical stability of FA by preparing FA/collagen biocomposites and studied their effect on osteoblast-like cell culture [322]. The researchers found an increased cellular activity in FA composites compared to HA composites. This finding was confirmed in another study, by means of variations in the fluoride content for FA-HA/PCL composites [323]. An interest-ing phenomenon of fractal growth of FA/gelatin composite crystals (Figure 7.3) was achieved by diffusion of calcium- and orthophosphate + fluoride-solutions

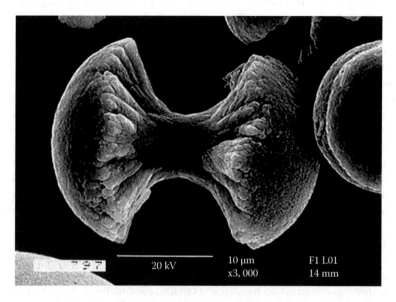

FIGURE 7.3 A biomimetically grown aggregate of FA that was crystallized in a gelatin matrix. Its shape can be explained and simulated by a fractal growth mechanism (scale bar: 10 μm). (Reprinted from Busch S. et al., *Eur. J. Inorg. Chem.*, 1643, 1999. With permission.)

from the opposite sides into a tube filled with a gelatin gel [324–333]. The reasons for this phenomenon are not quite clear yet; besides, up to now nothing has yet been reported on a possible biomedical application of such very unusual structural composites.

7.4.1.2 TCP-Based Formulations

Both α-TCP and β-TCP have higher solubility than HA (Table 7.3). Besides, they are faster resorbed in vivo (however, there are some reports about the lack of TCP biodegradation after implantation in calvarial defects [334]). Therefore, α-TCP and β-TCP were widely used instead of apatites to prepare completely biodegradable biocomposites [335–354]. For example, a biodegradable and osteoconductive biocomposite made of β-TCP particles and gelatin was proposed [342]. This material was tested in vivo with good results. It was found to be biocompatible, osteoconductive, and biodegradable with no need for a second surgical operation to remove the device after healing occurred. Both herbal extracts [343] and K₂HPO₄ [344] might be added to this formulation. Another research group prepared biocomposites of crosslinked gelatin with β-TCP and found both good biocompatibility and bone formation upon subcutaneous implantation in rats [345]. Yang et al. [349] extended this to porous (porosity ~75%) β-TCP/gelatin biocomposites, which also contained BMP-4. Furthermore, cell-compatible and possessive some osteoinductive properties porous β-TCP/alginate-gelatin hybrid scaffolds were prepared and successfully tested in vitro [346]. More to the point, biocomposites of β-TCP with PLLA [339–341] were prepared. Although β-TCP was able to counter the acidic degradation of the polyester to some extent, it did not prevent a pH drop down to ~6. α-TCP/gelatin formulations are known as well [352].

Based on the self-reinforcement concept, biocomposites of TCP with polylactides were prepared and studied using conventional mechanical testing [355]. Resorbable scaffolds were fabricated from such biocomposites [356]. Chitosan was also used as the matrix for the incorporation of β-TCP by a solid/liquid phase separation of the polymer solution and subsequent sublimation of the solvent. Due to complexation of the functional groups of chitosan with calcium ions of β-TCP, these biocomposites had high compressive modulus and strength [357]. PCL/β-TCP biocomposites were developed in other studies [358–361] and their in vitro degradation behavior was systematically monitored by immersion in simulated body fluid at 37°C [360]. To extend this topic further, PCL/β-TCP biocomposites might be loaded by drugs [361].

An in vitro study with primary rat calvarial osteoblasts showed an increased cellular activity in the BMP-loaded samples [349]. Other researchers investigated BMP-2-loaded porous β-TCP/gelatin biocomposites (porosity ~95%, average pore size 180–200 μm) [362] and confirmed the precious study. Biocomposites of β-TCP and glutaraldehyde crosslinked gelatin were manufactured and tested in vitro to measure the material cytotoxicity [345]. The experimental results revealed that the amount of glutaraldehyde crosslinking agent should be less than 8% to decrease the toxicity on the osteoblasts and to avoid inhibition of cellular growth caused by the release of residual or uncrosslinked glutaraldehyde. A long-term implantation study of PDLLA/α-TCP composites in a loaded sheep implant model showed good results after 12 months but a strong osteolytic reaction after 24 months. This was ascribed to the almost complete dissolution of α-TCP to this time and an adverse reaction of the remaining PDLLA [363].

More complex CaPO$_4$/polymer formulations are known as well. For example, a biocomposite consists of three interpenetrating networks: TCP, CDHA, and PLGA [364]. First, a porous TCP network was produced by coating a polyurethane foam by hydrolysable α-TCP slurry. Then, a CDHA network was derived from self-setting CaPO$_4$ formulations filled in the porous TCP network. Finally, the remaining open pore network in the CDHA/α-TCP structures was infiltrated with PLGA. This biocomposite consists of three phases with different degradation behavior. It was postulated that bone would grow on the fastest degrading network of PLGA, while the remaining CaPO$_4$ phases would remain intact thus maintaining their geometry and load-bearing capability [364].

7.4.1.3 Formulations Based on Other Calcium Orthophosphates

The number of research publications devoted to formulations based on other CaPO$_4$ is substantially lesser than the number of formulations devoted to apatites and TCP. Biphasic calcium phosphate (BCP), which is a solid composite of HA and β-TCP, appears to be most popular among the remaining CaPO$_4$. For example, collagen-coated BCP ceramics was studied and the biocompatibility toward osteoblasts was found to increase upon coating with collagen [365]. Another research group created porous PDLLA/BCP scaffolds and coated them with a hydrophilic PEG/vancomycin composite for both drug-delivery purposes and surface modification [366]. More to the point, both PLGA/BCP [367,368] and PLLA/BCP [369] biocomposites were fabricated and their cytotoxicity and fibroblast properties were found to be acceptable for natural bone tissue reparation, filling, and augmentation [370,371]. Besides, PCL/BCP [372] and gelatin/BCP [373,374] biocomposites are known as well.

A choice of DCPD-based biocomposites of DCPD, albumin, and duplex DNA was prepared by water/oil/water interfacial reaction method [205]. Core–shell type DCPD/chitosan biocomposite fibers were prepared by the wet spinning method in another study [375]. The energy-dispersive x-ray spectroscopy analysis indicated that Ca and P atoms were mainly distributed on the outer layer of the composite fibers; however, a little amount of P atoms remained inside the fibers. This indicated that the composite fibers formed a unique core–shell structure with the shell of CaPO$_4$ and the core of chitosan [375]. A similar formulation was prepared for further applications in self-setting biocomposites [376]. DCPA/ BSA (bovine serum albumin) biocomposites were synthesized through the co-precipitation of BSA on the nanodimensional particles of DCPA performed in ethanol [377]. Nanodimensional DCPA was synthesized and incorporated into dental resins to form dental biocomposites [378–380]. Although this is not to the point, it is interesting to mention that some DCPD/polymer composites could be used as proton conductors in battery devices [381,382]. Nothing has been reported on their biocompatibility, but, perhaps, the improved formulations will be used sometime to fabricate biocompatible batteries for implantable electronic devices.

Various ACP-based biocomposites and hybrid formulations for dental applications have been developed [383,384]. Besides, several ACP-based formulations were investigated as potential biocomposites for bone grafting [300,385–387] and drug delivery [388]. ACP/PPF biocomposites were prepared by in situ precipitation [386], while PHB/carbonated ACP and PHBHV/carbonated ACP biocomposites appeared to be well suited as slowly biodegradable bone substitution material [300]. Another example comprises hybrid nanodimensional capsules of ~50–70 nm in diameter, which were fabricated by ACP mineralization of shell crosslinked polymer micelles and nanosized cages [387]. These nanosized capsules consisted of a continuous ultrathin inorganic surface layer that infiltrated the outer crosslinked polymeric domains. They might be used as structurally robust, pH-responsive biocompatible hybrid nanostructures for drug delivery, bioimaging, and therapeutic applications [387].

7.4.2 INJECTABLE BONE SUBSTITUTES

With the development of minimally invasive surgical methods, for example, percutaneous surgery, directly injectable biomaterials are needed. The challenge is to place a biomaterial at the site of surgery by the least possible invasive method. In this regard, injectable bone substitutes (IBS) appear to be a convenient alternative to solid bone-filling materials. They represent ready-to-use suspensions of $CaPO_4$ microspheres [389,390], nanosized rods [391], or powder(s) in a liquid carrier phase. They look like opaque viscous pastes with rheological properties sufficient to inject them into bone defects by means of surgical syringes and needles. Besides, IBS could be easily produced in a sterile stage. Their stable composition and mechanical properties are suitable for reproducibility of the biological response [383].

IBS requires suitable rheological properties to ensure bonding of the mineral phase in situ with good cell permeability. Usually, the necessary level of viscosity is created by the addition of water-soluble polymers [392–394]. Therefore, the majority of $CaPO_4$-based IBS formulations might be considered a subgroup of $CaPO_4/$polymer biocomposites. For example, an IBS was described that involved a silanized hydroxyethylcellulose carrier with BCP (HA + β-TCP) [395]. The suspension is liquid at pH within 10–12, but gels quickly at pH <9. Similarly, Bennett et al. showed that a polydioxanone-co-glycolide-based biocomposite reinforced with HA or β-TCP could be used as an injectable or moldable putty [396]. During the crosslinking reaction following injection, carbon dioxide is released allowing the formation of interconnected pores. Furthermore, HA/poly(L-lactide-co-ε-caprolactone) biocomposite microparticles were fabricated as an injectable scaffold via the Pickering emulsion route in the absence of any molecular surfactants. A stable injectable oil-in-water emulsion was obtained using water-dispersed HA nanosized crystals as the particulate emulsifier and a dichloromethane solution of poly(L-lactide-co-ε-caprolactone) as an oil phase [397].

Daculsi et al. developed viscous IBS biocomposites based on BCP (60% HA + 40% β-TCP) and 2% aqueous solution of HPMC, which was said to be perfectly biocompatible, resorbable, and easily fitted bone defects (due to an initial plasticity)

[394–405]. The best ratio BCP/HPMC aqueous solution was found to be at ~65/35 w/w. To extend this subject further, IBS might be loaded by cells [406,407], radiopaque elements [408], or microparticles [409], as well as functionalized by nucleic acids [391]. The list of the commercially available $CaPO_4$-based IBS formulations is presented in Table 7.5 [410].

The advanced characteristics of IBS come from their good rheological properties and biocompatibility and the ease of tissue regeneration. Although the fabrication of IBS biocomposites in most cases improved the mechanical properties of the system and provided the material with resistance to fluids penetration, these achievements were limited by the amount of polymer that can be added to the paste. For instance, Mickiewicz et al. reported that after a critical concentration (that depended on the type and molecular weight of the polymer, but was always around 10%), the polymer started forming a thick coating on the crystal clusters, preventing them from interlocking, originating plastic flow, and, as a consequence, decreasing mechanical properties [411]. More to the point, Fujishiro et al. reported a decrease in mechanical properties with higher amounts of gel, which was attributed to the formation of pores due to the leaching of gelatin in solution [412]. Therefore, it seems that mechanical properties, although improved by the addition of polymers, are still a limitation for the application of $CaPO_4$-based IBS formulations in load-bearing sites [125]. Further details on IBS are available elsewhere [392].

7.5   BIOACTIVITY AND BIODEGRADATION OF CALCIUM ORTHOPHOSPHATE-BASED FORMULATIONS

The continuous degradation of an implant causes a gradual load transfer to the healing tissue, preventing stress-shielding atrophy, and stimulates the healing and remodeling of bones. Some requirements must be fulfilled by the ideal prosthetic biodegradable materials, such as biocompatibility, adequate initial strength and stiffness, retention of mechanical properties throughout sufficient time to assure its biofunctionality, and nontoxicity of the degradation byproducts [125]. Generally speaking, bioactivity (i.e., ability of bonding to bones) of biologically relevant $CaPO_4$ reinforced by other materials is usually lower than that of pure ones [17,413].

In general, both bioactivity and biodegradability of any biocomposite and/or hybrid biomaterial are determined by the same properties of the constituents. Both processes are very multifactorial because, during implantation, the surface of any graft contacts with biological fluids and, shortly afterward, is colonized by cells. Much more biology, than chemistry and material science altogether, is involved into these very complex processes and many specific details still remain unknown. In addition, biodegradation of all components of biocomposites occurs simultaneously and the obtained products might influence both the entire process and biodegradation of each component. For example, in the case of biocomposites prepared from polyesters and TCP, hydrolysis reactions of the ester bonds, acid dissociation of the carboxylic end groups, dissolution of TCP, and buffering reactions by the dissolved phosphate ions occur simultaneously [414]. Therefore, to simplify the task, biodegradation of the individual components should be considered independently. An in vitro biodegradation of the biologically relevant $CaPO_4$

TABLE 7.5

List of Some Commercial Nonsetting CaPO₄ IBS and Pastes with Indication of Producer, Product Name, Composition (When Available), and Form

Producer	Product Name	Composition	Form
ApaTech (UK)	Actifuse™	HA, polymer and aqueous solution	Pre-mixed
	Actifuse™ Shape Actifuse™ ABX	Si-substituted CaPO₄ and a polymer	pre-mixed
Baxter (US)	TricOs T TricOs	BCP (60% HA, 40% β-TCP) granules and Tissucol (fibrin glue)	To be mixed
Berkeley Advanced Biomaterials	Bi-Ostetic Putty	Not disclosed	Not disclosed
BioForm (US)	Calcium hydroxylapatite implant	HA powder embedded in a mixture of glycerine, water, and carboxymethylcellulose	Pre-mixed
Biomatlante (FR)	MBCP Gel®	BCP granules (60% HA, 40% β-TCP; 0.08–0.2 mm) and 2% HPMC	Pre-mixed
	Hydr'Os	BCP granules (60% HA, 40% β-TCP; micro- and nanosized particles) and saline solution	Pre-mixed
Degradable solutions (CH)	Easy graft™	β-TCP or BCP granules (0.45–1.0 mm) coated with 10 μm PLGA, N-methyl-2-pyrrolydone	To be mixed
Dentsply (US)	Pepgen P-15® flow	HA (0.25–0.42 mm), P-15 peptide and aqueous Na hyaluronate solution	To be mixed
DePuy Spine (US)	Healos® Fx	HA (20%–30%) and collagen	To be mixed
Fluidinova (P)	NanoXIM TCP	β-TCP (5% or 15%) and water	Pre-mixed
	NanoXIM HA	HA (5%, 15%, 30% or 40%) and water	Pre-mixed
Integra LifeSciences (US)	Mozaik Osteoconductive Scaffold	β-TCP (80%) and type 1 collagen (20%)	To be mixed
Mathys Ltd (CH)	Ceros® Putty/cyclOS® Putty	β-TCP granules (0.125–0.71 mm; 94%) and recombinant Na hyaluronate powder (6%)	To be mixed
Medtronic (US)	Mastergraft®	BCP (85% HA, 15% β-TCP) and bovine collagen	To be mixed
Osartis/AAP (GER)	Ostim®	Nanocrystalline HA (35%) and water (65%)	Pre-mixed
Smith & Nephew (US)	JAXTCP	β-TCP granules and an aqueous solution of 1.75% carboxymethylcellulose and 10% glycerol	To be mixed
Stryker (US)	Calstrux™	β-TCP granules and carboxymethylcellulose	To be mixed
Teknimed (FR)	Nanogel	HA (100–200 nm) (30%) and water (70%)	Pre-mixed
Therics (US)	Therigraft™ Putty	β-TCP granules and polymer	Pre-mixed
Zimmer (US)	Collagraft	BCP granules (65% HA, 35% β-TCP; 0.5–1.0 mm), bovine collagen, and bone marrow aspirate	To be mixed

Source: Bohner, M., *Eur. Cell Mater,* 20, 1, 2010.

might be described by their chemical dissolution in slightly acidic media (they are almost insoluble in alkaline solutions [75–78]), which, in the case of CDHA, might be described as a sequence of four successive chemical equations (7.1)–(7.4) [415,416]:

$$Ca_{10-x}(HPO_4)_x(PO_4)_{6-x}(OH)_{2-x} + (2-x)H^+$$

$$= Ca_{10-x}(HPO_4)_x(PO_4)_{6-x}(H_2O)_{2-x}^{(2-x)} \tag{7.1}$$

$$Ca_{10-x}(HPO_4)_x(PO_4)_{6-x}(H_2O)_{2-x}^{(2-x)+}$$

$$= 3Ca_3(PO_4)_2 + (1-x)Ca^{2+} + (2-x)H_2O \tag{7.2}$$

$$Ca_3(PO_4)_2 + 2H^+ = Ca^{2+} + 2CaHPO_4 \tag{7.3}$$

$$CaHPO_4 + H^+ = Ca^{2+} + H_2PO_4^- \tag{7.4}$$

Biodegradability of polymers generally depends on the following factors: (1) chemical stability of the polymer backbone, (2) hydrophobicity of the monomer, (3) morphology of the polymer, (4) initial molecular weight, (5) fabrication processes, (6) geometry of the implant, and (7) properties of the scaffold such as porosity and pore diameter [219]. A summary on degradation of PLA and PGA, as well as that of SEVA-C, is available in literature [Ref. 125, p. 798 and p. 803, respectively], where the interested readers are referred to.

Concerning in vivo studies, biodegradation of HA/PLLA and CDHA/PLLA biocomposite rods in subcutis and medullary cavities of rabbits was investigated mechanically and histologically; the degradation was found to be faster for the case of using uncalcinated CDHA instead of calcinated HA [417]. In a more detailed study, new bone formation was detected at 2 weeks after implantation, especially for formulations with a high HA content [418]. More to the point, a direct contact between bones and these composites without intervening fibrous tissue was detected in this case [418,419]. Both SEVA-C and SEVA-C/HA biocomposites were found to exhibit a noncytotoxic behavior [420,421], inducing a satisfactory tissue response when implanted, as shown by in vivo studies [421]. Furthermore, SEVA-C/HA biocomposites induce a positive response on osteoblast-like cells to what concerns cell adhesion and proliferation [420]. An in vivo study on biodegradation of microspheres (PLGA, gelatin, and poly(trimethylene carbonate) were used)/CaPO_4 biocomposites revealed that they exhibited microsphere degradation after 12 weeks of subcutaneous implantation, which was accompanied by compression strength decreasing [422]. Interestingly, but the amount of CaPO_4 in biocomposites was found to have a greater effect on the early stages of osteoblast behavior (cell attachment and proliferation) rather than the immediate and late stages (proliferation and differentiation) [423].

Both in vitro (the samples were immersed into 1% trypsin/phosphate-buffered saline solution at 37°C) biodegradation and in vivo (implantation of samples into the posterolateral lumbar spine of rabbits) biodegradation have been investigated for nanosized HA/collagen/PLA biocomposites [424]. The results demonstrated that weight loss increased continuously in vitro with a reduction in the mass of ~20% after 4 weeks. During the experimental period in vitro, a relative rate of reduction in the three components in this material was shown to differ greatly: collagen decreased the fastest from 40% by weight to ~20% in the composite; HA content increased from 45% to ~60%; while PLA changed little. In vivo, the collagen/HA ratio appeared to be slightly higher near the transverse process than in the central part of the intertransverse process [424]. Hasegawa et al. [425] performed an in vivo study, spanning over a period of 5–7 years, on high-strength HA/PLLA biocomposite rods for the internal fixation of bone fractures. In that work, both uncalcined CDHA and calcined HA were used as reinforcing phases in PLLA matrix. Those composites were implanted in the femur of 25 rabbits. It was found that the implanted materials were resorbed after 6 years of implantation. The presence of remodeled bone and trabecular bone bonding was the significant outcome. These data clearly demonstrate a biodegradation independence of various components of biocomposites.

7.6   CONCLUSION

All types of calcified tissues of humans and mammals appear to possess a complex hierarchical biocomposite structure. Their mechanical properties are outstanding (considering weak constituents from which they are assembled) and far beyond those, that can be achieved using the same synthetic materials with present technologies. This is because biological organisms produce biocomposites that are organized in terms of both composition and structure, containing both brittle $CaPO_4$ and ductile bioorganic components in very complex structures, hierarchically organized at the nano, micro, and meso levels. Additionally, the calcified tissues are always multifunctional: for example, bone provides structural support for the body plus blood cell formation. The third defining characteristic of biological systems, in contrast with current synthetic systems, is their self-healing ability, which is nearly universal in nature. These complex structures, which have risen from millions of years of evolution, inspire materials scientists in the design of novel biomaterials [426].

Obviously, no single-phase biomaterial is able to provide all the essential features of bones and/or other calcified tissues and, therefore, there is a great need to engineer multiphase biomaterials (biocomposites) with a structure and composition mimicking those of natural bones. The studies summarized in this review have shown that the proper combination of a ductile matrix with a brittle, hard, and bioactive $CaPO_4$ filler offers many advantages for biomedical applications. The desirable properties of some components can compensate for a poor mechanical behavior of $CaPO_4$ bioceramics, while in turn the desirable bioactive properties of $CaPO_4$ improve those of other phases, thus expanding the possible application of each material within the body [69,70]. However, the reviewed literature clearly indicates that among the possible types of $CaPO_4$/polymer biocomposites and hybrid biomaterials, only simple, complex, and graded ones, as well as fibrous, laminar, and particulate ones, have been investigated. Presumably, a future progress in this subject will require concentrating efforts on the elaboration and development of both hierarchical and hybrid biocomposites. Furthermore, following the modern tendency of tissue engineering, a novel generation of $CaPO_4$/polymer biocomposites and hybrid biomaterials should also contain a biological living part.

To conclude, the future of the $CaPO_4$/polymer biocomposites and hybrid biomaterials is now directly dependent on the formation of multidisciplinary teams composed of experts but primarily experts ready to collaborate in close collaboration with others and thus be able to deal efficiently with the complexity of the human organism. The physical chemistries of solids, solid surfaces, polymer dispersion, and solutions, as well as material–cell interactions are among the phenomena to be tackled. Furthermore, much work remains to be done on a long way from a laboratory to clinics and the success depends on the effective cooperation of clinicians, chemists, biologists, bioengineers, and materials scientists.

REFERENCES

1. Chau, A.M.T., Mobbs, R.J. Bone graft substitutes in anterior cervical discectomy and fusion. *Eur. Spine J.* 2009, 18, 449–464.
2. Kaveh, K., Ibrahim, R., Bakar, M.Z.A., Ibrahim, T.A. Bone grafting and bone graft substitutes. *J. Anim. Vet. Adv.* 2010, 9, 1055–1067.
3. Tazaki, J., Murata, M., Yuasa, T., Akazawa, T., Ito, K., Hino, J., Nida, A., Arisue, M., Shibata, T. Autograft of human tooth and demineralized dentin matrices for bone augmentation. *J. Ceram. Soc. Jpn.* 2010, 118, 442–445.
4. Conway, J.D. Autograft and nonunions: Morbidity with intramedullary bone graft versus iliac crest bone graft. Orthop. *Clin. North Am.* 2010, 41, 75–84.
5. Keller, E.E., Triplett, W.W. Iliac crest bone grafting: Review of 160 consecutive cases. *J. Oral Maxillofac. Surg.* 1987, 45, 11–14.
6. Schaaf, H., Lendeckel, S., Howaldt, H.P., Streckbein, P. Donor site morbidity after bone harvesting from the anterior iliac crest. *Oral Surg. Oral Med. Oral Pathol. Oral Radiol. Endod.* 2010, 109, 52–58.
7. Carlsen, A., Gorst-Rasmussen, A., Jensen, T. Donor site morbidity associated with autogenous bone harvesting from the ascending mandibular ramus. *Implant Dent.* 2013, 22, 503–506.
8. Fuchs, J.R., Nasseri, B.A., Vacanti, J.P. Tissue engineering: A 21st century solution to surgical reconstruction. *Ann. Thorac. Surg.* 2001, 72, 557–591.
9. Li, Z., Kawashita, M. Current progress in inorganic artificial biomaterials. *J. Artif. Organ.* 2011, 14, 163–170.
10. Pezzotti, G., Yamamoto, K. Artificial hip joints: The biomaterials challenge. *J. Mech. Behav. Biomed. Mater.* 2014, 31, 3–20.
11. Panchbhavi, V.K. Synthetic bone grafting in foot and ankle surgery. *Foot Ankle Clin.* 2010, 15, 559–576.
12. Bohner, M. Resorbable biomaterials as bone graft substitutes. *Mater. Today* 2010, 13, 24–30.
13. Lowenstam, H.A., Weiner, S. *On Biomineralization.* Oxford University Press: New York, 1989; 324pp.

14. Weiner, S., Wagner, H.D. The material bone: Structure-mechanical function relations. *Ann. Rev. Mater. Sci.* 1998, 28, 271–298.

15. Dorozhkin, S.V. *Calcium Orthophosphates: Applications in Nature, Biology, and Medicine.* Pan Stanford: Singapore, 2012; 854pp.

16. Suchanek, W., Yoshimura, M. Processing and properties of hydroxyapatite-based biomaterials for use as hard tissue replacement implants. *J. Mater. Res.* 1998, 13, 94–117.

17. Hench, L.L. Bioceramics. *J. Am. Ceram. Soc.* 1998, 81, 1705–1728.

18. Burr, D.B. The contribution of the organic matrix to bone's material properties. *Bone* 2002, 31, 8–11.

19. Thompson, J.B., Kindt, J.H., Drake, B., Hansma, H.G., Morse, D.E., Hansma, P.K. Bone indentation recovery time correlates with bond reforming time. *Nature* 2001, 414, 773–776.

20. Olszta, M.J., Cheng, X.G., Jee, S.S., Kumar, B.R., Kim, Y.Y., Kaufman, M.J., Douglas, E.P., Gower, L.B. Bone structure and formation: A new perspective. *Mater. Sci. Eng. R* 2007, 58, 77–116.

21. Fonseca, H., Moreira-Gonçalves, D., Coriolano, H.J.A., Duarte, J.A. Bone quality: The determinants of bone strength and fragility. *Sports Med.* 2014, 44, 37–53.

22. Murugan, R., Ramakrishna, S. Development of nanocomposites for bone grafting. *Compos. Sci. Technol.* 2005, 65, 2385–2406.

23. Vallet-Regi, M., Arcos, D. Nanostructured hybrid materials for bone tissue regeneration. *Curr. Nanosci.* 2006, 2, 179–189.

24. Bauer, T., Muschler, G. Bone grafts materials. An overview of the basic science. *Clin. Orthop. Rel. Res.* 2000, 371, 10–27.

25. Athanasiou, K.A., Zhu, C.F., Lanctot, D.R., Agrawal, C.M., Wang, X. Fundamentals of biomechanics in tissue engineering of bone. *Tissue Eng.* 2000, 6, 361–381.

26. Doblaré, M., Garcia, J.M., Gómez, M.J. Modelling bone tissue fracture and healing: A review. *Eng. Fract. Mech.* 2004, 71, 1809–1840.

27. Vallet-Regi, M. Revisiting ceramics for medical applications. *J. Chem. Soc. Dalton Trans.* 2006, 44, 5211–5220.

28. Huiskes, R., Ruimerman, R., van Lenthe, H.G., Janssen, J.D. Effects of mechanical forces on maintenance and adaptation of form in trabecular bone. *Nature* 2000, 405, 704–706.

29. Boccaccini, A.R., Blaker, J.J. Bioactive composite materials for tissue engineering scaffolds. *Expert Rev. Med. Dev.* 2005, 2, 303–317.

30. Durucan, C., Brown, P.W. Biodegradable hydroxyapatite-polymer composites. *Adv. Eng. Mater.* 2001, 3, 227–231.

31. Kim, H.W., Knowles, J.C., Kim, H.E. Hydroxyapatite/poly(ε-caprolactone) composite coatings on hydroxyapatite porous bone scaffold for drug delivery. *Biomaterials* 2004, 25, 1279–1287.

32. Hutmacher, D.W., Schantz, J.T., Lam, C.X.F., Tan, K.C., Lim, T.C. State of the art and future directions of scaffold-based bone engineering from a biomaterials perspective. *J. Tissue Eng. Regen. Med.* 2007, 1, 245–260.

33. Guarino, V., Causa, F., Ambrosio, L. Bioactive scaffolds for bone and ligament tissue. *Expert Rev. Med. Dev.* 2007, 4, 405–418.

34. Yunos, D.M., Bretcanu, O., Boccaccini, A.R. Polymer-bioceramic composites for tissue engineering scaffolds. *J. Mater. Sci.* 2008, 43, 4433–4442.

35. Hench, L.L., Polak, J.M. Third-generation biomedical materials. *Science* 2002, 295, 1014–1017.

36. Crane, G.M., Ishaug, S.L., Mikos, A.G. Bone tissue engineering. *Nat. Med.* 1995, 1, 1322–1324.

37. Mathijsen, A. *Nieuwe Wijze van Aanwending van het Gips-Verband bij Beenbreuken.* J.B. van Loghem: Haarlem, 1852.

38. Dreesman, H. Über Knochenplombierung. *Beitr. Klin. Chir.* 1892, 9, 804–810.

39. Wang, M. Developing bioactive composite materials for tissue replacement. *Biomaterials* 2003, 24, 2133–2151.
40. "Composite Material," Wikipedia, last modified July 3, 2015, http://en.wikipedia.org/wiki/Composite_material.
41. Gibson, R.F. A review of recent research on mechanics of multifunctional composite materials and structures. *Compos. Struct.* 2010, 92, 2793–2810.
42. Evans, S.L., Gregson, P.J. Composite technology in load-bearing orthopaedic implants. *Biomaterials* 1998, 19, 1329–1342.
43. Wan, Y.Z., Hong, L., Jia, S.R., Huang, Y., Zhu, Y., Wang, Y.L., Jiang, H.J. Synthesis and characterization of hydroxyapatite-bacterial cellulose nanocomposites. *Compos. Sci. Technol.* 2006, 66, 1825–1832.
44. Wan, Y.Z., Huang, Y., Yuan, C.D., Raman, S., Zhu, Y., Jiang, H.J., He, F., Gao, C. Biomimetic synthesis of hydroxyapatite/bacterial cellulose nanocomposites for biomedical applications. *Mater. Sci. Eng. C* 2007, 27, 855–864.
45. Ohtsuki, C., Kamitakahara, M., Miyazaki, T. Coating bone-like apatite onto organic substrates using solutions mimicking body fluid. *J. Tissue Eng. Regen. Med.* 2007, 1, 33–38.
46. Oyane, A. Development of apatite-based composites by a biomimetic process for biomedical applications. *J. Ceram. Soc. Jpn.* 2010, 118, 77–81.
47. Dorozhkin, S.V. Calcium orthophosphate coatings, films and layers. *Prog. Biomater.* 2012, 1, 1–40.
48. Surmenev, R.A., Surmeneva, M.A., Ivanova, A.A. Significance of calcium phosphate coatings for the enhancement of new bone osteogenesis—A review. *Acta Biomater.* 2014, 10, 557–579.
49. Dorozhkin, S.V. Calcium orthophosphate coatings on magnesium and its biodegradable alloys. *Acta Biomater.* 2014, 10, 2919–2934.
50. Planeix JM., Jaunky W., Duhoo T., Czernuszka, J.T., Hosseini, M.W., Brès, E.F. A molecular tectonics-crystal engineering approach for building organic-inorganic composites. Potential application to the growth control of hydroxyapatite crystals. *J. Mater. Chem.* 2003, 13, 2521–2524.
51. Zhao, J., Guo, L.Y., Yang, X.B., Weng, J. Preparation of bioactive porous HA/PCL composite scaffolds. *Appl. Surf. Sci.* 2008, 255, 2942–2946.
52. Dorozhkin, S., Ajaal, T. Toughening of porous bioceramic scaffolds by bioresorbable polymeric coatings. *Proc. Inst. Mech. Eng. H* 2009, 223, 459–470.
53. Woo, A.S., Jang, J.L., Liberman, R.F., Weinzweig, J. Creation of a vascularized composite graft with acellular dermal matrix and hydroxyapatite. *Plast. Reconstr. Surg.* 2010, 125, 1661–1669.
54. Zhao, J., Duan, K., Zhang, J.W., Lu, X., Weng, J. The influence of polymer concentrations on the structure and mechanical properties of porous polycaprolactone-coated hydroxyapatite scaffolds. *Appl. Surf. Sci.* 2010, 256, 4586–4590.
55. Dong, J., Uemura, T., Kojima, H., Kikuchi, M., Tanaka, J., Tateishi, T. Application of low-pressure system to sustain *in vivo* bone formation in osteoblast/porous hydroxyapatite composite. *Mater. Sci. Eng. C* 2001, 17, 37–43.
56. Zerbo, I.R., Bronckers, A.L.J.J., de Lange, G., Burger, E.H. Localisation of osteogenic and osteoclastic cells in porous β-tricalcium phosphate particles used for human maxillary sinus floor elevation. *Biomaterials* 2005, 26, 1445–1451.
57. Mikán, J., Villamil, M., Montes, T., Carretero, C., Bernal, C., Torres, M.L., Zakaria, F.A. Porcine model for hybrid material of carbonated apatite and osteoprogenitor cells. *Mater. Res. Innovat.* 2009, 13, 323–326.
58. Oe, K., Miwa, M., Nagamune, K., Sakai, Y., Lee, S.Y., Niikura, T., Iwakura, T., Hasegawa, T., Shibanuma, N., Hata, Y., Kuroda, R, Kurosaka, M. Nondestructive evaluation of cell numbers in bone marrow stromal cell/β-tricalcium phosphate composites using ultrasound. *Tissue Eng. C* 2010, 16, 347–353.

59. Krout, A., Wen, H.B., Hippensteel, E., Li, P. A hybrid coating of biomimetic apatite and osteocalcin. *J. Biomed. Mater. Res. A* 2005, 73A, 377–387.
60. Kundu, B., Soundrapandian, C., Nandi, S.K., Mukherjee, P., Dandapat, N., Roy, S., Datta, B.K., Mandal, T.K., Basu, D., Bhattacharya, R.N. Development of new localized drug delivery system based on ceftriaxone-sulbactam composite drug impregnated porous hydroxyapatite: A systematic approach for *in vitro* and *in vivo* animal trial. *Pharm. Res.* 2010, 27, 1659–1676.
61. Kickelbick, G. (Ed.) Hybrid materials. *Synthesis, Characterization, and Applications.* Wiley-VCH Verlag: Weinheim, Germany, 2007; 498pp.
62. Matthews, F.L., Rawlings, R.D. *Composite Materials: Engineering and Science.* CRC Press: Boca Raton, FL, 2000; 480pp.
63. Xia, Z., Riester, L., Curtin, W.A., Li, H., Sheldon, B.W., Liang, J., Chang, B., Xu, J.M. Direct observation of toughening mechanisms in carbon nanotube ceramic matrix composites. *Acta Mater.* 2004, 52, 931–944.
64. Tavares, M.I.B., Ferreira, O., Preto, M., Miguez, E., Soares, I.L., da Silva, E.P. Evaluation of composites miscibility by low field NMR. *Int. J. Polym. Mater.* 2007, 56, 1113–1118.
65. Kiran, E. Polymer miscibility, phase separation, morphological modifications and polymorphic transformations in dense fluids. *J. Supercrit. Fluids* 2009, 47, 466–483.
66. Šupová, M. Problem of hydroxyapatite dispersion in polymer matrices: A review. *J. Mater. Sci. Mater. Med.* 2009, 20, 1201–1213.
67. Böstman, O., Pihlajamäki, H. Clinical biocompatibility of biodegradable orthopaedic implants for internal fixation: A review. *Biomaterials* 2000, 21, 2615–2621.
68. John, M.J., Thomas, S. Biofibres and biocomposites. *Carbohydr. Polym.* 2008, 71, 343–364.
69. Rea, S.M., Bonfield, W. Biocomposites for medical applications. *J. Aust. Ceram. Soc.* 2004, 40, 43–57.
70. Tanner, K.E. Bioactive ceramic-reinforced composites for bone augmentation. *J. Roy. Soc. Interface* 2010, 7, S541–S557.
71. Gravitis, Y.A., Tééyaér, R.E., Kallavus, U.L., Andersons, B.A., Ozol'-Kalnin, V.G., Kokorevich, A.G., Érin'sh, P.P., Veveris, G.P. Biocomposite structure of wood cell membranes and their destruction by explosive autohydrolysis. *Mech. Compos. Mater.* 1987, 22, 721–725.
72. Bernard, S.L., Picha, G.J. The use of coralline hydroxyapatite in a 'biocomposite' free flap. *Plast. Reconstr. Surg.* 1991, 87, 96–107.
73. Hing, K.A. Bioceramic bone graft substitutes: Influence of porosity and chemistry. *Int. J. Appl. Ceram. Technol.* 2005, 2, 184–199.
74. Naqshbandi, A.R., Sopyan, I., Gunawan, Development of porous calcium phosphate bioceramics for bone implant applications: A review. *Rec. Pat. Mater. Sci.* 2013, 6, 238–252.
75. LeGeros, R.Z. Calcium phosphates in oral biology and medicine. *Monographs in Oral Science.* Myers, H.M. (Ed.); Karger: Basel, Switzerland, 1991; Vol. 15, 201pp.
76. Elliott, J.C. Structure and chemistry of the apatites and other calcium orthophosphates. In: *Studies in Inorganic Chemistry.* Elsevier: Amsterdam, the Netherlands, 1994; Vol. 18, 389pp.
77. Brown, P.W., Constantz, B. (Eds.) *Hydroxyapatite and Related Materials.* CRC Press: Boca Raton, FL, 1994; 343pp.
78. Amjad, Z. (Ed.) *Calcium Phosphates in Biological and Industrial Systems.* Kluwer: Boston, MA, 1997; 529pp.
79. Carraher, C.E., Jr. *Introduction to Polymer Chemistry*, 2nd edn., CRC Press: Boca Raton, FL, 2010; 534pp.
80. Young, R.J., Lovell, P.A. *Introduction to Polymers*, 3rd edn., CRC Press: Boca Raton, FL, 2011; 688pp.

81. Thomson, R.C., Ak, S., Yaszemski, M.J., Mikos, A.G. Polymer scaffold processing. In: *Principles of Tissue Engineering*, Academic Press: New York, 2000; pp. 251–262.
82. Ramakrishna, S., Mayer, J., Wintermantel, E., Leong, K.W. Biomedical applications of polymer-composite materials: A review. *Compos. Sci. Technol.* 2001, 61, 1189–1224.
83. Shastri, V.P. Non-degradable biocompatible polymers in medicine: Past, present and future. *Curr. Pharm. Biotechnol.* 2003, 4, 331–337.
84. Chen, H., Yuan, L., Song, W., Wu, Z., Li, D. Biocompatible polymer materials: Role of protein-surface interactions. *Prog. Polym. Sci.* 2008, 33, 1059–1087.
85. Langer, R., Vacanti, J.P. Tissue engineering. *Science* 1993, 260, 920–925.
86. Lanza, R.P., Hayes, J.L., Chick, W.L. Encapsulated cell technology. *Nat. Biotechnol.* 1996, 14, 1107–1111.
87. Shukla, S.C., Singh, A., Pandey, A.K., Mishra, A. Review on production and medical applications of ε-polylysine. *Biochem. Eng. J.* 2012, 65, 70–81.
88. Agrawal, C.M., Ray, R.B. Biodegradable polymeric scaffolds for musculoskeletal tissue engineering. *J. Biomed. Mater. Res.* 2001, 55, 141–150.
89. Kweon, H., Yoo, M., Park, I., Kim, T., Lee, H., Lee, S., Oh, J., Akaike, T., Cho, C. A novel degradable polycaprolactone network for tissue engineering. *Biomaterials* 2003, 24, 801–808.
90. Wang, Y.C., Zhang, P.H. Electrospun absorbable polycaprolactone (PCL) scaffolds for medical applications. *Adv. Mater. Res.* 2014, 906, 221–225.
91. Sartori, S., Chiono, V., Tonda-Turo, C., Mattu, C., Gianluca, C. Biomimetic polyurethanes in nano and regenerative medicine. *J. Mater. Chem. B* 2014, 2, 5128–5144.
92. Temenoff, J.S., Mikos, A.G. Injectable biodegradable materials for orthopedic tissue engineering. *Biomaterials* 2000, 21, 2405–2412.
93. Behravesh, E., Yasko, A.W., Engel, P.S., Mikos, A.G. Synthetic biodegradable polymers for orthopaedic applications. *Clin. Orthop. Rel. Res.* 1999, 367S, S118–S125.
94. Lewandrowski, K.U., Gresser, J.D., Wise, D.L., White, R.L., Trantolo, D.J. Osteoconductivity of an injectable and bioresorbable poly(propyleneglycol-*co*-fumaric acid) bone cement. *Biomaterials* 2000, 21, 293–298.
95. Peter, S.J., Miller, M.J., Yaszemski, M.J., Mikos, A.G. Poly(propylene fumarate). In: *Handbook of Biodegradable Polymers*, Domb, A.J., Kost, J., Wiseman, D.M. (Eds.); Harwood Academic: Amsterdam, the Netherlands, 1997; pp. 87–97.
96. Xu, J., Feng, E., Song, J. Renaissance of aliphatic polycarbonates: New techniques and biomedical applications. *J. Appl. Polym. Sci.* 2014, 131, 39822 (16 pages).
97. Boland, E.D., Coleman, B.D., Barnes, C.P., Simpson, D.G., Wnek, G.E., Bowlin, G.L. Electrospinning polydioxanone for biomedical applications. *Acta Biomater.* 2005, 1, 115–123.
98. Gilbert, J.L. Acrylics in biomedical engineering. In: *Encyclopedia of Materials: Science and Technology*, Elsevier: Amsterdam, the Netherlands, 2001; pp. 11–18.
99. Frazer, R.Q., Byron, R.T., Osborne, P.B., West, K.P. PMMA: An essential material in medicine and dentistry. *J. Long-Term Eff. Med. Implants* 2005, 15, 629–639.
100. Li, Y.W., Leong, J.C, Y., Lu, W.W., Luk, K.D, K., Cheung, K.M.C., Chiu, K.Y., Chow, S.P. A novel injectable bioactive bone cement for spinal surgery: A developmental and preclinical study. *J. Biomed. Mater. Res.* 2000, 52, 164–170.
101. Mckellop, H., Shen, F., Lu, B., Campbell, P., Salovey, R. Development of an extremely wear resistant UHMW polyethylene for total hip replacements. *J. Orthop. Res.* 1999, 17, 157–167.
102. Kurtz, S.M., Muratoglu, O.K., Evans, M., Edidin, A.A. Advances in the processing, sterilization and crosslinking of ultra-high molecular weight polyethylene for total joint arthroplasty. *Biomaterials* 1999, 20, 1659–1688.
103. Laurencin, C.T., Ambrosio, M.A., Borden, M.D., Cooper, J.A., Jr. Tissue engineering: Orthopedic applications. *Ann. Rev. Biomed. Eng.* 1999, 1, 19–46.

104. Meijer, G.J., Cune, M.S., van Dooren, M., de Putter, C., van Blitterswijk, C.A. A comparative study of flexible (Polyactive™) versus rigid (hydroxylapatite) permucosal dental implants. I. Clinical aspects. *J. Oral Rehabil.* 1997, 24, 85–92.

105. Meijer, G.J., Dalmeijer, R.A., de Putter, C., van Blitterswijk, C.A. A comparative study of flexible (Polyactive™) versus rigid (hydroxylapatite) permucosal dental implants. II. Histological aspects. *J. Oral Rehabil.* 1997, 24, 93–101.

106. Waris, E., Ashammakhi, N., Lehtimäki, M., Tulamo, R.M., Törmälä, P., Kellomäki, M., Konttinen, Y.T. Long-term bone tissue reaction to polyethylene oxide/polybutylene terephthalate copolymer (Polyactive®) in metacarpophalangeal joint reconstruction. *Biomaterials* 2008, 29, 2509–2515.

107. Svensson, A., Nicklasson, E., Harrah, T., Panilaitis, B., Kaplan, D.L., Brittberg, M., Gatenholm, P. Bacterial cellulose as a potential scaffold for tissue engineering of cartilage. *Biomaterials* 2005, 26, 419–431.

108. Rampinelli, G., di Landro, L., Fujii, T. Characterization of biomaterials based on microfibrillated cellulose with different modifications. *J. Reinforced Plastics Compos.* 2010, 29, 1793–1803.

109. Granja, P.L., Barbosa, M.A., Pouysége, L., de Jéso, B., Rouais, F., Baquuey, C. Cellulose phosphates as biomaterials. Mineralization of chemically modified regenerated cellulose hydrogels. *J. Mater. Sci.* 2001, 36, 2163–2172.

110. Granja, P.L., Jéso, B.D., Bareille, R., Rouais, F., Baquey, C., Barbosa, M.A. Cellulose phosphates as biomaterials. *In vitro* biocompatibility studies. *React. Funct. Polym.* 2006, 66, 728–739.

111. Thomas, V., Dean, D.R., Vohra, Y.K. Nanostructured biomaterials for regenerative medicine. *Curr. Nanosci.* 2006, 2, 155–177.

112. Dee, K.C., Bizios, R. Mini-review: Proactive biomaterials and bone tissue engineering. *Biotechnol. Bioeng.* 1996, 50, 438–442.

113. Ignjatovic, N., Tomic, S., Dakic, M., Miljkovic, M., Plavsic, M., Uskokovic, D. Synthesis and properties of hydroxyapatite/poly-L-lactide composite biomaterials. *Biomaterials* 1999, 20, 809–816.

114. Ignjatovic, N., Savic, V., Najman, S., Plavsic, M., Uskokovic, D. A study of HAp/PLLA composite as a substitute for bone powder using FT-IR spectroscopy. *Biomaterials* 2001, 22, 571–575.

115. Marra, K.G., Szem, J.W., Kumta, P.N., DiMilla, P.A., Weiss, L.E. *In vitro* analysis of biodegradable polymer blend/hydroxyapatite composites for bone tissue engineering. *J. Biomed. Mater. Res.* 1999, 47, 324–335.

116. Ashammakhi, N., Rokkanen, P. Absorbable polyglycolide devices in trauma and bone surgery. *Biomaterials* 1997, 18, 3–9.

117. Boyan, B., Lohmann, C., Somers, A., Neiderauer, G., Wozney, J., Dean, D., Carnes, D., Schwartz, Z. Potential of porous poly-D,L-lactide-*co*-glycolide particles as a carrier for recombinant human bone morphogenetic protein-2 during osteoinduction *in vivo*. *J. Biomed. Mater. Res.* 1999, 46, 51–59.

118. Hollinger, J.O., Leong, K. Poly(α-hydroxyacids): Carriers for bone morphogenetic proteins. *Biomaterials* 1996, 17, 187–194.

119. Griffith, L.G. Polymeric biomaterials. *Acta Mater.* 2000, 48, 263–277.

120. Peter, S.J., Miller, M.J., Yasko, A.W., Yaszemski, M.J., Mikos, A.G. Polymer concepts in tissue engineering. *J. Biomed. Mater. Res.* 1998, 43, 422–427.

121. Ishuang, S.L., Payne, R.G., Yaszemski, M.J., Aufdemorte, T.B., Bizios, R., Mikos, A.G. Osteoblast migration on poly(α-hydroxy esters). *Biotechnol. Bioeng.* 1996, 50, 443–451.

122. Shikinami, Y., Okuno, M. Bioresorbable devices made of forged composites of hydroxyapatite (HA) particles and poly-L-lactide (PLLA): Part I. Basic characteristics. *Biomaterials* 1999, 20, 859–877.

123. Rezwana, K., Chena, Q.Z., Blakera, J.J., Boccaccini, A.R. Biodegradable and bio-active porous polymer/inorganic composite scaffolds for bone tissue engineering. *Biomaterials* 2006, 27, 3413–3431.

124. Seal, B.L., Otero, T.C., Panitch, A. Polymeric biomaterials for tissue and organ regeneration. *Mater. Sci. Eng. R* 2001, 34, 147–230.

125. Mano, J.F., Sousa, R.A., Boesel, L.F., Neves, N.M., Reis, R.L. Bioinert, biodegradable and injectable polymeric matrix composites for hard tissue replacement: State of the art and recent developments. *Compos. Sci. Technol.* 2004, 64, 789–817.

126. Middleton, J., Tipton, A. Synthetic biodegradable polymers as orthopedic devices. *Biomaterials* 2000, 21, 2335–2346.

127. Coombes, A.G., Meikle, M.C. Resorbable synthetic polymers as replacements for bone graft. *Clin. Mater.* 2004, 17, 35–67.

128. de las Heras Alarcón, C., Pennadam, S., Alexander, C. Stimuli responsive polymers for biomedical applications. *Chem. Soc. Rev.* 2005, 34, 276–285.

129. Kohane, D.S., Langer, R. Polymeric biomaterials in tissue engineering. *Pediatr. Res.* 2008, 63, 487–491.

130. Okada, M. Chemical syntheses of biodegradable polymers. *Prog. Polym. Sci.* 2002, 27, 87–133.

131. Jordan, J., Jacob, K.I., Tannenbaum, R., Sharaf, M.A., Jasiuk, I. Experimental trends in polymer nanocomposites—A review. *Mater. Sci. Eng. A* 2005, 393, 1–11.

132. Converse, G.L., Yue, W., Roeder, R.K. Processing and tensile properties of hydroxyapatite-whisker-reinforced polyetheretherketone. *Biomaterials* 2007, 28, 927–935.

133. Yue, W., Roeder, R.K. Micromechanical model for hydroxyapatite whisker reinforced polymer biocomposites. *J. Mater. Res.* 2006, 21, 2136–2145.

134. Converse, G.L., Roeder, R.K. Tensile properties of hydroxyapatite whisker reinforced polyetheretherketone. *Mater. Res. Soc. Symp. Proc.* 2005, 898, 44–49.

135. Mizutani, Y., Hattori, M., Okuyama, M., Kasuga, T., Nogami, M. Preparation of porous composites with a porous framework using hydroxyapatite whiskers and poly(L-lactic acid) short fibers. *Key Eng. Mater.* 2006, 309–311, 1079–1082.

136. Choi, W.Y., Kim, H.E., Kim, M.J., Kim, U.C., Kim, J.H., Koh, Y.H. Production and characterization of calcium phosphate (CaP) whisker-reinforced poly(ε-caprolactone) composites as bone regenerative. *Mater. Sci. Eng. C* 2010, 30, 1280–1284.

137. Watanabe, T., Ban, S., Ito, T., Tsuruta, S., Kawai, T., Nakamura, H. Biocompatibility of composite membrane consisting of oriented needle-like apatite and biodegradable copolymer with soft and hard tissues in rats. *Dent. Mater. J.* 2004, 23, 609–612.

138. Li, H., Chen, Y., Xie, Y. Photo-crosslinking polymerization to prepare polyanhydride/needle-like hydroxyapatite biodegradable nanocomposite for orthopedic application. *Mater. Lett.* 2003, 57, 2848–2854.

139. Peng, Q., Weng, J., Li, X., Gu, Z. Manufacturing porous blocks of nano-composite of needle-like hydroxyapatite crystallites and chitin for tissue engineering. *Key Eng. Mater.* 2005, 288–289, 199–202.

140. Kasuga, T., Ota, Y., Nogami, M., Abe, Y. Preparation and mechanical properties of polylactic acid composites containing hydroxyapatite fibers. *Biomaterials* 2000, 22, 19–23.

141. Smith, L. Ceramic-plastic material as a bone substitute. *Arch. Surg.* 1963, 87, 653–661.

142. Bonfield, W., Grynpas, M.D., Tully, A.E., Bowman, J., Abram, J. Hydroxyapatite reinforced polyethylene—A mechanically compatible implant material for bone replacement. *Biomaterials* 1981, 2, 185–189.

143. Bonfield, W., Bowman, J., Grynpas, M.D. Composite material for use in orthopaedics. UK Patent 8032647, 1981.

144. Bonfield, W. Composites for bone replacement. *J. Biomed. Eng.* 1988, 10, 522–526.

145. Guild, F.J., Bonfield, W. Predictive character of hydroxyapatite-polyethelene HAPEX™ composite. *Biomaterials* 1993, 14, 985–993.

146. Huang, J., di Silvio, L., Wang, M., Tanner, K.E., Bonfield, W. *In vitro* mechanical and biological assessment of hydroxyapatite-reinforced polyethylene composite. *J. Mater. Sci. Mater. Med.* 1997, 8, 775–779.

147. Wang, M., Joseph, R., Bonfield, W. Hydroxyapatite-polyethylene composites for bone substitution: Effect of ceramic particle size and morphology. *Biomaterials* 1998, 19, 2357–2366.

148. Ladizesky, N.H., Ward, I.M., Bonfield, W. Hydroxyapatite/high-performance polyethylene fiber composites for high load bearing bone replacement materials. *J. Appl. Polym. Sci.* 1997, 65, 1865–1882.

149. Nazhat, S.N., Joseph, R., Wang, M., Smith, R., Tanner, K.E., Bonfield, W. Dynamic mechanical characterisation of hydroxyapatite reinforced polyethylene: Effect of particle size. *J. Mater. Sci. Mater. Med.* 2000, 11, 621–628.

150. Guild, F.J., Bonfield, W. Predictive modelling of the mechanical properties and failure processes of hydroxyapatite-polyethylene (HAPEX™) composite. *J. Mater. Sci. Mater. Med.* 1998, 9, 497–502.

151. Wang M., Ladizesky NH., Tanner, K.E., Ward IM., Bonfield, W. Hydrostatically extruded HAPEX™. *J. Mater. Sci.* 2000, 35, 1023–1030.

152. That PT., Tanner, K.E., Bonfield, W. Fatigue characterization of a hydroxyapatite-reinforced polyethylene composite. I. Uniaxial fatigue. *J. Biomed. Mater. Res.* 2000, 51, 453–460.

153. That PT., Tanner, K.E., Bonfield, W. Fatigue characterization of a hydroxyapatite-reinforced polyethylene composite. II. Biaxial fatigue. *J. Biomed. Mater. Res.* 2000, 51, 461–468.

154. Bonner M., Saunders LS., Ward IM., Davies GW., Wang M., Tanner, K.E., Bonfield, W. Anisotropic mechanical properties of oriented HAPEX™. *J. Mater. Sci.* 2002, 37, 325–334.

155. di Silvio, L., Dalby, M.J., Bonfield, W. Osteoblast behaviour on HA/PE composite surfaces with different HA volumes. *Biomaterials* 2002, 23, 101–107.

156. Dalby, M.J., Kayser, M.V., Bonfield, W., di Silvio, L. Initial attachment of osteoblasts to an optimised HAPEX™ topography. *Biomaterials* 2002, 23, 681–690.

157. Zhang, Y., Tanner, K.E., Gurav, N., di Silvio, L. *In vitro* osteoblastic response to 30 vol% hydroxyapatite-polyethylene composite. *J. Biomed. Mater. Res. A* 2007, 81A, 409–417.

158. Rea, S.M., Brooks, R.A., Schneider, A., Best, S.M., Bonfield, W. Osteoblast-like cell response to bioactive composites-surface-topography and composition effects. *J. Biomed. Mater. Res. B Appl. Biomater.* 2004, 70B, 250–261.

159. Salernitano, E., Migliaresi, C. Composite materials for biomedical applications: A review. *J. Appl. Biomater. Biomech.* 2003, 1, 3–18.

160. Pandey, A., Jan, E., Aswath, P.B. Physical and mechanical behavior of hot rolled HDPE/HA composites. *J. Mater. Sci.* 2006, 41, 3369–3376.

161. Bonner M., Ward IM., McGregor W., Tanner, K.E., Bonfield, W. Hydroxyapatite/polypropylene composite: A novel bone substitute material. *J. Mater. Sci. Lett.* 2001, 20, 2049–2052.

162. Suppakarn, N., Sanmaung, S., Ruksakulpiwa, Y., Sutapun, W. Effect of surface modification on properties of natural hydroxyapatite/polypropylene composites. *Key Eng. Mater.* 2008, 361–363, 511–514.

163. Younesi, M., Bahrololoom, M.E. Formulating the effects of applied temperature and pressure of hot pressing process on the mechanical properties of polypropylene-hydroxyapatite bio-composites by response surface methodology. *Mater. Des.* 2010, 31, 4621–4630.

164. Sousa, R.A., Reis, R.L., Cunha, A.M., Bevis, M.J. Processing and properties of bone-analogue biodegradable and bioinert polymeric composites. *Compos. Sci. Technol.* 2003, 63, 389–402.

165. Wang, M., Deb, S., Bonfield, W. Chemically coupled hydroxyapatite-polyethylene composites: Processing and characterisation. *Mater. Lett.* 2000, 44, 119–124.

166. Wang, M., Bonfield, W. Chemically coupled hydroxyapatite-polyethylene composites: Structure and properties. *Biomaterials* 2001, 22, 1311–1320.

167. Homaeigohar, S.S., Shokrgozar, M.A., Khavandi, A., Sadi, A.Y. *In vitro* biological evaluation of β-TCP/HDPE—A novel orthopedic composite: A survey using human osteoblast and fibroblast bone cells. *J. Biomed. Mater. Res. A* 2008, 84A, 491–499.

168. Downes, R.N., Vardy, S., Tanner, K.E., Bonfield, W. Hydroxyapatite-polyethylene composite in orbital surgery. *Bioceramics* 1991, 4, 239–246.

169. Dornhoffer, H.L. Hearing results with the dornhoffer ossicular replacement prostheses. *Laryngoscope* 1998, 108, 531–536.

170. Swain, R.E., Wang, M., Beale, B., Bonfield, W. HAPEX™ for otologic applications. *Biomed. Eng. Appl. Basis Commun.* 1999, 11, 315–320.

171. Yi, Z., Li, Y., Jidong, L., Xiang, Z., Hongbing, L., Yuanyuan, W., Weihu, Y. Novel biocomposite of hydroxyapatite reinforced polyamide and polyethylene: Composition and properties. *Mater. Sci. Eng. A* 2007, 452–453, 512–517.

172. Unwin, A.P., Ward, I, M., Ukleja, P., Weng, J. The role of pressure annealing in improving the stiffness of polyethylene/hydroxyapatite composites. *J. Mater. Sci.* 2001, 36, 3165–3177.

173. Fang, L.M., Leng, Y., Gao, P. Processing and mechanical properties of HA/UHMWPE nanocomposites. *Biomaterials* 2006, 27, 3701–3707.

174. Fang, L.M., Gao, P., Leng, Y. High strength and bioactive hydroxyapatite nano-particles reinforced ultrahigh molecular weight polyethylene. *Composites B* 2007, 38, 345–351.

175. Fang, L.M., Leng, Y., Gao, P. Processing of hydroxyapatite reinforced ultrahigh molecular weight polyethylene for biomedical applications. *Biomaterials* 2005, 26, 3471–3478.

176. Selvin, T.P., Seno, J., Murukan, B., Santhosh, A.A., Sabu, T., Weimin, Y., Sri, B. Poly(ethylene-*co*-vinyl acetate)/calcium phosphate nanocomposites: Thermo mechanical and gas permeability measurements. *Polym. Compos.* 2010, 31, 1011–1019.

177. Sousa, R.A., Reis, R.L., Cunha, A.M., Bevis, M.J. Structure development and interfacial interactions in high-density polyethylene/hydroxyapatite (HDPE/HA) composites molded with preferred orientation. *J. Appl. Polym. Sci.* 2002, 86, 2873–2886.

178. Reis, R.L., Cunha, A.M., Oliveira, M.J., Campos, A.R., Bevis, M.J. Relationship between processing and mechanical properties of injection molded high molecular mass polyethylene + hydroxyapatite composites. *Mater. Res. Inn.* 2001, 4, 263–272.

179. Donners, J.J.J.M., Nolte, R.J.M., Sommerdijk, N.A, J.M. Dendrimer-based hydroxyapatite composites with remarkable materials properties. *Adv. Mater.* 2003, 15, 313–316.

180. Schneider, O.D., Stepuk, A., Mohn, D., Luechinger, N.A., Feldman, K., Stark, W.J. Light-curable polymer/calcium phosphate nanocomposite glue for bone defect treatment. *Acta Biomater.* 2010, 6, 2704–2710.

181. Ignjatovic, N.L., Plavsic, M., Miljkovic, M.S., Zivkovic, L.M., Uskokovic, D.P. Microstructural characteristics of calcium hydroxyapatite/poly-L-lactide based composites. *J. Microsc.* 1999, 196, 243–248.

182. Skrtic, D., Antonucci, J.M., Eanes, E.D. Amorphous calcium phosphate-based bioactive polymeric composites for mineralized tissue regeneration. *J. Res. Natl. Inst. Stand. Technol.* 2003, 108, 167–182.

183. Rizzi, S.C., Heath, D.J., Coombes, A.G, A., Bock, N., Textor, M., Downes, S. Biodegradable polymer/hydroxyapatite composites: surface analysis and initial attachment of human osteoblasts. *J. Biomed. Mater. Res.* 2001, 55, 475–486.

184. Kato, K., Eika, Y., Ikada, Y. In situ hydroxyapatite crystallization for the formation of hydroxyapatite/polymer composites. *J. Mater. Sci.* 1997, 32, 5533–5543.

185. Navarro, M., Planell, J.A. Bioactive composites based on calcium phosphates for bone regeneration. *Key Eng. Mater.* 2010, 441, 203–233.

186. Zhang, R.Y., Ma, P.X. Porous poly(L-lactic acid)/apatite composites created by biomimetic process. *J. Biomed. Mater. Res.* 1999, 45, 285–293.
187. Liu, Q., de Wijn, J.R., van Blitterswijk, C.A. Composite biomaterials with chemical bonding between hydroxyapatite filler particles and PEG/PBT copolymer matrix. *J. Biomed. Mater. Res.* 1998, 40, 490–497.
188. Cerrai, P., Guerra, G.D., Tricoli, M., Krajewski, A., Ravaglioli, A., Martinetti, R., Dolcini, L. Fini, M., Scarano, A., Piattelli, A. Periodontal membranes from composites of hydroxyapatite and bioresorbable block copolymers. *J. Mater. Sci. Mater. Med.* 1999, 10, 677–682.
189. Roeder, R.K., Sproul, M.M., Turner, C.H. Hydroxyapatite whiskers provide improved mechanical properties in reinforced polymer composites. *J. Biomed. Mater. Res. A* 2003, 67A, 801–812.
190. Wagoner Johnson, A.J., Herschler, B.A. A review of the mechanical behavior of CaP and CaP/polymer composites for applications in bone replacement and repair. *Acta Biomater.* 2011, 7, 16–30.
191. Hutmacher, D.W. Scaffolds in tissue engineering bone and cartilage. *Biomaterials* 2000, 21, 2529–2543.
192. Mathieu, L.M., Bourban, P.E., Manson, J.A.E. Processing of homogeneous ceramic/polymer blends for bioresorbable composites. *Compos. Sci. Technol.* 2006, 66, 1606–1614.
193. Redepenning, J., Venkataraman, G., Chen, J., Stafford, N. Electrochemical preparation of chitosan/hydroxyapatite composite coatings on titanium substrates. *J. Biomed. Mater. Res. A* 2003, 66A, 411–416.
194. Rhee, S.H., Tanaka, J. Synthesis of a hydroxyapatite/collagen/chondroitin sulfate nanocomposite by a novel precipitation method. *J. Am. Ceram. Soc.* 2001, 84, 459–461.
195. Pezzotti, G., Asmus, S.M.F. Fracture behavior of hydroxyapatite/polymer interpenetrating network composites prepared by in situ polymerization process. *Mater. Sci. Eng. A* 2001, 316, 231–237.
196. Weickmann, H., Gurr, M., Meincke, O., Thomann, R., Mülhaupt, R. A versatile solvent-free "one-pot" route to polymer nanocomposites and the in situ formation of calcium phosphate/layered silicate hybrid nanoparticles. *Adv. Funct. Mater.* 2010, 20, 1778–1786.
197. Aryal, S., Bhattarai, S.R., Bahadur, K.C.R., Khil, M.S., Lee, D.R., Kim, H.Y. Carbon nanotubes assisted biomimetic synthesis of hydroxyapatite from simulated body fluid. *Mater. Sci. Eng. A* 2006, 426, 202–207.
198. Kealley, C., Ben-Nissan, B., van Riessen, A., Elcombe, M. Development of carbon nanotube reinforced hydroxyapatite bioceramics. *Key Eng. Mater.* 2006, 309–311, 597–600.
199. Kealley, C., Elcombe, M., van Riessen, A., Ben-Nissan, B. Development of carbon nanotube reinforced hydroxyapatite bioceramics. *Physica B* 2006, 385–386, 496–498.
200. Aryal, S., Bahadur, K.C.R., Dharmaraj, N., Kim, K.W., Kim, H.Y. Synthesis and characterization of hydroxyapatite using carbon nanotubes as a nano-matrix. *Scr. Mater.* 2006, 54, 131–135.
201. Rautaray, D., Mandal, S., Sastry, M. Synthesis of hydroxyapatite crystals using amino acid-capped gold nanoparticles as a scaffold. *Langmuir* 2005, 21, 5185–5191.
202. Wang, X.J., Li, Y., Wei, J., de Groot, K. Development of biomimetic nano-hydroxyapatite/poly(hexamethylene adipamide) composites. *Biomaterials* 2002, 23, 4787–4791.
203. Wei, J., Li, Y. Tissue engineering scaffold material of nano-apatite crystals and polyamide composite. *Eur. Polym. J.* 2004, 40, 509–515.
204. Memoto, R., Nakamura, S., Isobe, T., Senna, M. Direct synthesis of hydroxyapatite-silk fibroin nano-composite sol via a mechano-chemical route. *J. Sol Gel Sci. Technol.* 2001, 21, 7–12.

205. Fujiwara, M., Shiokawa, K., Morigaki, K., Tatsu, Y., Nakahara, Y. Calcium phosphate composite materials including inorganic powders, BSA or duplex DNA prepared by W/O/W interfacial reaction method. *Mater. Sci. Eng. C* 2008, 28, 280–288.

206. Nagata, F., Miyajima, T., Yokogawa, Y. A method to fabricate hydroxyapatite/poly(lactic acid) microspheres intended for biomedical application. *J. Eur. Ceram. Soc.* 2006, 26, 533–535.

207. Russias, J., Saiz, E., Nalla, R.K., Tomsia, A.P. Microspheres as building blocks for hydroxyapatite/polylactide biodegradable composites. *J. Mater. Sci.* 2006, 41, 5127–5133.

208. Khan, Y.M., Cushnie, E.K., Kelleher, J.K., Laurencin, C.T. *In situ* synthesized ceramic-polymer composites for bone tissue engineering: Bioactivity and degradation studies. *J. Mater. Sci.* 2007, 42, 4183–4190.

209. Kim, H.W., Knowles, J.C., Kim, H.E. Hydroxyapatite and gelatin composite foams processed via novel freeze-drying and crosslinking for use as temporary hard tissue scaffolds. *J. Biomed. Mater. Res. A* 2005, 72A, 136–145.

210. Sinha, A., Das, G., Sharma, B.K., Roy, R.P., Pramanick, A.K., Nayar, S. Poly(vinyl alcohol)-hydroxyapatite biomimetic scaffold for tissue regeneration. *Mater. Sci. Eng. C* 2007, 27, 70–74.

211. Sugawara, A., Yamane, S., Akiyoshi, K. Nanogel-templated mineralization: Polymer-calcium phosphate hybrid nanomaterials. *Macromol. Rapid Commun.* 2006, 27, 441–446.

212. Kickelbick, G. Concepts for the incorporation of inorganic building blocks into organic polymers on a nanoscale. *Prog. Polym. Sci.* 2003, 28, 83–114.

213. Liu, Q., de Wijn, J.R., van Blitterswijk, C.A. Nanoapatite/polymer composites: Mechanical and physicochemical characteristics. *Biomaterials* 1997, 18, 1263–1270.

214. Uskokovic, P.S., Tang, C.Y., Tsui, C.P., Ignjatovic, N., Uskokovic, D.P. Micromechanical properties of a hydroxyapatite/poly-L-lactide biocomposite using nanoindentation and modulus mapping. *J. Eur. Ceram. Soc.* 2007, 27, 1559–1564.

215. Todo, M., Kagawa, T. Improvement of fracture energy of HA/PLLA biocomposite material due to press processing. *J. Mater. Sci.* 2008, 43, 799–801.

216. Woo, K.M., Seo, J., Zhang, R.Y., Ma, P.X. Suppression of apoptosis by enhanced protein adsorption on polymer/hydroxyapatite composite scaffolds. *Biomaterials* 2007, 28, 2622–2630.

217. Ma, P.X., Zhang, R., Xiao, G., Franceschi, R. Engineering new bone tissue *in vitro* on highly porous poly(α-hydroxyl acids)/hydroxyapatite composite scaffolds. *J. Biomed. Mater. Res.* 2001, 54, 284–293.

218. Wang, M., Chen, L.J., Ni, J., Weng, J., Yue, C.Y. Manufacture and evaluation of bioactive and biodegradable materials and scaffolds for tissue engineering. *J. Mater. Sci. Mater. Med.* 2001, 12, 855–860.

219. Baji, A., Wong, S.C., Srivatsan, T.S., Njus, G.O., Mathur, G. Processing methodologies for polycaprolactone-hydroxyapatite composites: A review. *Mater. Manuf. Process.* 2006, 21, 211–218.

220. Wei, G., Ma, P.X. Macroporous and nanofibrous polymer scaffolds and polymer/bone-like apatite composite scaffolds generated by sugar spheres. *J. Biomed. Mater. Res. A* 2006, 78A, 306–315.

221. Guan, L., Davies, J.E. Preparation and characterization of a highly macroporous biodegradable composite tissue engineering scaffold. *J. Biomed. Mater. Res. A* 2004, 71A, 480–487.

222. Sun, F., Zhou, H., Lee, J. Various preparation methods of highly porous hydroxyapatite/polymer nanoscale biocomposites for bone regeneration. *Acta Biomater.* 2011, 7, 3813–3828.

223. Teng, X.R., Ren, J., Gu, S.Y. Preparation and characterization of porous PDLLA/HA composite foams by supercritical carbon dioxide technology. *J. Biomed. Mater. Res. B Appl. Biomater.* 2007, 81B, 185–193.

224. Ren, J., Zhao, P., Ren, T., Gu, S., Pan, K. Poly (D,L-lactide)/nano-hydroxyapatite composite scaffolds for bone tissue engineering and biocompatibility evaluation. *J. Mater. Sci. Mater. Med.* 2008, 19, 1075–1082.

225. Wang, M., Yue, C.Y., Chua, B. Production and evaluation of hydroxyapatite reinforced polysulfone for tissue replacement. *J. Mater. Sci. Mater. Med.* 2001, 12, 821–826.

226. Chlopek, J., Rosol, P., Morawska-Chochol, A. Durability of polymer-ceramics composite implants determined in creep tests. *Compos. Sci. Technol.* 2006, 66, 1615–1622.

227. Robinson, P., Wilson, C., Mecholsky, J. Processing and mechanical properties of hydroxyapatite-polysulfone laminated composites. *J. Eur. Ceram. Soc.* 2014, 34, 1387–1396.

228. You, C., Miyazaki, T., Ishida, E., Ashizuka, M., Ohtsuki, C., Tanihara, M. Fabrication of poly(vinyl alcohol)-apatite hybrids through biomimetic process. *J. Eur. Ceram. Soc.* 2007, 27, 1585–1588.

229. Xu, F., Li, Y., Yao, X., Liao, H., Zhang, L. Preparation and *in vivo* investigation of artificial cornea made of nano-hydroxyapatite/poly (vinyl alcohol) hydrogel composite. *J. Mater. Sci. Mater. Med.* 2007, 18, 635–640.

230. Xu, F., Li, Y., Deng, Y., Xiong, G. Porous nano-hydroxyapatite/poly(vinyl alcohol) composite hydrogel as artificial cornea fringe: Characterization and evaluation *in vitro*. *J. Biomater. Sci. Polym. Edn.* 2008, 19, 431–439.

231. Nayar, S., Pramanick, A.K., Sharma, B.K., Das, G., Kumar, B.R., Sinha, A. Biomimetically synthesized polymer-hydroxyapatite sheet like nano-composite. *J. Mater. Sci. Mater. Med.* 2008, 19, 301–304.

232. Poursamar, S.A., Orang, F., Bonakdar, S., Savar, M.K. Preparation and characterisation of poly vinyl alcohol/hydroxyapatite nanocomposite via in situ synthesis: A potential material as bone tissue engineering scaffolds. *Int. J. Nanomanuf.* 2010, 5, 330–334.

233. Guha, A., Nayar, S., Thatoi, H.N. Microwave irradiation enhances kinetics of the biomimetic process of hydroxyapatite nanocomposites. *Bioinspir. Biomim.* 2010, 5, 024001 (5 pages).

234. Bigi, A., Boanini, E., Gazzano, M., Rubini, K. Structural and morphological modifications of hydroxyapatite-polyaspartate composite crystals induced by heat treatment. *Cryst. Res. Technol.* 2005, 40, 1094–1098.

235. Bertoni, E., Bigi, A., Falini, G., Panzavolta, S., Roveri, N. Hydroxyapatite polyacrylic acid nanocrystals. *J. Mater. Chem.* 1999, 9, 779–782.

236. Qiu, H.J., Yang, J., Kodali, P., Koh, J., Ameer, G.A. A citric acid-based hydroxyapatite composite for orthopedic implants. *Biomaterials* 2006, 27, 5845–5854.

237. Greish, Y.E., Brown, P.W. Chemically formed HAp-Ca poly(vinyl phosphonate) composites. *Biomaterials* 2001, 22, 807–816.

238. Greish, Y.E., Brown, P.W. Preparation and characterization of calcium phosphate-poly(vinyl phosphonic acid) composites. *J. Mater. Sci. Mater. Med.* 2001, 12, 407–411.

239. Greish, Y.E., Brown, P.W. Formation and properties of hydroxyapatite-calcium poly(vinyl phosphonate) composites. *J. Am. Ceram. Soc.* 2002, 85, 1738–1744.

240. Nakahira, A., Tamai, M., Miki, S., Pezotti, G. Fracture behavior and biocompatibility evaluation of nylon-infiltrated porous hydroxyapatite. *J. Mater. Sci.* 2002, 37, 4425–4430.

241. Sailaja, G.S., Velayudhan, S., Sunny, M.C., Sreenivasan, K., Varma, H.K., Ramesh, P. Hydroxyapatite filled chitosan-polyacrylic acid polyelectrolyte complexes. *J. Mater. Sci.* 2003, 38, 3653–3662.

242. Zhang, H., Xu, J.J., Chen, H.Y. Electrochemically deposited 2D nanowalls of calcium phosphate-PDDA on a glassy carbon electrode and their applications in biosensing. *J. Phys. Chem. C* 2007, 111, 16564–16570.

243. Piticescu, R.M., Chitanu, G.C., Albulescu, M., Giurginca, M., Popescu, M.L., Łojkowski, W. Hybrid HAp-maleic anhydride copolymer nanocomposites obtained by in-situ functionalisation. *Solid State Phenomena* 2005, 106, 47–56.

244. Enlow, D., Rawal, A., Kanapathipillai, M., Schmidt-Rohr, K., Mallapragada, S., Lo, C.T., Thiyagarajan, P., Akin, M. Synthesis and characterization of self-assembled block copolymer templated calcium phosphate nanocomposite gels. *J. Mater. Chem.* 2007, 17, 1570–1578.

245. Kaito, T., Myoui, A., Takaoka, K., Saito, N., Nishikawa, M., Tamai, N., Ohgushi, H., Yoshikawa H. Potentiation of the activity of bone morphogenetic protein-2 in bone regeneration by a PLA-PEG/hydroxyapatite composite. *Biomaterials* 2005, 26, 73–79.

246. Fan, J.P., Tsui, C.P., Tang, C.Y., Chow, C.L. Modeling of the mechanical behavior of HA/PEEK biocomposite under quasi-static tensile load. *Biomaterials* 2004, 25, 5363–5373.

247. Abu Bakar, M.S., Cheng, M.H.W., Tang, S.M., Yu, S.C., Liao, K., Tan, C, T., Khor, K.A., Cheang, P. Tensile properties, tension-tension fatigue and biological response of polyetheretherketone-hydroxyapatite composites for load-bearing orthopedic implants. *Biomaterials* 2003, 24, 2245–2250.

248. Abu Bakar, M.S., Cheang, P., Khor, K.A. Mechanical properties of injection molded hydroxyapatite-polyetheretherketone biocomposites. *Compos. Sci. Technol.* 2003, 63, 421–425.

249. Abu Bakar, M.S., Cheang, P., Khor, K.A. Tensile properties and microstructural analysis of spheroidized hydroxyapatite-poly(etheretherketone) biocomposites. *Mater. Sci. Eng. A* 2003, 345, 55–63.

250. Fan, J.P., Tsui, C.P., Tang, C.Y. Modeling of the mechanical behavior of HA/PEEK biocomposite under quasi-static tensile load. *Mater. Sci. Eng. A* 2004, 382, 341–350.

251. Yu, S., Hariram, K.P., Kumar, R., Cheang, P., Aik, K.K. *In vitro* apatite formation and its growth kinetics on hydroxyapatite/polyetheretherketone biocomposites. *Biomaterials* 2005, 26, 2343–2352.

252. Gong, X.H., Tang, C.Y., Hu, H.C., Zhou, X.P. Improved mechanical properties of HIPS/hydroxyapatite composites by surface modification of hydroxyapatite via in situ polymerization of styrene. *J. Mater. Sci. Mater. Med.* 2004, 15, 1141–1146.

253. Wang, L., Weng, L., Song, S., Sun, Q. Mechanical properties and microstructure of polyetheretherketone-hydroxyapatite nanocomposite materials. *Mater. Lett.* 2010, 64, 2201–2204.

254. Laurencin, C.T., Attawia, M.A., Lu, L.Q., Borden, M.D., Lu, H.H., Gorum, W.J., Lieberman, J.R. Poly(lactide-*co*-glycolide)/hydroxyapatite delivery of BMP-2-producing cells: A regional gene therapy approach to bone regeneration. *Biomaterials* 2001, 22, 1271–1277.

255. Kim, S.S., Ahn, K.M., Park, M.S., Lee, J.H., Choi, C.Y., Kim, B.S. A poly(lactide-*co*-glycolide)/hydroxyapatite composite scaffold with enhanced osteoconductivity. *J. Biomed. Mater. Res. A* 2007, 80A, 206–215.

256. Oliveira, J., Miyazaki, T., Lopes, M., Ohtsuki, C., Santos, J. Bonelike®/PLGA hybrid materials for bone regeneration: Preparation route and physicochemical characterization. *J. Mater. Sci. Mater. Med.* 2005, 16, 253–259.

257. Kim, S., Kim, S.S., Lee, S.H., Ahn, S.E., Gwak, S.J., Song, J.H., Kim, B.S., Chung, H.M. *In vivo* bone formation from human embryonic stem cell-derived osteogenic cells in poly(D,L-lactic-*co*-glycolic acid)/hydroxyapatite composite scaffolds. *Biomaterials* 2008, 29, 1043–1053.

258. Petricca, S.E., Marra, K.G., Kumta, P.N. Chemical synthesis of poly(lactic-*co*-glycolic acid)/hydroxyapatite composites for orthopaedic applications. *Acta Biomater.* 2006, 2, 277–286.

259. Sato, M., Slamovich, E.B., Webster, T.J. Enhanced osteoblast adhesion on hydrothermally treated hydroxyapatite/titania/poly(lactide-*co*-glycolide) sol-gel titanium coatings. *Biomaterials* 2005, 26, 1349–1357.

260. Gu, S.Y., Zhan, H., Ren, J., Zhou, X.Y. Sol-gel synthesis and characterisation of nano-sized hydroxyapatite powders and hydroxyapatite/poly(D,L-lactide-*co*-glycolide) composite scaffolds. *Polymers & Polym. Compos.* 2007, 15, 137–144.

261. Aboudzadeh, N., Imani, M., Shokrgozar, M.A., Khavandi, A., Javadpour, J., Shafieyan, Y., Farokhi, M. Fabrication and characterization of poly(D,L-lactide-*co*-glycolide)/hydroxyapatite nanocomposite scaffolds for bone tissue regeneration. *J. Biomed. Mater. Res. A* 2010, 94A, 137–145.

262. Zhou, H., Lawrence, J.G., Bhaduri, S.B. Fabrication aspects of PLA-CaP/PLGA-CaP composites for orthopedic applications: A review. *Acta Biomater.* 2012, 8, 1999–2016.

263. Hoekstra, J.W.M., Ma, J., Plachokova, A.S., Bronkhorst, E.M., Bohner, M., Pan, J., Meijer, G.J., Jansen, J.A., van den Beucken, J.J.J.P. The *in vivo* performance of CaP/PLGA composites with varied PLGA microsphere sizes and inorganic compositions. *Acta Biomater.* 2013, 9, 7518–7526.

264. Dawes, E., Rushton, N. The effects of lactic acid on PGE2 production by macrophages and human synovial fibroblasts: A possible explanation for problems associated with the degradation of poly(lactide) implants? *Clin. Mater.* 1994, 17, 157–163.

265. Verheyen, C.C.P.M., Klein, C.P.A.T., de Blieck-Hogervorst, J.M.A., Wolke, J.G.C., de Wijin, J.R., van Blitterswijk, C.A., de Groot, K. Evaluation of hydroxylapatite poly(L-lactide) composites-physicochemical properties. *J. Mater. Sci. Mater. Med.* 1993, 4, 58–65.

266. Li, H., Chang, J. pH-compensation effect of bioactive inorganic fillers on the degradation of PLGA. *Compos. Sci. Technol.* 2005, 65, 2226–2232.

267. Agrawal, C.M., Athanasiou, K.A. Technique to control pH in vicinity of biodegrading PLA-PGA implants. *J. Biomed. Mater. Res. Appl. Biomater.* 1997, 38, 105–114.

268. Peter, S.J., Miller, S.T., Zhu, G., Yasko, A.W., Mikos, A.G. *In vivo* degradation of a poly(propylene fumarate)/β-tricalcium phosphate injectable composite scaffold. *J. Biomed. Mater. Res.* 1998, 41, 1–7.

269. Ara, M., Watanabe, M., Imai, Y. Effect of blending calcium compounds on hydrolitic degradation of poly(D,L-lactic acid-*co*-glycolic acid). *Biomaterials* 2002, 23, 2479–2483.

270. Linhart, W., Peters, F., Lehmann, W., Schwarz, K., Schilling, A., Amling, M., Rueger, J.M., Epple, M. Biologically and chemically optimized composites of carbonated apatite and polyglycolide as bone substitution materials. *J. Biomed. Mater. Res.* 2001, 54, 162–171.

271. Schiller, C., Epple, M. Carbonated apatites can be used as pH-stabilizing filler for biodegradable polyesters. *Biomaterials* 2003, 24, 2037–2043.

272. Schiller, C., Rasche, C., Wehmöller, M., Beckmann, F., Eufinger, H., Epple, M., Weihe, S. Geometrically structured implants for cranial reconstruction made of biodegradable polyesters and calcium phosphate/calcium carbonate. *Biomaterials* 2004, 25, 1239–1247.

273. Shikinami, Y., Okuno, M. Bioresorbable devices made of forged composites of hydroxyapatite (HA) particles and poly L-lactide (PLLA). Part II: Practical properties of miniscrews and miniplates. *Biomaterials* 2001, 22, 3197–3211.

274. Russias, J., Saiz, E., Nalla, R.K., Gryn, K., Ritchie, R.O., Tomsia, A.P. Fabrication and mechanical properties of PLA/HA composites: A study of *in vitro* degradation. *Mater. Sci. Eng. C* 2006, 26, 1289–1295.

275. Kim, H.W., Lee, H.H., Knowles, J.C. Electrospinning biomedical nanocomposite fibers of hydroxyapaite/poly(lactic acid) for bone regeneration. *J. Biomed. Mater. Res. A* 2006, 79A, 643–649.

276. Gross, K.A., Rodríguez-Lorenzo, L.M. Biodegradable composite scaffolds with an interconnected spherical network for bone tissue engineering. *Biomaterials* 2004, 25, 4955–4962.

277. Zhang, H., Chen, Z. Fabrication and characterization of electrospun PLGA/MWNTs/ hydroxyapatite biocomposite scaffolds for bone tissue engineering. *J. Bioact. Compat. Polym.* 2010, 25, 241–259.

278. Durucan, C., Brown, P.W. Low temperature formation of calcium-deficient hydroxyapatite-PLA/PLGA composites. *J. Biomed. Mater. Res.* 2000, 51, 717–725.

279. Durucan, C., Brown, P.W. Calcium-deficient hydroxyapatite-PLGA composites: Mechanical and microstructural investigation. *J. Biomed. Mater. Res.* 2000, 51, 726–734.

280. Ignjatovic, N., Suljovrujic, E., Biudinski-Simendic, J., Krakovsky, I., Uskokovic, D. Evaluation of hot-presses hydroxyapatite/poly-L-lactide composite biomaterial characteristics. *J. Biomed. Mater. Res. B Appl. Biomater.* 2004, 71B, 284–294.

281. Nazhat, S.N., Kellomäki, M., Törmälä, P., Tanner, K.E., Bonfield, W. Dynamic mechanical characterization of biodegradable composites of hydroxyapatite and polylactides. *J. Biomed. Mater. Res.* 2001, 58, 335–343.

282. Hasegawa, S., Tamura, J., Neo, M., Goto, K., Shikinami, Y., Saito, M., Kita, M., Nakamura, T. *In vivo* evaluation of a porous hydroxyapatite/poly-D,L-lactide composite for use as a bone substitute. *J. Biomed. Mater. Res. A* 2005, 75A, 567–579.

283. Hasegawa, S., Neo, M., Tamura, J., Fujibayashi, S., Takemoto, M., Shikinami, Y., Okazaki, K., Nakamura, T. *In vivo* evaluation of a porous hydroxyapatite/poly-D,L-lactide composite for bone tissue engineering. *J. Biomed. Mater. Res. A* 2007, 81A, 930–938.

284. Reis, R.L., Cunha, A.M. New degradable load-bearing biomaterials composed of reinforced starch based blends. *J. Appl. Med. Polym.* 2000, 4, 1–5.

285. Sousa, R.A., Mano, J.F., Reis, R.L., Cunha, A.M., Bevis, M.J. Mechanical performance of starch based bioactive composites moulded with preferred orientation for potential medical applications. *Polym. Eng. Sci.* 2002, 42, 1032–1045.

286. Marques, A.P., Reis, R.L. Hydroxyapatite reinforcement of different starch-based polymers affects osteoblast-like cells adhesion/spreading and proliferation. *Mater. Sci. Eng. C* 2005, 25, 215–229.

287. Reis, R.L., Cunha, A.M., Allan, P.S., Bevis, M.J. Structure development and control of injection-molded hydroxylapatite-reinforced starch/EVOH composites. *J. Polym. Adv. Tech.* 1997, 16, 263–277.

288. Vaz, C.M., Reis, R.L., Cunha, A.M. Use of coupling agents to enhance the interfacial interactions in starch-EVOH/hydroxylapatite composites. *Biomaterials* 2002, 23, 629–635.

289. Leonor, I.B., Ito, A., Onuma, K., Kanzaki, N., Reis, R.L. *In vitro* bioactivity of starch thermoplastic/hydroxyapatite composite biomaterials: An in situ study using atomic force microscopy. *Biomaterials* 2003, 24, 579–585.

290. Vaz, C.M., Reis, R.L., Cunha, A.M. Degradation model of starch-EVOH+HA composites. *Mater. Res. Innovat.* 2001, 4, 375–380.

291. Boeree, N., Dove, J., Cooper, J.J., Knowles, J.C., Hastings, G.W. Development of a degradable composite for orthopaedic use – Mechanical evaluation of an hydroxyapatite-polyhydroxybutyrate composite materials. *Biomaterials* 1993, 14, 793–796.

292. Doyle, C., Tanner, E.T., Bonfield, W. *In vitro* and *in vivo* evaluation of polyhydroxybutyrate and of polyhydroxybutyrate reinforced with hydroxyapatite. *Biomaterials* 1991, 12, 841–847.

293. Ni, J., Wang, M. *In vitro* evaluation of hydroxyapatite reinforced polyhydroxybutyrate composite. *Mater. Sci. Eng. C* 2002, 20, 101–109.

294. Knowles, J.C., Hastings, G.W., Ohta, H., Niwa, S., Boeree, N. Development of a degradable composite for orthopedic use – *In vivo* biomechanical and histological evaluation of two bioactive degradable composites based on the polyhydroxybutyrate polymer. *Biomaterials* 1992, 13, 491–496.

295. Luklinska, Z.B., Bonfield, W. Morphology and ultrastructure of the interface between hydroxyapatite-polybutyrate composite implant and bone. *J. Mater. Sci. Mater. Med.* 1997, 8, 379–383.

296. Reis, E.C.C., Borges, A.P.B., Fonseca, C.C., Martinez, M.M.M., Eleotério, R.B., Morato, G.O., Oliveira, P.M. Biocompatibility, osteointegration, osteoconduction, and biodegradation of a hydroxyapatite-polyhydroxybutyrate composite. *Braz. Arch. Biol. Technol.* 2010, 53, 817–826.

297. Chen, D.Z., Tang, C.Y., Chan, K.C., Tsui, C.P., Yu, P.H.F., Leung, M.C.P., Uskokovic, P.S. Dynamic mechanical properties and *in vitro* bioactivity of PHBHV/HA nanocomposite. *Compos. Sci. Technol.* 2007, 67, 1617–1626.

298. Rai, B., Noohom, W., Kithva, P.H., Grøndahl, L., Trau, M. Bionanohydroxyapatite/poly(3-hydroxybutyrate-*co*-3-hydroxyvalerate) composites with improved particle dispersion and superior mechanical properties. *Chem. Mater.* 2008, 20, 2802–2808.

299. Wang, Y.W., Wu, Q., Chen, J., Chen, G.Q. Evaluation of three-dimensional scaffolds made of blends of hydroxyapatite and poly(3-hydroxybutyrate-*co*-3-hydroxyhexanoate) for bone reconstruction. *Biomaterials* 2005, 26, 899–904.

300. Linhart, W., Lehmann, W., Siedler, M., Peters, F., Schilling, A.F., Schwarz, K., Amling, M., Rueger, J.M., Epple, M. Composites of amorphous calcium phosphate and poly(hydroxybutyrate) and poly(hydroxybutyrate-*co*-hydroxyvalerate) for bone substitution: assessment of the biocompatibility. *J. Mater. Sci.* 2006, 41, 4806–4813.

301. Azevedo, M., Reis, R.L., Claase, M., Grijpma, D., Feijen, J. Development and properties of polycaprolactone/hydroxyapatite composite biomaterials. *J. Mater. Sci. Mater. Med.* 2003, 14, 103–107.

302. Choi, D., Marra, K.G., Kumta, P.N. Chemical synthesis of hydroxyapatite/poly(ε-caprolactone) composites. *Mater. Res. Bull.* 2004, 39, 417–432.

303. Hao, J., Yuan, M., Deng, X. Biodegradable and biocompatible nanocomposites of poly(ε-caprolactone) with hydroxyapatite nanocrystals: Thermal and mechanical properties. *J. Appl. Polym. Sci.* 2003, 86, 676–683.

304. Walsh, D., Furuzono, T., Tanaka, J. Preparation of porous composite implant materials by *in situ* polymerization of porous apatite containing ε-caprolactone or methyl methacrylate. *Biomaterials* 2001, 22, 1205–1212.

305. Verma, D., Katti, K., Katti, D. Bioactivity in in situ hydroxyapatite-polycaprolactone composites. *J. Biomed. Mater. Res. A* 2006, 78A, 772–780.

306. Kim, H.W. Biomedical nanocomposites of hydroxyapatite/polycaprolactone obtained by surfactant mediation. *J. Biomed. Mater. Res. A* 2007, 83A, 169–177.

307. Guerra, G.D., Cerrai, P., Tricoli, M., Krajewski, A., Ravaglioli, A., Mazzocchi, M., Barbani, N. Composites between hydroxyapatite and poly(ε-caprolactone) synthesized in open system at room temperature. *J. Mater. Sci. Mater. Med.* 2006, 17, 69–79.

308. Bianco, A., di Federico, E., Moscatelli, I., Camaioni, A., Armentano, I., Campagnolo, L., Dottori, M., Kenny, J.M., Siracusa, G., Gusmano, G. Electrospun poly(ε-caprolactone)/Ca-deficient hydroxyapatite nanohybrids: Microstructure, mechanical properties and cell response by murine embryonic stem cells. *Mater. Sci. Eng. C.* 2009, 29, 2063–2071.

309. Heo, S.J., Kim, S.E., Wei, J., Hyun, Y.T., Yun, H.S., Kim, D.H., Shin, J.W., Shin, J.W. Fabrication and characterization of novel nano- and micro-HA/PCL composite scaffolds using a modified rapid prototyping process. *J. Biomed. Mater. Res. A* 2009, 89A, 108–116.

310. Chuenjitkuntaworn, B., Inrung, W., Damrongsri, D., Mekaapiruk, K., Supaphol, P., Pavasant, P. Polycaprolactone/hydroxyapatite composite scaffolds: Preparation, characterization, and *in vitro* and *in vivo* biological responses of human primary bone cells. *J. Biomed. Mater. Res. A* 2010, 94A, 241–251.

311. di Foggia, M., Corda, U., Plescia, E., Taddei, P., Torreggiani, A. Effects of sterilisation by high-energy radiation on biomedical poly-(ε-caprolactone)/hydroxyapatite composites. *J. Mater. Sci. Mater. Med.* 2010, 21, 1789–1797.

312. Lebourg, M., Antón, J.S., Ribelles, J.L.G. Hybrid structure in PCL-HAp scaffold resulting from biomimetic apatite growth. *J. Mater. Sci. Mater. Med.* 2010, 21, 33–44.

313. Makarov, C., Gotman, I., Jiang, X., Fuchs, S., Kirkpatrick, C.J., Gutmanas, E.Y. *In situ* synthesis of calcium phosphate-polycaprolactone nanocomposites with high ceramic volume fractions. *J. Mater. Sci. Mater. Med.* 2010, 21, 1771–1779.

314. Causa, F., Netti, P.A., Ambrosio, L., Ciapetti, G., Baldini, N., Pagani, S., Martini, D., Giunti, A. Poly-ε-caprolactone/hydroxyapatite composites for bone regeneration: *In vitro* characterization and human osteoblast response. *J. Biomed. Mater. Res. A* 2006, 76A, 151–162.

315. Thomas, V., Jagani, S., Johnson, K., Jose, M.V., Dean, D.R., Vohra, Y.K., Nyairo, E. Electrospun bioactive nanocomposite scaffolds of polycaprolactone and nanohydroxyapatite for bone tissue engineering. *J. Nanosci. Nanotechol.* 2006, 6, 487–493.

316. Dunn, A., Campbell, P., Marra, K.G. The influence of polymer blend composition on the degradation of polymer/hydroxyapatite biomaterials. *J. Mater. Sci. Mater. Med.* 2001, 12, 673–677.

317. Calandrelli, L., Immirzi, B., Malinconico, M., Volpe, M., Oliva, A., Ragione, F. Preparation and characterization of composites based on biodegradable polymers for *in vivo* application. *Polymer* 2000, 41, 8027–8033.

318. Chen, B., Sun, K. Poly(ε-caprolactone)/hydroxyapatite composites: Effects of particle size, molecular weight distribution and irradiation on interfacial interaction and properties. *Polym. Test.* 2005, 24, 64–70.

319. Ural, E., Kesenci, K., Fambri, L., Migliaresi, C., Piskin, E. Poly(D,L-lactide/ε-caprolactone)/hydroxyapatite composites. *Biomaterials* 2000, 21, 2147–2154.

320. Takayama, T., Todo, M. Improvement of fracture properties of hydroxyapatite particle filled poly(L-lactide)/poly(ε-caprolactone) biocomposites using lysine tri-isocyanate. *J. Mater. Sci.* 2010, 45, 6266–6270.

321. Shokrollahi, P., Mirzadeh, H., Scherman, O.A., Huck, W.T.S. Biological and mechanical properties of novel composites based on supramolecular polycaprolactone and functionalized hydroxyapatite. *J. Biomed. Mater. Res. A* 2010, 95A, 209–221.

322. Yoon, B.H., Kim, H.W., Lee, S.H., Bae, C.J., Koh, Y.H., Kong, Y.M., Kim, H.E. Stability and cellular responses to fluorapatite-collagen composites. *Biomaterials* 2005, 26, 2957–2963.

323. Kim, H.W., Lee, E.J., Kim, H.E., Salih, V., Knowles, J.C. Effect of fluoridation of hydroxyapatite in hydroxyapatite/polycaprolactone composites on osteoblast activity. *Biomaterials* 2005, 26, 4395–4404.

324. Busch, S., Dolhaine, H., DuChesne, A., Heinz, S., Hochrein, O., Laeri, F., Podebrad, O., Vietze, U., Weiland, T., Kniep R. Biomimetic morphogenesis of fluorapatite-gelatin composites: Fractal growth, the question of intrinsic electric fields, core/shell assemblies, hollow spheres and reorganization of denatured collagen. *Eur. J. Inorg. Chem.* 1999, 1999, 1643–1653.

325. Busch, S., Schwarz, U., Kniep, R. Chemical and structural investigations of biomimetically grown fluorapatite-gelatin composite aggregates. *Adv. Funct. Mater.* 2003, 13, 189–198.

326. Simon, P., Carrillo-Cabrera, W., Formanek, P., Göbel, C., Geiger, D., Ramlau, R., Tlatlik, H., Buder, J., Kniep, R. On the real-structure of biomimetically grown hexagonal pristamic seed of fluoroapatite-gelatin-composites: TEM investigations along [001]. *J. Mater. Chem.* 2004, 14, 2218–2224.

327. Göbel, C., Simon, P., Buder, J., Tlatlik, H., Kniep, R. Phase formation and morphology of calcium phosphate-gelatin-composites grown by double diffusion technique: The influence of fluoride. *J. Mater. Chem.* 2004, 14, 2225–2230.

328. Simon, P., Schwarz, U., Kniep, R. Hierarchical architecture and real structure in a biomimetic nano-composite of fluorapatite with gelatine: A model system for steps in dentino- and osteogenesis? *J. Mater. Chem.* 2005, 15, 4992–4996.

329. Tlatlik, H., Simon, P., Kawska, A., Zahn, D., Kniep, R. Biomimetic fluorapatite-gelatin nanocomposites: pre-structuring of gelatin matrices by ion impregnation and its effect on form development. *Angew. Chem. Int. Ed. Engl.* 2006, 45, 1905–1910.
330. Simon, P., Zahn, D., Lichte, H., Kniep, R. Intrinsic electric dipole fields and the induction of hierarchical form developments in fluorapatite-gelatin nanocomposites: A general principle for morphogenesis of biominerals? *Angew. Chem. Int. Ed. Engl.* 2006, 45, 1911–1915.
331. Kniep, R., Simon, P. Fluorapatite-gelatin-nanocomposites: Self-organized morphogenesis, real structure and relations to natural hard materials. In: *Biomineralization I, Crystallization and Self-Organization Process*, Naka, K. (Ed.); *Topics in Current Chemistry,* Springer: Berlin, Germany, 2007; Vol. 270, pp. 73–125.
332. Kniep, R., Simon, P. "Hidden" hierarchy of microfibrils within 3D-periodic fluorapatite-gelatin nanocomposites: Development of complexity and form in a biomimetic system. *Angew. Chem. Int. Ed. Engl.* 2008, 47, 1405–1409.
333. Brickmann, J., Paparcone, R., Kokolakis, S., Zahn, D., Duchstein, P., Carrillo-Cabrera, W., Simon, P., Kniep, R. Fluorapatite-gelatine nanocomposite superstructures: new insights into a biomimetic system of high complexity. *Chem. Phys. Chem.* 2010, 11, 1851–1853.
334. Handschel, J., Wiesmann, H.P., Stratmann, U., Kleinheinz, J., Meyer, U., Joos, U. TCP is hardly resorbed and not osteoconductive in a non-loading calvarial model. *Biomaterials* 2002, 23, 1689–1695.
335. Wang, M., Wang, J., Ni, J. Developing tricalcium phosphate/polyhydroxybutyrate composite as a new biodegradable material for clinical applications. *Biomechanics* 2000, 192, 741–744.
336. Kikuchi, M., Koyama, Y., Takakuda, K., Miyairi, H., Shirahama, N., Tanaka, J. *In vitro* change in mechanical strength of β-tricalcium phosphate/copolymerized poly-L-lactide composites and their application for guided bone regeneration. *J. Biomed. Mater. Res.* 2002, 62, 265–272.
337. Ignatius, A.A., Augat, P., Claes, L.E. Degradation behaviour of composite pins made of tricalcium phosphate and poly(L, D,L-lactide). *J. Biomater. Sci. Polym. Edn.* 2001, 12, 185–194.
338. Ignatius, A.A., Wolf, S., Augat, P., Claes, L.E. Composites made of rapidly resorbable ceramics and poly(lactide) show adequate mechanical properties for use as bone substitute materials. *J. Biomed. Mater. Res.* 2001, 57, 126–131.
339. Kikuchi, M., Tanaka, J. Chemical interaction in β-tricalcium phosphate/copolymerized poly-L-lactide composites. *J. Ceram. Soc. Jpn.* 2000, 108, 642–645.
340. Aunoble, S., Clement, D., Frayssinet, P., Harmand, MF., le Huec, J.C. Biological performance of a new β-TCP/PLLA composite material for applications in spine surgery: *In vitro* and *in vivo* studies. *J. Biomed. Mater. Res. A* 2006, 78A, 416–422.
341. Haaparanta, A.M., Haimi, S., Ellä, V., Hopper, N., Miettinen, S., Suuronen, R., Kellomäki, M. Porous polylactide/β-tricalcium phosphate composite scaffolds for tissue engineering applications. *J. Tissue Eng. Regen. Med.* 2010, 4, 366–373.
342. Chen, T.M., Yao, C.H., Wang, H.J., Chou, G.H., Lee, T.W., Lin, F.H. Evaluation of a novel malleable, biodegradable osteoconductive composite in a rabbit cranial defect model. *Mater. Chem. Phys.* 1998, 55, 44–50.
343. Dong, G.C., Chen, H.M., Yao, C.H. A novel bone substitute composite composed of tricalcium phosphate, gelatin and drynaria fortunei herbal extract. *J. Biomed. Mater. Res. A* 2008, 84A, 167–177.
344. Ji, J., Yuan, X., Xia, Z., Liu, P., Chen, J. Porous β-tricalcium phosphate composite scaffold reinforced by K₂HPO₄ and gelatin. *Key Eng. Mater.* 2010, 434–435, 620–623.
345. Yao, C.H., Liu, B.S., Hsu, S.H., Chen, Y.S., Tsai, C.C. Biocompatibility and biodegradation of a bone composite containing tricalcium phosphate and genipin crosslinked gelatin. *J. Biomed. Mater. Res. A* 2004, 69A, 709–717.

346. Eslaminejad, M.B., Mirzadeh, H., Mohamadi, Y., Nickmahzar, A. Bone differentiation of marrow-derived mesenchymal stem cells using β-tricalcium phosphate-alginate-gelatin hybrid scaffolds. *J. Tissue Eng. Regen. Med.* 2007, 1, 417–424.

347. Takahashi, Y., Yamamoto, M., Tabata, Y. Osteogenic differentiation of mesenchymal stem cells in biodegradable sponges composed of gelatin and β-tricalcium phosphate. *Biomaterials* 2005, 26, 3587–3596.

348. Bigi, A., Cantelli, I., Panzavolta, S., Rubini, K. α-tricalcium phosphate-gelatin composite cements. *J. Appl. Biomater. Biomech.* 2004, 2, 81–87.

349. Yang, S.H., Hsu, C.K., Wang, K.C., Hou, S.M., Lin, F.H. Tricalcium phosphate and glutaraldehyde crosslinked gelatin incorporating bone morphogenetic protein—A viable scaffold for bone tissue engineering. *J. Biomed. Mater. Res. B Appl. Biomater.* 2005, 74B, 468–475.

350. Kato, M., Namikawa, T., Terai, H., Hoshino, M., Miyamoto, S., Takaoka, K. Ectopic bone formation in mice associated with a lactic acid/dioxanone/ethylene glycol copolymer-tricalcium phosphate composite with added recombinant human bone morphogenetic protein-2. *Biomaterials* 2006, 27, 3927–3933.

351. Muramatsu, K., Oba, K., Mukai, D., Hasegawa, K., Masuda, S., Yoshihara, Y. Subacute systemic toxicity assessment of β-tricalcium phosphate/carboxymethyl-chitin composite implanted in rat femur. *J. Mater. Sci. Mater. Med.* 2007, 18, 513–522.

352. Panzavolta, S., Fini, M., Nicoletti, A., Bracci, B., Rubini, K., Giardino, R., Bigi, A. Porous composite scaffolds based on gelatin and partially hydrolyzed α-tricalcium phosphate. *Acta Biomater.* 2009, 5, 636–643.

353. Uchino, T., Kamitakahara, M., Otsuka, M., Ohtsuki, C. Hydroxyapatite-forming capability and mechanical properties of organic-inorganic hybrids and α-tricalcium phosphate porous bodies. *J. Ceram. Soc. Jpn.* 2010, 118, 57–61.

354. Boguń, M., Rabiej, S. The influence of fiber formation conditions on the structure and properties of nanocomposite alginate fibers containing tricalcium phosphate or montmorillonite. *Polym. Compos.* 2010, 31, 1321–1331.

355. Bleach, N.C., Tanner, K.E., Kellomäki, M., Törmälä, P. Effect of filler type on the mechanical properties of self-reinforced polylactide-calcium phosphate composites. *J. Mater. Sci. Mater. Med.* 2001, 12, 911–915.

356. Liu, L., Xiong, Z., Yan, Y.N., Hu, Y.Y., Zhang, R.J., Wang, S.G. Porous morphology, porosity, mechanical properties of poly(α-hydroxy acid)-tricalcium phosphate composite scaffolds fabricated by low-temperature deposition. *J. Biomed. Mater. Res. A* 2007, 82A, 618–629.

357. Zhang, Y., Zhang, M.Q. Synthesis and characterization of macroporous chitosan/calcium phosphate composite scaffolds for tissue engineering. *J. Biomed. Mater. Res.* 2001, 55, 304–312.

358. Rai, B., Teoh, S.H., Hutmacher, D.W., Cao, T., Ho, K.H. Novel PCL-based honeycomb scaffolds as drug delivery systems for rhBMP-2. *Biomaterials* 2005, 26, 3739–3748.

359. Rai, B., Teoh, S.H., Ho, K.H., Hutmacher, D.W., Cao, T., Chen, F., Yacob, K. The effect of rhBMP-2 on canine osteoblasts seeded onto 3D bioactive polycaprolactone scaffolds. *Biomaterials* 2004, 25, 5499–5506.

360. Lei, Y., Rai, B., Ho, K.H., Teoh, S.H. *In vitro* degradation of novel bioactive polycaprolactone – 20% tricalcium phosphate composite scaffolds for bone engineering. *Mater. Sci. Eng. C* 2007, 27, 293–298.

361. Miyai, T., Ito, A., Tamazawa, G., Matsuno, T., Sogo, Y., Nakamura, C., Yamazaki, A., Satoh, T. Antibiotic-loaded poly-ε-caprolactone and porous β-tricalcium phosphate composite for treating osteomyelitis. *Biomaterials* 2008, 29, 350–358.

362. Takahashi, Y., Yamamoto, M., Tabata, Y. Enhanced osteoinduction by controlled release of bone morphogenetic protein-2 from biodegradable sponge composed of gelatin and β-tricalcium phosphate. *Biomaterials* 2005, 26, 4856–4865.

363. Ignatius, A.A., Betz, O., Augat, P., Claes, L.E. *In vivo* investigations on composites made of resorbable ceramics and poly(lactide) used as bone graft substitutes. *J. Biomed. Mater. Res. Appl. Biomater.* 2001, 58, 701–709.

364. Miao, X., Lim, W.K., Huang, X., Chen, Y. Preparation and characterization of interpenetrating phased TCP/HA/PLGA composites. *Mater. Lett.* 2005, 59, 4000–4005.

365. Brodie, J.C., Goldie, E., Connel, G., Merry, J., Grant, M.H. Osteoblast interactions with calcium phosphate ceramics modified by coating with type I collagen. *J. Biomed. Mater. Res. A* 2005, 73A, 409–421.

366. Zhang, L.F., Sun, R., Xu, L., Du, J., Xiong, Z.C., Chen, H.C., Xiong, C.D. Hydrophilic poly (ethylene glycol) coating on PDLLA/BCP bone scaffold for drug delivery and cell culture. *Mater. Sci. Eng. C* 2008, 28, 141–149.

367. Ignjatovic, N., Ninkov, P., Ajdukovic, Z., Konstantinovic, V., Uskokovic, D. Biphasic calcium phosphate/poly-(D,L-lactide-*co*-glycolide) biocomposite as filler and blocks for reparation of bone tissue. *Mater. Sci. Forum* 2005, 494, 519–524.

368. Ignjatovic, N., Ninkov, P., Ajdukovic, Z., Vasiljevic-Radovic, D., Uskokovic, D. Biphasic calcium phosphate coated with poly-D,L-lactide-*co*-glycolide biomaterial as a bone substitute. *J. Eur. Ceram. Soc.* 2007, 27, 1589–1594.

369. Yang, W., Yin, G., Zhou, D., Gu, J., Li, Y. *In vitro* characteristics of surface-modified biphasic calcium phosphate/poly(L-Lactide) biocomposite. *Adv. Eng. Mater.* 2010, 12, B128-B132.

370. Ignjatovic, N., Ninkov, P., Kojic, V., Bokurov, M., Srdic, V., Krnojelac, D., Selakovic, S., Uskokovic, D. Cytotoxicity and fibroblast properties during *in vitro* test of biphasic calcium phosphate/poly-D,L-lactide-*co*-glycolide biocomposites and different phosphate materials. *Microsc. Res. Techniq.* 2006, 69, 976–982.

371. Ajdukovic, Z., Ignjatovic, N., Petrovic, D., Uskokovic, D. Substitution of osteoporotic alveolar bone by biphasic calcium phosphate/poly-D,L-lactide-*co*-glycolide biomaterials. *J. Biomater. Appl.* 2007, 21, 317–328.

372. Kim, H.W., Knowles, J.C., Kim, H.E. Effect of biphasic calcium phosphates on drug release and biological and mechanical properties of poly(ε-caprolactone) composite membranes. *J. Biomed. Mater. Res. A* 2004, 70A, 467–479.

373. Bakhtiari, L., Rezai, H.R., Hosseinalipour, S.M., Shokrgozar, M.A. Investigation of biphasic calcium phosphate/gelatin nanocomposite scaffolds as a bone tissue engineering. *Ceram. Int.* 2010, 36, 2421–2426.

374. Bakhtiari, L., Rezai, H.R., Hosseinalipour, S.M., Shokrgozar, M.A. Preparation of porous biphasic calcium phosphate-gelatin nanocomposite for bone tissue engineering. *J. Nano Res.* 2010, 11, 67–72.

375. Matsuda, A., Ikoma, T., Kobayashi, H., Tanaka, J. Preparation and mechanical property of core-shell type chitosan/calcium phosphate composite fiber. *Mater. Sci. Eng. C* 2004, 24, 723–728.

376. Rattanachan, S., Lorprayoon, C., Boonphayak, P. Synthesis of chitosan/brushite powders for bone cement composites. *J. Ceram. Soc. Jpn.* 2008, 116, 36–41.

377. Ohsawa, H., Ito, A., Sogo, Y., Yamazaki, A., Ohno, T. Synthesis of albumin/DCP nanocomposite particles. *Key Eng. Mater.* 2007, 330–332, 239–242.

378. Xu, H.H.K., Sun, L., Weir, M.D., Antonucci, J.M., Takagi, S., Chow, L.C., Peltz, M. Nano DCPA-whisker composites with high strength and Ca and PO_4 release. *J. Dent. Res.* 2006, 85, 722–727.

379. Xu, H.H.K., Weir, M.D., Sun, L., Takagi, S., Chow, L.C. Effects of calcium phosphate nanoparticles on Ca-PO_4 composite. *J. Dent. Res.* 2007, 86, 378–383.

380. Xu, H.H.K., Weir, M.D., Sun, L. Nanocomposites with Ca and PO_4 release: Effects of reinforcement, dicalcium phosphate particle size and silanization. *Dent. Mater.* 2007, 23, 1482–1491.

381. Tortet, L., Gavarri, J.R., Nihoul, G., Dianoux, A.J. Proton mobilities in brushite and brushite/polymer composites. *Solid State Ionics* 1997, 97, 253–256.
382. Tortet, L., Gavarri, J.R., Musso, J., Nihoul, G., Sarychev, A.K. Percolation and modeling of proton conduction in polymer/brushite composites. *J. Solid State Chem.* 1998, 141, 392–403.
383. Dorozhkin, S.V. Amorphous calcium orthophosphates: Nature, chemistry and biomedical applications. *Int. J. Mater. Chem.* 2012, 2, 19–46.
384. Dorozhkin, S.V. Calcium orthophosphates in dentistry. *J. Mater. Sci. Mater. Med.* 2013, 24, 1335–1363.
385. Gutierrez, M.C., Jobbágy, M., Ferrer, M.L., del Monte, F. Enzymatic synthesis of amorphous calcium phosphate-chitosan nanocomposites and their processing into hierarchical structures. *Chem. Mater.* 2008, 20, 11–13.
386. Hakimimehr, D., Liu, D.M., Troczynski, T. In-situ preparation of poly(propylene fumarate) – hydroxyapatite composite. *Biomaterials* 2005, 26, 7297–7303.
387. Perkin, K.K., Turner, J.L., Wooley, K.L., Mann, S. Fabrication of hybrid nanocapsules by calcium phosphate mineralization of shell cross-linked polymer micelles and nanocages. *Nano Lett.* 2005, 5, 1457–1461.
388. Wang, K.W., Zhu, Y.J., Chen, F., Cao, S.W. Calcium phosphate/block copolymer hybrid porous nanospheres: Preparation and application in drug delivery. *Mater. Lett.* 2010, 64, 2299–2301.
389. Jacoveila, P.F. Use of calcium hydroxylapatite (Radiesse®) for facial augmentation. *Clin. Interv. Aging* 2008, 3, 161–174.
390. Lizzul, P.F., Narurkar, V.A. The role of calcium hydroxylapatite (Radiesse®) in nonsurgical aesthetic rejuvenation. *J. Drugs Dermatol.* 2010, 9, 446–450.
391. Klesing, J., Chernousova, S., Kovtun, A., Neumann, S., Ruiz, L., Gonzalez-Calbet, J.M., Vallet-Regi, M., Heumann, R., Epple, M. An injectable paste of calcium phosphate nanorods, functionalized with nucleic acids, for cell transfection and gene silencing. *J. Mater. Chem.* 2010, 20, 6144–6148.
392. Low, K.L., Tan, S.H., Zein, S.H.S., Roether, J.A., Mouriño, V., Boccaccini, A.R. Calcium phosphate-based composites as injectable bone substitute materials. *J. Biomed. Mater. Res. B Appl. Biomater.* 2010, 94B, 273–286.
393. Weiss, P., Gauthier, O., Bouler, J.M., Grimandi, G., Daculsi, G. Injectable bone substitute using a hydrophilic polymer. *Bone* 1999, 25, Suppl. 2, 67S–70S.
394. Daculsi, G., Weiss, P., Bouler, J.M., Gauthier, O., Millot, F., Aguado, E. Biphasic calcium phosphate/hydrosoluble polymer composites: A new concept for bone and dental substitution biomaterials. *Bone* 1999, 25, Suppl. 2, 59S–61S.
395. Turczyn, R., Weiss, P., Lapkowski, M., Daculsi, G. In situ self-hardening bioactive composite for bone and dental surgery. *J. Biomater. Sci. Polym. Edn.* 2000, 11, 217–223.
396. Bennett, S., Connolly, K., Lee, D.R., Jiang, Y., Buck, D., Hollinger, J.O., Gruskin, E.A. Initial biocompatibility studies of a novel degradable polymeric bone substitute that hardens in situ. *Bone* 1996, 19, 101S–107S.
397. Liu, X., Okada, M., Maeda, H., Fujii, S., Furuzono, T. Hydroxyapatite/biodegradable poly(L-lactide-*co*-ε-caprolactone) composite microparticles as injectable scaffolds by a Pickering emulsion route. *Acta Biomater.* 2011, 7, 821–828.
398. Daculsi, G., Rohanizadeh, R., Weiss, P., Bouler, J.M. Crystal polymer interaction with new injectable bone substitute; SEM and HrTEM study. *J. Biomed. Mater. Res.* 2000, 50, 1–7.
399. Grimande, G., Weiss, P., Millot, F., Daculsi, G. *In vitro* evaluation of a new injectable calcium phosphate material. *J. Biomed. Mater. Res.* 1998, 39, 660–666.
400. Weiss, P., Lapkowski, M., LeGeros, R.Z., Bouler, J.M., Jean, A., Daculsi, G. FTIR spectroscopic study of an organic/mineral composite for bone and dental substitute materials. *J. Mater. Sci. Mater. Med.* 1997, 8, 621–629.

401. Weiss, P., Bohic, S., Lapkowski, M., Daculsi, G. Application of FTIR microspectroscopy to the study of an injectable composite for bone and dental surgery. *J. Biomed. Mater. Res.* 1998, 41, 167–170.

402. Schmitt, M., Weiss, P., Bourges, X., del Valle, G.A., Daculsi, G. Crystallization at the polymer/calcium-phosphate interface in a sterilized injectable bone substitute IBS. *Biomaterials* 2002, 23, 2789–2794.

403. Gauthier, O., Müller, R., von Stechow, D., Lamy, B., Weiss, P., Bouler, J.M., Aguado, E., Daculsi, G. *In vivo* bone regeneration with injectable calcium phosphate biomaterial: A three-dimensional micro-computed tomographic, biomechanical and SEM study. *Biomaterials* 2005, 26, 5444–5453.

404. Weiss, P., Layrolle, P., Clergeau, L.P., Enckel, B., Pilet, P., Amouriq, Y., Daculsi, G., Giumelli, B. The safety and efficacy of an injectable bone substitute in dental sockets demonstrated in a human clinical trial. *Biomaterials* 2007, 28, 3295–3305.

405. Fatimi, A., Tassin, J.F., Axelos, M.A.V., Weiss, P. The stability mechanisms of an injectable calcium phosphate ceramic suspension. *J. Mater. Sci. Mater. Med.* 2010, 21, 1799–1809.

406. Trojani, C., Boukhechba, F., Scimeca, J.C., Vandenbos, F., Michiels, J.F., Daculsi, G., Boileau, P., Weiss, P., Carle, G.F., Rochet, N. Ectopic bone formation using an injectable biphasic calcium phosphate/Si-HPMC hydrogel composite loaded with undifferentiated bone marrow stromal cells. *Biomaterials* 2006, 27, 3256–3264.

407. Zhang, S.M., Lü, G. Clinical application of compound injectable bone substitutes in bone injury repair. *J. Clin. Rehabil. Tissue Eng. Res.* 2009, 13, 10117–10120.

408. Daculsi, G., Uzel, P.A., Bourgeois, N., le François, T., Rouvillain, J.L., Bourges, X., Baroth, S. New injectable bone substitute using reversible thermosensitive hydrogel and BCP granules: *In vivo* rabbit experiments. *Key Eng. Mater.* 2009, 396–398, 457–460.

409. Iooss, P., le Ray, A.M., Grimandi, G., Daculsi, G., Merle, C. A new injectable bone substitute combining poly(ε-caprolactone) microparticles with biphasic calcium phosphate granules. *Biomaterials* 2001, 22, 2785–2794.

410. Bohner, M. Design of ceramic-based cements and putties for bone graft substitution. *Eur. Cell Mater.* 2010, 20, 1–12.

411. Mickiewicz, R.A., Mayes, A.M., Knaack, D. Polymer—Calcium phosphate cement composites for bone substitutes. *J. Biomed. Mater. Res.* 2002, 61, 581–592.

412. Fujishiro, Y., Takahashi, K., Sato, T. Preparation and compressive strength of α-tricalcium phosphate/gelatin gel composite cement. *J. Biomed. Mater. Res.* 2001, 54, 525–230.

413. Kasuga, T., Yoshida, M., Ikushima, A.J., Tuchiya, M., Kusakari, H. Bioactivity of zirconia-toughened glass-ceramics. *J. Am. Ceram. Soc.* 1992, 75, 1884–1888.

414. Pan, J., Han, X., Niu, W., Cameron, R.E. A model for biodegradation of composite materials made of polyesters and tricalcium phosphates. *Biomaterials* 2011, 32, 2248–2255.

415. Dorozhkin, S.V. Inorganic chemistry of the dissolution phenomenon: The dissolution mechanism of calcium apatites at the atomic (ionic) level. *Comments Inorg. Chem.* 1999, 20, 285–299.

416. Dorozhkin, S.V. Dissolution mechanism of calcium apatites in acids: A review of literature. *World J. Methodol.* 2012, 2, 1–17.

417. Furukawa, T., Matsusue, Y., Yasunaga, T., Shikinami, Y., Okuno, M., Nakamura, T. Biodegradation behavior of ultra-high strength hydroxyapatite/poly(L-lactide) composite rods for internal fixation of bone fractures. *Biomaterials* 2000, 21, 889–898.

418. Furukawa, T., Matsusue, Y., Yasunaga, T., Nakagawa, Y., Okada, Y., Shikinami, Y., Okuno, M., Nakamura, T. Histomorphometric study on high-strength hydroxyapatite/poly(L-lactide) composite rods for internal fixation of bone fractures. *J. Biomed. Mater. Res.* 2000, 50, 410–419.

419. Yasunaga, T., Matsusue, Y., Furukawa, T., Shikinami, Y., Okuno, M., Nakamura, T. Bonding behaviour of ultrahigh strength unsintered hydroxyapatite particles/poly(L-lactide) composites to surface of tibial cortex in rabbits. *J. Biomed. Mater. Res.* 1999, 47, 412–419.

420. Marques, A.P., Reis, R.L., Hunt, J.A. *In vitro* evaluation of the biocompatibility of novel starch based polymeric and composite material. *Biomaterials* 2002, 6, 1471–1478.
421. Mendes, S.C., Bovell, Y.P., Reis, R.L., Cunha, A.M., de Bruijn, J.D., van Blitterswijk, C.A. Biocompatibility testing of novel starch-based materials with potential application in orthopaedic surgery. *Biomaterials* 2001, 22, 2057–2064.
422. Habraken, W.J.E.M., Liao, H.B., Zhang. Z., Wolke, J.G.C., Grijpma, D.W., Mikos, A.G., Feijen, J., Jansen, J.A. *In vivo* degradation of calcium phosphate cement incorporated into biodegradable microspheres. *Acta Biomater.* 2010, 6, 2200–2211.
423. Ngiam, M., Liao, S., Patil, A.J., Cheng, Z., Chan, C.K., Ramakrishna, S. The fabrication of nano-hydroxyapatite on PLGA and PLGA/collagen nanofibrous composite scaffolds and their effects in osteoblastic behavior for bone tissue engineering. *Bone* 2009, 45, 4–16.
424. Liao, S.S., Cui, F.Z. *In vitro* and *in vivo* degradation of the mineralized collagen based composite scaffold: Nanohydroxyapatite/collagen/poly(L-lactide). *Tissue Eng.* 2004, 10, 73–80.
425. Hasegawa, S., Ishii, S., Tamura, J., Furukawa, T., Neo, M., Matsusue, Y., Shikinami, Y., Okuno, M., Nakamura, T. A 5–7 year *in vivo* study of high-strength hydroxyapatite/poly(L-lactide) composite rods for the internal fixation of bone fractures. *Biomaterials* 2006, 27, 1327–1332.
426. Meyers, M.A., Lin, A.Y.M., Seki, Y., Chen, P.Y., Kad, B.K., Bodde, S. Structural biological composites: An overview. *JOM* 2006, 58, 36–43.

8 Curcumin-Loaded Polymeric Nanoparticle

A Promising Route for the Treatment of Cancer

Chinmayee Saikia, Mandip Sarmah, Monoj K. Das, Anand Ramteke, and Tarun K. Maji

CONTENTS

8.1   INTRODUCTION

8.1.1   Cancer: A Threat to Humans

Cancer is one of the alarmingly increasing diseases in the world and stands second among the causes for disease-related deaths after cardiovascular disease. There are 14.1 million new cancer cases, 8.2 million cancer deaths, and 32.6 million people living with cancer worldwide, and the number is increasing every day. Its ever-increasing mortality rates estimate that 84 million people will die of cancer between 2005 and 2015 without intervention. More than 70% of the cases present for diagnosis and treatment services in the advanced stages of the disease, which has led to poor survival and high mortality rates.[1]

Many factors are implicated in the development and progression of this pathological state that broadly includes chemical, physical, and biological agents. All these agents, separately or in combination, alter normal cellular functions and thus contribute to the disease state. Surgery, radiation, and chemotherapy have been the mainstay of treatment for human malignancies for more than 40 years. Each of these treatment modules is restricted by its own set of limitations owing to factors including location, size, and stage of malignancy present, along with the age and medical condition of the patient. Surgery is the best option when the tumor is localized, but in advance stages, this option becomes unviable. Chemotherapy and radiotherapy are mainly limited by dose-associated side effects. Chemotherapy being a systemic approach impacts a wide range of tissues, whereas radiotherapy has comparatively a more localized effect.[2]

As the current anticancer therapies like radiotherapy and chemotherapy are often met with the burden of high cost, serious side effects, toxicity, and tumor relapse, approaches that are safe, nontoxic, cost-effective, and easily available are desired to control and manage tumor growth and progression. Plant-derived natural compounds as novel anticancer agents have gained impetus in the recent past. Phytochemicals isolated from plants can inhibit the action of various carcinogens or can act as blocking agents to activate detoxification, induce antioxidant enzymes, reduce inflammatory response, and decrease tumor cell growth by inducing apoptosis and/or cell cycle arrest. They can act as suppressing agents to restrain tumor cells from promotion and progression by destroying one or more cell signaling pathways. These agents also have the potential to reverse the process of carcinogenesis before progress to the invasive stage.[3,4] Importantly, these phytochemicals of plant origin have no or less toxicity, high efficiency, capability of oral administration, and low cost. Due to continuous efforts over the years, several anticancer drugs have come out but the main problem with these agents is the associated toxicity and the lack of specificity as these agents also kill the surrounding normal cells. Hence, there is a need for site-specific delivery of anticancer agents to achieve the highest therapeutic value.

8.1.2   Curcumin: Its Origin, History, and Applications

Although a number of drugs are available for the treatment of cancer nowadays, they have limited potential as they are either inefficient in treatment or toxic or very expensive. Some of the widely used drugs include cyclophosphamide, doxorubicin, cisplatin, epirubicin, etc. Therefore, to get rid of these disadvantages, the search for new types of drugs continues. Curcumin is one such type of phytochemical that is able to overcome most of these limitations. Curcumin, a hydrophobic polyphenol, is an orange crystalline powder derived from the herb *Curcuma longa* (commonly known as turmeric). The turmeric plant, perennial herb, belonging to the ginger family is extensively cultivated in India and Eastern Asia. The rhizome (or root) is the most useful part of the plant, which contains most medicinal values; it contains 2%–5% curcumin. Traditionally, curcumin has a variety of uses: as spice, pigment/coloring agent in foods and textiles, in cosmetics, and as medicine.[5,6] In traditional Indian and Chinese medicine, curcumin is used in the treatment of anorexia, cough, biliary diseases, diabetic wounds, rheumatism, hepatic disorders, sore throat, and sinusitis.[7] Its medicinal uses are widely described in Ayurveda. In India, turmeric paste in slaked lime is a popular home remedy for the treatment of local inflammation and wound healing. The pharmacological safety of curcumin is well accepted as it has been consumed as a dietary spice at a dose of up to 100 mg per day for centuries.[8] In the United States, curcumin is used as a coloring agent in cheese, mustard, pickles, ice cream, soups, etc.

Curcumin was first isolated in 1815 by Vogel,[9] and then its crystalline form was isolated in 1870 by Daube, identified as 1,6-heptadiene-3,5-dione-1,7-bis(4-hydroxy-3-methoxy phenyl)-(1E,6E) or diferuloylmethane.[10] Later on, Lampe in 1910 confirmed the feruloylmethane skeleton of curcumin.[11] Curcumin is insoluble in water and ether, but soluble in ethanol, dimethylsulfoxide, and acetone. Its molecular symbol is $C_{21}H_{20}O_6$ and molecular weight is 368.37 g/mole. Chemically, it is a bis-α, β- unsaturated β- diketone exhibiting a melting point of 183°C.

Turmeric contains curcumin along with other chemical constituents, commonly known as *Curcuminoids*.[12] The major curcuminoids present are demethoxycurcumin (curcumin II), bisdemethoxycurcumin (curcumin III), and cyclocurcumin (Figure 8.1). The curcuminoid complex is commonly known as Indian saffron, yellow ginger, or *kacha haldi*. The commercial curcumin contains about 77% curcumin I, 17% curcumin II, and 3% curcumin III as its major components.

Extensive research has been done on the medicinal significance of curcumin. It has been found to exhibit antioxidant,[13] antiviral,[14] antibacterial,[15] antifungal,[16] and anti-inflammatory activities,[17] among others (Figure 8.2). Subsequently, curcumin has the potential to cure various diseases like asthma, diabetes,[18] cataract formation,[19] neurodegenerative disease like Alzeimer's,[20] arthritis,[21] allergies,[22] atherosclerosis,[23] etc. Moreover, the most important character found in curcumin is its potential in the prevention and treatment of a variety of cancers: blood,[24] skin,[25] oral cavity,[26] lung,[27] pancreas,[28] prostate,[29] and intestinal tract.[30] Another promising advantage of curcumin is its minimal side effects in clinical application as a drug.[31]

8.1.3 Anticancer Potential of Curcumin

Curcumin has been in use for treatment of multiple carcinomas including colon,[32] prostate, head and neck,[33] breast, pancreatic, ovarian, lung, liver, and many others. The potentialities of curcumin are multidirectional from its proficiency

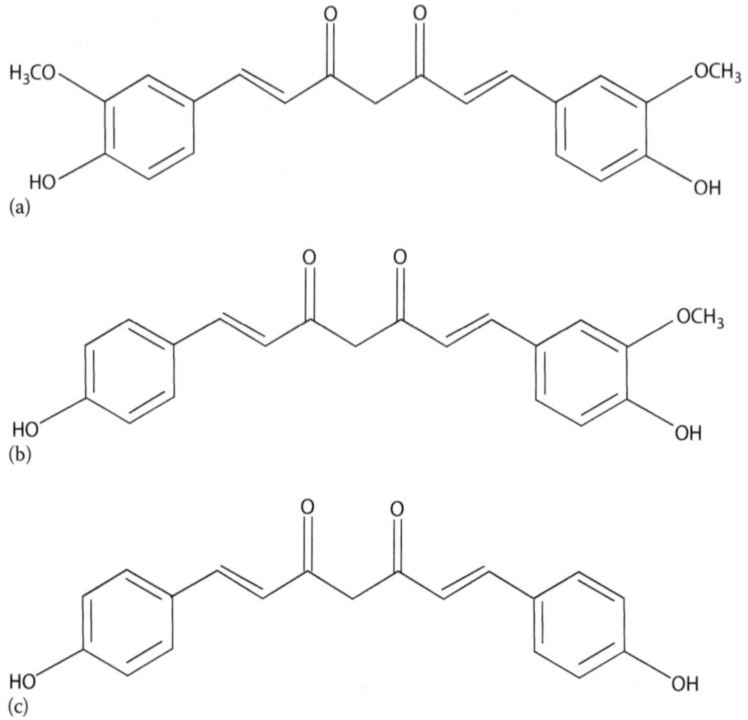

FIGURE 8.1 Structure of curcuminoids: (a) curcumin I, (b) curcumin II, and (c) curcumin III.

of chemoprevention and anticancer activity by interfering with almost all bio-chemical pathways. It suppresses proliferation and downregulates different transcription factors (NF-κB, AP-1, and Egr-1) and the expression of different cancer-inducing genes and their products (COX2, LOX, NOS, MMP-9, uPA, TNF, chemokines, cell surface adhesion molecules cyclin D1), including growth factor receptors.[34] Curcumin has also been reported as a potent antioxidant and anti-inflammatory molecule and is shown to be a mediator of chemoresistance and radioresistance in almost all stages of cancer through suppression of tumor from initiation, promotion, and metastasis.[35] The modulatory potential of cur-cumin on phase I and II xenobiotic metabolizing enzymes, antioxidants, and free radical scavenging properties plays a role in the first line of action against carcinogenesis through carcinogen bioactivation via the suppression of specific cytochrome P450 isozymes and induces the activity or expression of phase II carcinogen detoxifying enzymes, which may account for its cancer chemopre-ventive effects. Cyclin D1 is a proto-oncogene that is overexpressed as a result of gene amplification or translocation in many cancers, including breast,[36] esopha-gus,[37] lung,[38] liver,[39] and head and neck.[40] Recent findings suggest that curcumin downregulates cyclin D1 expression through the activation of both transcrip-tional and post-transcriptional modifications, which may contribute to the antip-roliferative effects of curcumin.

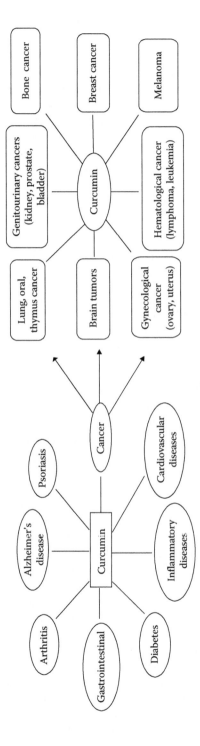

FIGURE 8.2 Different applications of curcumin, with emphasis on its application in different cancer treatments.

Curcumin is also known to suppress the proliferation of human vascular endothelial cells in vitro[41] and to abolish the FGF-2-induced angiogenic response in vivo[42] suggesting that curcumin also performs antiangiogenic activities. Tumor suppressor genes p53, PTEN, and RB1[43–45] regulate the various cellular and molecular pathways and prevents cancer formation. Numerous in vivo and in vitro reports showed that turmeric and its constituents have a significant role in cancer prevention or inhibition by regulating the expression of tumor suppression genes along with other important associated genes—egr-1, cmyc, and bcl-XL in B cells.[46] The combination of curcumin along with drugs plays a very diverse role on the chemosensitization of drugs by decreasing the P-glycoprotein function and expression and the promotion of caspase-3 activation along with decreased IC50 value against different types of cancers. Current reports also suggest that curcumin, in combination with radiation, inhibits TNF-α-mediated NF-κB activity, resulting in bcl-2 protein downregulation, which make it a potent radiosensitizer.

8.1.4 Shortcomings of Curcumin and Their Remedy

In spite of all these qualities of curcumin, different studies on absorption, distribution, metabolism, and excretion exposed its poor solubility and relatively low bioavailability. The low bioavailability of curcumin is because of its poor absorption, low serum level, limited tissue distribution, rapid metabolism, and rapid elimination.[46] Wahlstrem and Blennow first reported extremely low serum curcumin level in the blood plasma of Sprague–Dawley rats.[47] Later studies showed that the serum level of curcumin in rats and human is not directly comparable. In rats, when curcumin was given orally at a dose of 2 g/kg, a maximum serum concentration of 1.35 ± 0.23 µg/mL was observed at time 0.8 h, whereas in human the same dose resulted in either undetectable or extremely low serum level, that is, 0.006 ± 0.005 µg/mL at 1 h.[48] The route of administration also impacts the bioavailability of curcumin. Works of Yang et al. showed that when 10 mg/kg of curcumin administrated intravenously (i.v.) in rats, the maximum serum curcumin level was 0.36 ± 0.05 µg/mL, but when a 50-fold higher curcumin dose was given orally, only 0.06 ± 0.01 µg/mL maximum serum curcumin level was observed in rats.[49] Another limitation associated with curcumin is its poor tissue distribution. However, this has not yet been studied much. Pan et al. administrated curcumin in a mouse model via intraperitoneal (i.p.) route at a dose of 0.1 g/kg, and after 1 h found a maximum amount of 117 µg/g curcumin in intestine while 26.9 µg/g in liver, 26.1 µg/g in spleen, 7.5 µg/g in kidney, and only a trace amount of 0.4 µg/g in brain tissues.[50] Garcea et al. examined curcumin level in the colorectum and its pharmacodynamics consequences in colorectal cancer patients. When 3600 mg of curcumin was given to the patients via i.p. route, the concentration of curcumin in normal and malignant colorectal tissues were 12.7 ± 5.7 and 7.7 ± 1.8 mmol/g, respectively, and these doses showed pharmacological activity in colorectum.[51] When patients were given 450–3600 mg of curcumin daily for 1 week as dietary intake, no curcumin was found in their liver tissues.[52] From these results, it was suggested that the pharmacokinetics of curcumin observed in tissues when administered intraperitoneally cannot directly be compared with those observed after dietary intake. Half-life, that is, systematic elimination or clearance of curcumin from the body, determines its relative biological activity. Studies have shown that due to its rapid intestinal and hepatic metabolism, about 60%–70% of an oral dose of curcumin gets eliminated in the feces.[50] As mentioned, although curcumin is extremely safe via oral administration even at very high dose (which is not found in case of other drugs), its use is limited owing to its poor bioavailability, low solubility, and rapid degradation and metabolism. For these reasons, it is considered as a class II drug in the Biopharmaceutics Classification System.[53]

Consequently, continuous efforts have been made over the past three decades to overcome these disadvantages and to increase the efficacy of curcumin. Numerous strategies have been formulated to enhance the therapeutic efficiency of curcumin. Different types of formulations have been evaluated to gain the fullest advantages of curcumin. These formulations include adjuvants,[54] liposomes,[55] micelles,[56] phospholipid complexes,[46] and nanoparticles. The schematic representations of these formulations are shown in Figure 8.3. The intention behind preparing these formulations is primarily to increase the absorption of curcumin by tissues.

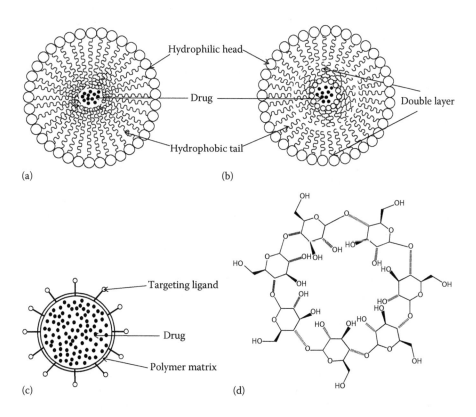

FIGURE 8.3 Schematic representation of (a) micelle, (b) liposome, (c) nanoparticle, and (d) cyclodextrin.

8.1.4.1 Adjuvants

Adjuvants are one of the major premises being used to improve the bioavailability of curcumin. They can block the metabolic pathways of curcumin and thereby modulate its activity. For example, when genistein was combined with curcumin, it showed a synergistic inhibitory effect against cellular proliferation of the breast cancer cell line MCF-7 induced by estrogenic pesticides.[57] This inhibitory effect was superior to individual effects of either curcumin or genistein. Similarly, several other adjuvants were evaluated in order to improve the bioavalability of curcumin. Shoba et al. reported that piperine, in combination with curcumin found to increase serum curcumin level and enhance curcumin bioavailability.[48] Again, Eugenol and terpenol are two agents that in combination with curcumin enhanced skin curcumin absorption.[58]

8.1.4.2 Liposomes, Micelles, and Phospholipid Complexes

These are other promising novel formulations that can reduce the hydrophobicity of curcumin and also can increase the permeability of membrane barriers by interacting with membrane components. Liposomes have the advantages of loading both hydrophilic and hydrophobic drugs. Dhule et al. investigated the in vitro and in vivo antitumor activity of liposomal curcumin against osteosarcoma cells and demonstrated that liposomal curcumin exhibits significant anticancer potential on KHOS osteosarcoma cell lines and MCF-7 breast cancer cell lines.[59] They encapsulated curcumin in cyclodextrin followed by second encapsulation within liposomes. The induced apoptosis by these liposomal curcumin was further confirmed by in vivo studies on xenograft OS mice models. A recent study on solid lipid complex with 134 nm and 84% encapsulation reported high oral bioavailability in the plasma of male Wistar rats. With this formulation, the serum level of curcumin was found to be greatly enhanced in comparison to free curcumin.[60] Micelles and phospholipid complexes can improve the gastrointestinal absorption of natural drugs, resulting in higher plasma levels and lower kinetic elimination that in turn result in improved bioavailability. Pharmacokinetic studies of Ma et al. established that polymeric micellar curcumin offered a 60-fold higher biological half-life for curcumin in rats compared to curcumin solubilized in a mixture of DMA, poly(ethylene glycol) (PEG), and dextrose.[61]   Methoxypoly(ethyleneglycol)-b-poly(ε-caprolactone-co-p-dioxanone), MPEG-P(CL-co-PDO) micelles loaded with curcumin with >95% encapsulation efficiency found to inhibit the growth of PC-3 human prostate cancer in a dose-dependent manner.[62] In vivo studies of curcumin–phospholipid complex in Sprague–Dawley male rats showed significant enhancement in plasma curcumin level along with a 1.5-fold increase in curcumin half-life over free curcumin.[63]

8.1.4.3 Derivatives

Various curcumin derivatives and analogs have been developed in order to enhance the metabolic stability and anticancer activity of curcumin. Mosley et al. reviewed different studies on the biological activity of curcumin and its derivatives.[64] Their studies reported a curcumin analogue designated as EF24, which showed increased antitumor activity in vitro and in vivo compared to curcumin. The bioavailability of this curcumin analogue oral and i.p. was found to be 60% and 35%, respectively. Many other groups investigated the effect of curcumin in combination with other promising drugs. For example, curcumin in combination with paclitaxel causes a significant reduction in tumor growth when studied in MDA-MB-231 xenograft models.[65] Another route to improve its bioavailability was to chelate curcumin with metals. The presence of two phenolic groups and one active methylene group make curcumin an excellent ligand for chelation. Several studies have been conducted on the biological activity of curcumin metal chelates. For example, curcumin copper complex,[66] curcumin vanadyl complex,[67] etc., have shown superior anticancer activity than curcumin; curcumin boron complex has a 10-fold in vitro inhibitory effect against HIV-1 and HIV-2 protease than curcumin[68]; curcumin manganese complex exhibited more potent neuroprotective activity than curcumin both in vitro and in vivo.[69] These results suggested their better biological activity over curcumin. However, more research is needed to prove they are safe therapeutics.

8.1.4.4 Cyclodextrin

Cyclodextrins (CD) are a family of compounds made up of sugar molecules bound together in a ring. They have a hydrophilic outer surface and hydrophobic central cavity. Therefore, they are used to enhance the solubility and bioavailability of hydrophobic drugs. The hydrophobic cavity thus protects the hydrophobic drug molecule from aqueous environments, while the polar outer surface of the CD molecule provides the solubilizing effect. The commonly used cyclodextrins in pharmaceutical applications are α, β, and γ-CD, and their derivatives such as hydroxypropyl-β-CD (HPβCD) and methyl β-CD (MβCD). Yadav et al. prepared solid inclusion complexes with HPβCD and MβCD complexes by solvent evaporation methods.[70] The ability to increase the solubility of curcumin by CD is found to increase in the order HPβCD > MβCD > γCD > βCD. Curcumin molecules seemed to fit better in HPβCD than into the cavities of MβCD, thereby exhibiting similar solubility. The results showed at 12 h 97.82% of curcumin was released with HPβCD complex as compared to 68.75% release with MβCD and 16.12% with the pure drug. They have correlated these higher release rates with improved in vivo bioavailability of curcumin–HPβCD complexes as compared to curcumin alone while studying rat colitis models. Rahman et al. reported the preparation of β-CD–curcumin inclusion complexes and its entrapment within liposomes followed by subsequent assessment of in vitro cytotoxicity using model lung and colon cancer cell lines. All the formulations showed preferential anticancer activity.[71]

8.1.4.5 Nanoparticles

Nanoparticle-based formulations have caught the attention of researchers recently due to their capacity to penetrate membrane barriers because of their small size.[72] Nanoparticles offer various benefits, including membrane penetration, binding and stabilization of proteins, and lysosomal escape after endocytosis. Most of the biological systems and nanomaterials share the same range of sizes that offer better interaction between the two (Figure 8.4). Besides this, their prospective for being modified for targeting specific organs makes them excellent drug carriers. Targeted drug delivery system based on nanoparticles appears to deliver curcumin with better permeability, longer circulation, and stronger resistance to metabolic processes. Various aspects of nanoparticles in curcumin delivery are discussed next.

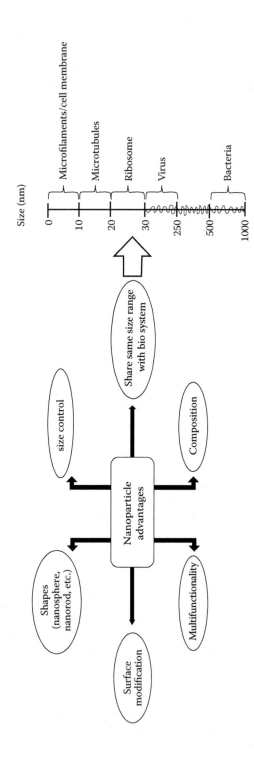

FIGURE 8.4 Advantages of nanoparticles as drug delivery systems.

8.2 NANOTECHNOLOGY: AN AUSPICIOUS TOOL IN CURCUMIN DELIVERY

Nanotechnology has gained immense popularity in the development of advanced therapeutic systems. One of the most active research areas of nanotechnology is nanomedicine, where nanotechnology is applied to highly specific medical interference for the diagnosis, prevention, and treatment of diseases. A *nanoparticle* is a microscopic particle with at least one dimension less than 100 nm. The properties of the material changes as the percentage of atoms of the material become significant. Due to this, nanoparticles show a number of special properties relative to larger particles. They have very high surface area to volume ratio and this provides a tremendous driving force for diffusion. Nanoparticles can easily enter biological membranes, cells, tissues, and organs, which is not possible for larger sized particles.[73] This characteristic optimizes their potential for interaction with biomolecules. Hence, the development of nanomaterials has allowed to better understand molecular biology.

The particle size, shape, and surface of nanoparticles should be essentially manipulated to achieve both passive and active drug targeting through various routes of administration. Many important properties of nanoparticles like circulation time, targeting, internalization, clearance, etc., depend on their size. Therefore, cellular uptake of nanoparticles with different sizes has been extensively studied in recent years.[74,75] Studies on cellular uptake of different sized polystyrene nanoparticles on human colon adenocarcinoma cells showed that particles with 100 nm displayed most efficient cellular uptake compared to those with sizes of 50, 200, 500, and 1000 nm.[76] The surface charge of nanoparticles has much importance in their efficacy and pathways of uptake since biological systems contain numerous biomolecules with various charges. Positively charged nanoparticles showed significant cellular uptake followed by negatively charged ones, whereas neutral nanoparticles showed lowest internalization than that of positively and negatively charged nanoparticles. The shape of nanoparticles also plays an important role in their affinity to interact with biological systems. The effect of nanomaterial shape has been demonstrated in recent studies on cellular uptake.[77] Nanorods exhibit highest uptake in human cervical cancer cells, followed by spheres, cylinders, and cubes. The intracellular uptake efficiency of rod-shaped and spherical nanoparticles have been investigated on many types of cells.[78]

Nanostructured biomaterials alter and improve the pharmacokinetic and pharmacodynamics properties of various types of drugs. Drugs are incorporated into the nanoparticles either through physical entrapment, adsorption, or chemical conjugation, thereby significantly improving the therapeutic index of the drugs compared to free drug counterparts. Nanoparticles-based drug delivery systems have potential to enhance the safety, solubility, and bioavailability of drugs. They are specially designed to absorb or encapsulate a drug and thereby protect them from enzymatic degradation, enabling their controlled release and prolonged blood circulation. Moreover, these systems provide targeted delivery of the active agents to tissues or cells, decreasing their toxicity and hence limiting their nonspecific uptake. In these systems, the controlled release of encapsulated drug and the particle degradation features can be readily modulated by the choice of matrix components.

Although numerous strategies have been formulated to enhance the bioavailability of curcumin, only its application in the field of nanotechnology has considerably enhanced its therapeutic effects. Many types of nanoformulations such as liposomes,[79] micelles,[56] solid lipid nanoparticles,[80] protiens,[81] nanoemulsions,[82] polymeric nanoparticles,[83] etc., have been established as curcumin delivery carriers. These nanoparticulate drug delivery systems seem to be a promising approach for the delivery of curcumin. Among these diverse drug delivery approaches, currently significant research effort is being made on curcumin delivery using polymeric nanoparticles.

8.3   POLYMER NANOPARTICLES: PROMISING MATERIAL IN CURCUMIN DELIVERY

Polymer nanoparticles include polymeric micelles, nanocapsules, and also nanospheres. Polymeric micelle possesses a hydrophobic core, which acts as a pool for hydrophobic drugs, and a hydrophilic covering that stabilizes the hydrophobic core and makes the whole system water soluble. Hence, the aqueous solubility of curcumin can be increased by encapsulating within polymeric micelle system.[84] Nanocapsules can be defined as a vesicular system that can encapsulate water-soluble drugs in a polymer membrane. On the other hand, nanospheres can be defined as a matrix system that is able to distribute drugs uniformly within the polymer matrix. Hence, nanospheres are most suitable for incorporating water-insoluble curcumin. The importance on polymeric nanoparticles lies due to their stable structure; tailor-made property, such as size; zeta potential; drug release profiles, etc., that can be tuned by altering polymer length, selecting surfactants, cross-linking agents, fillers, solvents, etc., during the synthesis process. The functional groups present on the surface of polymeric nanoparticles can also be chemically modified with targeting ligands to get better therapeutics.[85,86] The drug can be absorbed to the nanocapsule during the synthesis process or covalently conjugated to the surface of the nanoparticles. Once they are at the target site, the drug may be released from the nanoparticle by diffusion, swelling, erosion, degradation, or in response to the input of an external energy such as a magnetic field, light, or ultrasound. Degradation and drug release kinetic can be specifically controlled by different physicochemical properties of polymer: molecular weight, polydispersity index, hydrophobicity, and crystallinity.

Polymeric nanoparticles as the carriers of curcumin can boost the drug's efficacy by targeting definite cells or tissues.[87] Subsequently, their toxicity reduces as fewer drugs accumulate in healthy tissues, and hence, occasionally, higher doses also can be administrated. Polymeric nanoparticle–based systems can provide efficient solubilization, stabilization, and controlled delivery of curcumin for cancer therapy. The *controlled delivery* technique is used for the purpose of achieving more effective therapies while eliminating the potential for both under- and over-dosing. It can be defined as a technique in which the drug is made available to a specific target at a rate and duration necessary to accomplish an anticipated effect. Numerous experiments have been done time to time to develop such systems. For example, some controlled release systems have been evaluated in such a way that they can respond to changes in biological environment and deliver the drug accordingly. Controlled delivery has become an important factor in designing efficient drug delivery systems. The next generation of controlled delivery systems are *targeted delivery* systems, which allow the transport of drug directly to the site of disease under various conditions and thereby treat it deliberately with no side effects on the patient's body. In cancer therapy, both controlled and targeted delivery of the anticancer agent to the site of action is highly necessary for maximizing the killing effect during tumor growth phase and hence to avoid drug exposure to healthy tissues, thereby reducing toxicity. It is also necessary to maintain a fixed rate of infusion of the drug into the tumor to maximize exposure to dividing cells, resulting in tumor regression. Therefore, owing to all the advantages of controlled release technique, curcumin-loaded, pH-sensitive, and thermosensitive polymer nanoparticles have been prepared for the treatment of various types of cancers.[88,89]

Both synthetic and natural biodegradable and biocompatible polymers have been employed in the preparation of nanoparticle-based drug delivery systems. The most explored polymers include poly(ethylene glycol), poly(lactic acid-co-glycolic acid) (PLGA), chitosan, dextran, and starch. The polymeric nanoparticle surface can be sterically stabilized by grafting, conjugating, or adsorbing hydrophilic polymers to its surface, which can reduce hepatic uptake and improve the half-life circulation of the nanoparticles.

8.3.1 DIFFERENT TECHNIQUES FOR POLYMER NANOPARTICLE PREPARATION

In the case of polymer nanoparticles, the preparation technique plays a key role in achieving the desired properties. Properties like size, surface size, permeability, drug encapsulation, drug solubility, drug release, biocompatibility, toxicity, antigenicity, etc., are very much dependent on the polymer structure, that is, indirectly on the preparation methods. These can be accomplished by different techniques. Some of these techniques are defined next and schematically presented in Figure 8.5.

8.3.1.1 Nanoprecipitation

Nanoprecipitation is also known as the solvent displacement method. This method involves the precipitation of a preformed polymer from an organic solution and the diffusion of the organic solvent in the aqueous medium in the presence or absence of a surfactant. The polymer is dissolved in a water-miscible solvent with intermediate polarity, which is then injected into an aqueous solution containing a stabilizer/surfactant, under stirring condition. Nanoparticles are formed instantaneously by rapid solvent diffusion. The remaining solvent is removed from the suspension under reduced pressure. This method is basically applicable to poorly soluble drugs. Different properties of the nanoparticles like particle size, drug release, and yield are found to be effectively organized by amending the preparation parameters. The particle size is found to depend on the rate of addition of the organic phase into the aqueous phase. As the rate of mixing of the two phases increases, both particle size and drug entrapment decrease. Particle size also depends on the polymer concentration in the organic phase.

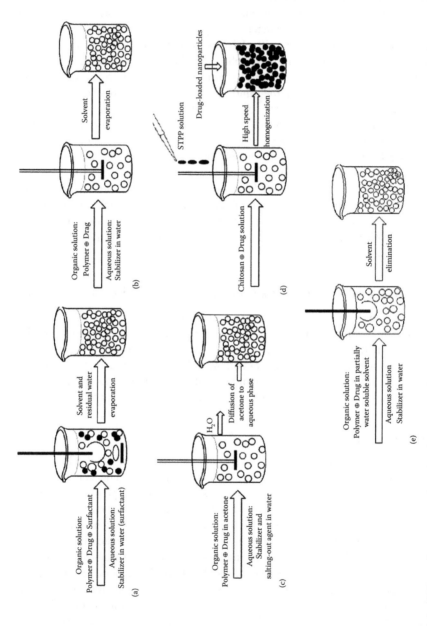

FIGURE 8.5   Schematic representation of different techniques of nanoparticle synthesis: (a) nanoprecipitation, (b) solvent evaporation, (c) salting out, (d) ionic gelation or coacervation, and (e) emulsification.

8.3.1.2 Solvent Evaporation

It is the first method and also most frequently used method to prepare polymer nanoparticles. It includes initial preparation of polymer solutions in volatile solvent to formulate emulsions. The emulsion is then converted into a nanoparticle suspension on evaporation of the solvent, which is permitted to diffuse through the continuous phase of the emulsion. Two types of emulsions can be prepared: a single emulsion, oil-in-water (o/w), or a double emulsion, (water-in-oil)-in-water (w/o/w). The method employs high-speed homogenization or ultrasonication, followed by evaporation of the solvent either by continuous magnetic stirring at room temperature or under reduced pressure. The nanoparticles are then collected by ultracentrifugation and washed with water to remove stabilizer residue or any free drug and finally it is lyophilized. Particle size has been found to be controlled by the type and concentration of the stabilizer, speed of the homogenizer, ultrasonication time, and polymer concentration. The nanoparticles PLA,[90] PLGA,[91] cellulose acetate phthalate, PCL,[92] etc., are formulated by this technique.

8.3.1.3 Salting Out

The salting out method is based on the separation of a water-miscible solvent from aqueous solution via a salting out effect. It can be considered as a modification of the emulsification- solvent diffusion technique. In this method, polymer and drugs are dissolved in a solvent (e.g., acetone), which is subsequently emulsified into an aqueous gel containing the salting agent and a colloidal stabilizer. Electrolytes such as magnesium chloride and calcium chloride or non electrolytes like sucrose can be used as salting out agents, whereas polyvinylpyrrolidine or hydroxycellulose are used as colloidal stabilizers. The resultant oil/water emulsion is then diluted with a sufficient volume of water or aqueous solution to increase the diffusion of the solvent into the aqueous phase, thus inducing the formation of nanospheres. Here the selection of the salting out agent is crucial as it plays an important role in the encapsulation efficiency of the drug. Different parameters can be varied such as stirring rate, polymer concentration in the organic phase, types of electrolytes, and types of stabilizers in the aqueous phase to get the desired properties in the nanoparticles. PLA, poly(methacrylic) acid, ethyl cellulose nanosphere with high encapsulation efficiency is reported to be prepared by this technique. But this method involves limited use of lipophilic drugs and extensive nanoparticle washing steps.

8.3.1.4 Ionic Gelation or Coacervation

The coacervation technique is basically used for the preparation of polymer nanoparticles using any biodegradable hydrophilic polymers, for example, chitosan, gelatin, and sodium alginate. Coacervation is defined as the separation of two liquid phases in a colloidal system. The phase more concentrated in a colloid component is the coacervate and the other phase is the equilibrium solution. Banik et al. prepared isoniazid-loaded chitosan nanoparticles by this method.[93] The method involves a mixture of two aqueous phases, of which one is the chitosan polymer and the drug and the other is poly anion sodium tripolyphosphate. In this technique, negatively charged amino groups of chitosan chains interact with positively charged tripolyphosphate to form coacervate in the nanometer size range. The application of surfactants was found to be useful to control the particle size. Hence, coacervates are formed as a result of the electrostatic interaction between two aqueous phases while ionic gelation includes the material undergoing transition from liquid to gel due to ionic interaction conditions at room temperature.

8.3.1.5 Emulsification

It is one of the fastest techniques for nanoparticle preparation. Based on the application of an organic or aqueous continuous phase, the emulsification technique can be classified into two categories. The continuous organic phase procedure involves the dispersion of monomer into an emulsion or inverse microemulsion, or into a material in which the monomer is not soluble. But this procedure uses toxic organic solvents, surfactants, and initiators due to which its application has limitations. Lowe et al. reported the synthesis of polyacrylamide nanospheres by using this technique.[94] In the continuous aqueous phase, the monomer is dissolved in the continuous aqueous solution. This method does not require any surfactant or emulsifier. The polymerization process initiates by using an initiator molecule that might be anionic or a free radical. Phase separation and formation of solid particles takes place before or after the termination of the reaction. Lescure et al. formulated poly(alkylcyanoacrylate) nanoparticles and found that the initiator concentration and pH of the medium influenced different properties of the nanoparticles.[95]

8.3.2 Parameter and Property Studies of Nanoparticles

The size of nanoparticles plays a very important role in controlling various other properties of the nanoparticles including stability, drug loading, drug release, and toxicity. Again, surface charge affects stability and surface modification along with in vivo performance of the nanoparticles, for example, cellular uptake, cellular target, and cytotoxicity. Generally, positively charged nanoparticles seem to show improved efficacy of drug delivery, cellular uptake, and imaging but in contrast lead to higher cytotoxicity. Therefore, characterization of the nanoparticles is necessary in terms of their size, surface morphology, and surface charge by using scanning electron microscopy (SEM), transmission electron microscopy (TEM), dynamic light scattering (DLS), zeta potential, etc.

SEM gives information about the surface morphology and size of the nanoparticles. However, it can give only limited information about size. Dry powdered nanoparticles should be coated with a conductive metal such as platinum or gold for SEM characterization. Information on drug encapsulation, distribution, crosslinking effect on surface, exfoliation of clay layer inside nanoparticles, etc., can be drawn from SEM analysis. TEM gives information about size, shape, and size distribution of the nanoparticles. Sample preparation for TEM is more complex and time consuming in comparison to SEM. The samples have to be exposed to liquid nitrogen. The size distribution can be better analyzed by DLS method. The samples are analyzed in solution state for this technique. The size distribution data derived from TEM and DLS differ as TEM analyzes the nanoparticles in a dry state. Particle size can be accurately analyzed further by atomic force microscopy (AFM), which offers ultrahigh resolution in particle size. Furthermore, AFM has the advantage of analyzing nonconducting samples (e.g., biological/polymeric nanoparticles), without any specific treatment. It is a very useful technique for analysing biological particles.

Zeta potential is determined in order to get information about colloidal stability and surface charge of the nanoparticles. High zeta potential values, either positive or negative, indicate good stability and minimal aggregation of nanoparticles. It also provides information about the coating material of the nanoparticles.

Drug loading and drug release are the two basic important properties that signify the success of a drug delivery system. High drug loading capacity reduces the quantity of the carrier for administration. Drug can be loaded into the nanoparticles in two different ways: either by incorporating it at the time of nanoparticle synthesis or by adsorbing the drug after the formation of nanoparticles. The first method has been found to be more useful compared to the latter. In the case of the entrapment method, many factors, for example, the concentration of polymer, cross-linker, and surfactant and the presence of clay particles[96–98] play a crucial role in governing the drug loading capacity. Drug loading efficiency of nanoparticles is calculated by using the following formula:

$$\text{Loading efficiency \%} = (\text{Total amount of drug} - \text{free amount of drug}) \times 100/\text{Weight of dry NPs}$$

Drug loading of the nanoparticles can be determined by UV-visible spectroscopy or high-performance liquid chromatography (HPLC) after centrifugal ultrafiltration. The same techniques are used for the determination of drug release for definite time periods. Drug release from nanoparticles depends on various factors like rate of diffusion through the nanoparticles matrix, desorption of surface-bound drug molecules, nanoparticle erosion, etc.

To analyze cytotoxicity of the nanoparticles, various techniques have been followed. One of the widely used techniques is MTT assay, which is a colorimetric assay for measuring the activity of cellular enzymes that reduce the tetrazolium dye, MTT (3-(4,5-Dimethylthiazol-2-yl)-2,5-diphenyltetrazolium bromide), to its insoluble formazan, giving a purple color. A solubilization solution, usually dimethyl sulfoxide, is added to dissolve the insoluble formazan product into a colored solution. The absorbance of that colored solution can be quantified by using a spectrophotometer at a certain wavelength. Some of the other tetrazolium dyes are MTS, XTT, and WTS. XTS assay is considered superior to MTT assay due to higher sensitivity and higher dynamic range. In this technique, the formed formazan dye is water soluble, hence does not require the final solubilizing step. WSTs (water-soluble tetrazolium) are a series of water-soluble dyes in the MTT assay that give different absorption spectra for the formed formazans. This technique can be performed directly (no need for the solubilizing step) and it produces a more effective signal than MTT.

Another important parameter of nanoparticles for drug delivery application is their cellular uptake. The uptake capacity of the nanoparticles in definite cancer cell lines can be evaluated by using either phase contrast, laser scanning confocal, fluorescence microscope, or TEM. Cell uptake (internalization) measures the stability of a nanoformulation.

8.3.3 DIFFERENT POLYMERIC NANOPARTICLE
FORMULATIONS FOR CURCUMIN DELIVERY

8.3.3.1 Poly(lactide-co-glycolide)

PLGA polymer nanoparticles have attracted great interest from researchers due to their excellent biocompatibility, biodegradability, and mechanical strength.[99] Studies on these PLGA nanoparticles have enhanced therapeutic efficiency against metastatic, ovarian, breast, and prostate cancer. Consequently, efforts are being made to formulate different types of PLGA nanoparticles for curcumin encapsulation in order to achieve a safe biomedical device. A simple solid-oil-water solvent evaporation method has been used to prepare curcumin-encapsulated PLGA nanoparticles.[100] The particle size of the nanoparticles can be controlled by varying the surfactant concentration and sonication time. The nanoprecipitation technique has also been used to prepare curcumin-loaded PLGA nanoparticles in the presence of polyvinylalcohol and ploy-L-lysine as stabilizers.[101] This system was found to be very stable with enhanced cellular drug uptake and retention capacity along with sustained release of curcumin. The nanoparticles have also shown a greater inhibitory effect on the growth of metastatic, ovarian, and breast cancer cells in comparison to free curcumin. Cetyl trimethylammonium bromide (CTAB) or PVA or PEG-5000 was used as stabilizer in emulsion diffusion evaporation methods for the preparation of curcumin-loaded PLGA nanoparticles.[102] The prepared nanoparticles showed significant cellular uptake, in vitro bioactivity and superior in vivo bioavailability in comparison to native curcumin. These types of nanoformulations have high potential in adjuvant therapies for prostate cancer.[100] Works of Anand et al. on PLGA–curcumin nanoparticles showed that curcumin serum level in curcumin-loaded nanoparticles almost doubled compared to curcumin alone.[103] Excellent in vivo bioavailability was also observed in this study. Besides these, the half-life of curcumin–nanoparticles combination was also significantly increased than those of curcumin alone, indicating their bioavailability in animals. Their noticeable anticancer efficacy was observed in nude mice xenograft model as well.[104]

To achieve any desired property like increase in drug retention time in blood, reduction in nonspecific distribution, or targeting tissues or specific cells, surface functionalization or modification of nanoparticles is necessary. In order to gain mucoadhesive property, Grabovac and Bernkop formulated modified PLGA nanoparticles with thiolated chitosan.[105] Bis(sulfosuccinimidyl)suberate (BS3) has been used for surface modification of PLGA nanoparticles to facilitate conjugation of annexin A2, which turned out to be an efficient target delivery of curcumin to annexin A2 positive MDA-MB-231 cancer cells.[106] This formulation increased the half-life of curcumin from 2.32 to 19.9 min in the cerebral cortex and from 7.56 to 16.7 min in the hippocampus. Along with these, retention time values of the cerebral cortex and the hippocampus were also increased about 2- and 1.8-fold, respectively. The curcumin plasma levels were found to be slightly higher with this system. Shahani et al. prepared a PLGA nanoparticles–based drug delivery system that showed a 10-fold increase in the concentration of curcumin in blood, lungs, and brain in comparison to PEG-400-curcumin formulation.[104] The system also showed a better curcumin loading capacity. Punfa et al. conjugated anti-P-glycoprotein onto PLGA nanoparticles to get better cellular uptake to target on the surface of cervical cancer cells KB-V1.[107] They used modified pluronic F127 as a stabilizer for the preparation of curcumin-PLGA-APgp nanoparticles via the nanoprecipitation technique. Both specific binding and cytotoxicity of the prepared nanoparticles were significantly higher than those of curcumin and curcumin-PLGA nanoparticles. Overall, studies have shown the potential of PLGA nanoparticles as an attractive delivery system for increasing the therapeutic antitumor effect of curcumin while minimizing side effects.

8.3.3.2 Polyethylene Glycol

PEG is a well-known synthetic polymer used in many biomedical devices. It is recognized as a safe material owing to its hydrophilicity, nontoxicity, biocompatibility, negligible antigenicity, and immunogenicity.[108,109] Because of these qualities PEG now has been widely used in drug delivery systems to increase the therapeutic efficacy of curcumin. The anticancer activity of PEG-curcumin conjugation has been studied on human prostate, colon, esophageal, and pancreatic cancer cells.[110] Works of Kim et al. showed their anticancer action against adipose tissues also.[111] PEG conjugation to curcumin improved the antiadipogenic function of curcumin in cultured adipocytes 3T3-L1 cells. PEG improved the water solubility and retention of curcumin making it a useful delivery device for curcumin in preadipocytes. A number of amphiphilic systems have been developed using PEG polymer for drug delivery applications. Sahu et al. prepared a novel polymer amphiphile based on methyl poly(ethylene glycol) (mPEG) as the hydrophilic segment and palmitate as the hydrophobic segment.[112] Palmitate, a hydrophobic, naturally occurring fatty acid in animals can be solubilized with curcumin in the core of the formulation while hydrophilic PEG helps to prolong the circulation time and biodistribution of curcumin. In vitro experiment with HeLa cell lines showed enzyme mediated degradation and release of encapsulated curcumin from mPEG-PA system (by cleaving the ester linkage of mPEG- PA). The nanocarrier showed good cellular uptake and cytotoxicity against HeLa cells.[113] Poly(caprolactone) is another widely studied synthetic biodegradable polymer in various biomedical applications. It is generally used to formulate block copolymer where it constitutes the hydrophobic segment with good drug encapsulation efficiency. It is conjugated with methyl PEG to encapsulate curcumin within mPEG- PCL nanoparticles for studying their cytotoxicity against C6 glioma cell lines.[114] The copolymer was prepared via ring opening copolymerization technique while the curcumin-loaded nanoparticles were synthesized by a simple coprecipitation method. The high affinity between curcumin and PCL leads to increased encapsulation efficiency and provides better sustained release of curcumin from the nanoparticles. Curcumin loaded in nanoparticles showed enhanced cellular uptake and cytotoxicity in malignant gloima cells compared to native curcumin. These nanoparticles were found effective against human lung cancer also, as evident from in vivo evaluation in A549 Xenograft mice models.[115] They showed little toxicity to normal tissues including bone marrow, liver, and kidney in therapeutic dose. Feng et al. prepared curcumin-loaded PCL-PEG-PCL triblock copolymeric nanoparticles.[116] The nanoparticles showed excellent controlled release of the drug, with only

55% release after 96 h and also effectively prolonged the retention of curcumin. The in vivo experiments on Wistar rats proved that curcumin-loaded PCL-PEG-PCL nanoparticles were suitable candidates for in vivo delivery of curcumin in rats via intravenous injection.

8.3.3.3 Chitosan

Chitosan, an abundant cationic polymer obtained by N-deacetylation of chitin, is mainly composed of N-acetyl-D-glucosamine and D-glucose amine.[117] Because of its nontoxicity, biocompatibility, biodegradability, bioadherence, antimicrobial activity, etc., chitosan has been widely used in different biomedical applications such as in drug delivery, gene therapy, wound dressing, and tissue engineering.[118,119] Mucoadhesivity of chitosan has been broadly explored due to its capacity to interact with negatively charged mucosal surfaces. Chitosan can facilitate in opening the tight junctions between mucosal cells for enhanced drug absorption.[120] Therefore, it is proved to be a suitable material for oral drug delivery and has attracted attention in cancer therapy as well. Mazzarino et al. prepared curcumin-loaded chitosan nanoparticles via nanoprecipitation method to study their mucoadhesive potential on mucin from bovine submaxillary glands. These nanoparticles showed excellent loading efficiency at 99%.[121] In vitro studies on curcumin-encapsulated chitosan nanoparticles showed that this nanoformulation was nontoxic to normal cell lines and had worthy cellular uptake and anticancer activity on human breast cancer cell lines T47D.[122] Kar et al. patented a chitosan–curcumin nanoparticle system that was proved to be safe in rat and mice studies at a dose of 40 and 4 mg of formulations, respectively, for 14 days.[123] Although chitosan has many favorable qualities for drug delivery applications, it also has some drawbacks such as limited solubility, poor initial loading for hydrophobic drugs, and burst release characteristics. Therefore, chemical modification of chitosan is required to improve polymer processability, solubility, drug release pattern, and the ability to interact with other substances. Anitha et al. prepared carboxymethyled chitosan (CMC) for improving its solubility at neutral and alkaline pH.[124] Curcumin-loaded CMC nanoparticles were prepared by employing simple ionotropic gelation method using TPP (sodium tripolyphosphate). The curcumin-loaded nanoparticle system showed significant toxicity against cancer cell lines MCF-7 (breast cancer cell) and PC-3 (prostate cancer cell) as compared to normal cell lines L929. The cancer cells showed a higher uptake of curcumin-N, O-chitosan nanoparticles than that of normal cells, thereby indicating more cellular internalization of curcumin-loaded nanoparticles within cancer cells. In another study with the same formulation, FACS (fluorescence activated cell sorting) was done to confirm the cellular uptake of the nanoparticles by MCF-7 and normal cells.[125] Shelma and Sharma have encapsulated curcumin within lauryl-sulfated chitosan and studied its oral bioavailability.[126] These nanoparticles showed enhanced toxicity toward C6 cell lines (fibroblast glioma cell) than native curcumin. The pharmacokinetic studies of nanoparticles showed enhanced plasma curcumin level, indicating its tremendous pharmacological availability.

A number of amphiphilic systems with chitosan polymer have been synthesized for effective curcumin delivery. Dextran sulfate, a biocompatible polyanionic polymer, was conjugated with chitosan to get a controlled release and pH-dependent delivery system for curcumin delivery.[127] This type of nanoparticle can be used for oral delivery of insulin[128] and intravenous delivery of anti-angiogenesis peptide.[129] The nanoparticles showed good stability and did not require any cross-linker. These nanoparticles showed good anticancer activity against human breast cancer cells (MCF-7), prostate cancer cells (PC-3), and osteosarcoma cells (MG-63). The activity was more prominent in MG-63 cells compared to other cell lines.[116] In another study, chitosan was modified with the naturally occurring anionic polysaccharide, alginate.[130] Pluronic F127 has been used to enhance the solubility of curcumin, that is, to enhance the encapsulation and dispersion of curcumin into the alginate–chitosan nanoparticles. A marked difference in encapsulation efficiency was found in alginate–chitosan nanoparticles with and without PF127. Moreover, these nanoparticles showed considerable cellular internalization and anticancer activity against human cervical cancer cell line, HeLA.

PF127 itself is a vital nontoxic copolymer highly used in drug delivery for its capability to increase the solubility of drugs and stabilizing properties. It comprises of polyoxyethylene (PEO) unit and polyoxypropylene (PPO); in aqueous solution it tends to aggregate into spherical micelle.[131] This micellar structure can be used for incorporation of both hydrophilic and hydrophobic drugs and prolongation of drug release.[132,133] But the main problem associated with it is its stability, which can be modified by coating with another suitable polymer. From this perspective, chitosan/PF127 nanoparticles were prepared for curcumin delivery by Le et al. However, the cellular uptake of these nanoparticles in HEK293 cells (human embryonic kidney cell) was not up to the mark.[134] The chitosan cover can protect the active agent from hydrolysis, thereby enhancing its circulation, and once targeted, the uptake of the nanoparticles can occur through an endocytosis process. The micelle will break down by the degradation of the chitosan cover by lysozyme, hence releasing curcumin into the nucleus.

In vitro drug release studies on curcumin-encapsulated polyelectrolyte complex of N-trimethyl chitosan and alginate showed controlled release of curcumin both in SGF and SIF medium.[135] Chitosan can be used to coat hydrophobic polymers, which were unable to form nanoparticles easily. By considering this, Liu et al. employed chitosan to prepare curcumin-loaded polycaprolactone-chitosan nanoparticles using a simple nano-coprecipitation technique.[136] These nanoparticles have pronounced cellular uptake and anticancer activity on HeLA cells and OCM-1 cells. Overall, the results indicated that the conjugation of hydrophobic PCL nanoparticles with mucoadhesive chitosan polymer enhanced drug loading and release, cellular interaction, and in vitro anticancer activity of the nanoparticles make them suitable for curcumin delivery.

A number of studies have been done on grafting of different polymers onto chitosan to gain desirable properties in drug delivery applications. PCL was grafted onto galactosylated chitosan backbone to prepare curcumin-loaded PCL–chitosan nanoparticles to achieve a hepatocyte targeted system.[137] PCL played a crucial role in enhancing the controlled release of curcumin from the nanoparticles while galactolysation of nanoparticles improved cellular uptake. The cellular uptake study of PCL–chitosan nanoparticles with and without galactolysation on the HepG2 cell line showed higher uptake of the galactolysed nanoparticles compared to PCL–chitosan nanoparticles, which was attributed to the interaction between asialoglycoprotein (ASGP) receptors on HepG2 cells and the galactose ligands on the surface of the nanoparticles. Studies on thermosensitive polymer nanoparticle systems like chitosan grafted with poly(N-isopropylacrylamide) nanoparticles and chitosan-g-poly(N-vinylcaprolactam) nanoparticles prepared for curcumin delivery have shown specific cytotoxicity against MCF-7, KB, and PC-3 cancer cell lines.[83,138]

8.3.3.4   Guar Gum

Another natural biodegradable polymer applicable in curcumin delivery is guar gum. It is a natural polysaccharide composed of two types of glucose: galactose and mannose. The structure contains a straight chain of D mannose units, linked by β-(1–4) glycoside linkages and bearing a single D-galactose unit on approximately every alternate mannose, joined by an α-(1–6) glycoside linkage. It shows stability in solutions in the pH range 5–7 and therefore it has been generally used for colon targeted drug delivery. Efforts have been made to improve the solubility and bioavailability of curcumin by incorporating it within hydrophilic guar gum. Curcumin-loaded guar gum nanoparticles, prepared by wet granulation method, showed good drug release in controlled manner, indicating its future potential.[139,140] However, very few studies have reported the use of this polymer for delivery of curcumin.

Chahatray et al. prepared guar gum–blended sodium alginate nanocomposite for curcumin delivery. The drug release characteristics of the nanocomposites were greatly improved by the incorporation of nanoclay cloisite 30B.[141] Clay minerals, synthetic or natural, have gained much attention recently in controlled release of drugs due to their unique swelling, intercalation, adsorption, and ion exchange properties. They are nontoxic for transdermal and oral applications. Use of clay in drug delivery systems offers intercalation of drugs into the interlayer gallery of clay minerals to accomplish controlled release.

8.3.3.5   Magnetic Nanoparticles

The major drawback in most chemotherapeutic approaches to cancer treatment is their nonspecificity, hence leading to severe side effects. To overcome this disadvantage, magnetic nanoparticles can be used. Magnetic nanoparticles have been extensively investigated as the next generation of targeted drug delivery due to their capability of functioning both at the cellular and molecular level of biological interactions.[142,143] Drug-loaded magnetic nanoparticles are being developed to be delivered to the tumor site under the influence of external magnetic field. But these nanoparticles must be magnetic only under external magnetic field otherwise they should be inactive once the magnetic field is removed. *Superparamagnetic* nanoparticles are an example. Magnetite (Fe_3O_4) is a natural mineral that is widely used as *superparamagnetic* nanoparticles for diverse biological applications like MRI, magnetic separation, magnetic drug delivery, etc.[144] However, their use is limited due to their tendency for aggregation, which can be minimized by engineering the surface of the magnetic nanoparticles by using polymer coating. A number of polymers have been explored for coating purposes such as dextran, chitosan, starch PEG, etc.[145] Yallapu et al. reported a preferential cellular uptake of cyclodextrin-PF68-coated iron oxide magnetic nanoparticles in MDA-MB-231 breast cancer cells.[146] Cyclodextrin has the ability to bind to the iron oxide nanoparticle surface with their -OH groups along with inclusion of curcumin through the hydrophobic cavity. Further coating with PF68 provides hydrophobic chain to bind hydrophobic cavities of cyclodextrin and the hydrophilic chain provides additional hydrophilicity and stability to the particles. Dual coating resulted in a significant loading and slow, sustained release of curcumin. Additionally, this formulation exhibited enhanced MRI properties, and its magnetic targeting facilitated an enhanced delivery of curcumin to the cancer cells. The unique autoflourescent property of curcumin offers opportunities to study its cellular uptake through fluorescence imaging. Tran et al. showed that chitosan-coated magnetic nanoparticles exhibited excellent cellular uptake as revealed by florescence microscope.[147] Thus, magnetic nanoparticles–based systems appear to have substantial potential in delivering curcumin to specific targets.

8.4   CONCLUSION AND FUTURE SCOPE

Curcumin is one of the most explored natural, plant-derived compounds in the treatment and prevention of cancer. However, curcumin has achieved limited success due to its poor bioavailability, rapid metabolism, and elimination. Efforts for development of advanced drug delivery systems to utilize this natural compound for its chemopreventive potential continue even today. In recent years, the application of nanotechnology in facilitating the practice of curcumin in the field of cancer therapy has experienced a constant growth. Nanoparticles reduce toxicity and side effects of drugs, and also enrich solubility and stability of drugs like curcumin. The importance of nanoparticles lies on their prospects for designing and tuning properties, which is not possible in other types of therapeutic means. Nanocarriers derived from a varieties of materials—lipid, protein, liposome, gold nanoparticles, polymer nanoparticles, iron oxide nanoparticles, etc.—are regulated to deliver the drug in a controlled and targeted manner to make them efficient drug delivery systems. Among these materials, polymer (natural or synthetic biodegradable) has been a widespread choice in the production of a variety of biomedical devices owing to their biodegradability, biocompatibility, and tunable characteristics. The incorporation of clay particles inside polymer matrix paves a new method for improving drug release properties of such systems. Researches relating to drug delivery formulations based on magnetic nanoparticles along with suitable polymer coating for improving biocompatibility, stability in biological environment, high therapeutic drug loading property, and intercellular uptake by cancer cells are in progress. These nanoparticles have been utilized in MRI, hyperthermia, magnetic targeting, etc. Again, the inclusion of targeting ligands such as peptide, folic acid, etc., to these systems is also one of the emerging techniques that expand the horizon of drug delivery systems. Along with their numerous advantages, nanoparticles are limited in their stability, tendency for agglomeration, and cytotoxicity. Consequently, improvement in stability and biocompatibility are the main concerns of nanotechnology research. Although oral curcumin is believed to be safe, intravenous nanoformulations of curcumin is considered risky as it might increase side effects. Hence, the preparation of effective intravenous curcumin is now highlighted as a future challenge. Altogether, these studies specify that nanotechnology-based drug delivery formulations hold great promise in cancer therapy that may enhance the solubility, bioavailability, and medicinal value, along with controlled and targeting delivery of this molecule from Mother Nature.

REFERENCES

1. International Agency for Research on Cancer. GLOBOCAN 2012: Estimated cancer incidence, mortality and prevalence worldwide in 2012. World Health Organization, Lyon, France. http://globocan.iarc.fr/Pages/fact_sheets_cancer.aspx. Accessed on August 4, 2015.
2. Casanovas, O. 2012. Limitations of therapies exposed. *Nature* 484:44–46.
3. Kelloff, J.G., Crowell, A.J., Steele, E.V., Lubet, A.R., Malone, A.W., Boone, W.C., Kopelovich, L. et al. 2000. Progress in cancer chemoprevention: Development of diet derived chemopreventive agents. *J. Nutr.* 130:467s–471s.
4. Dasgupta, T., Rao, A.R., Yadava, P.K. 2003. Modulatory effect of Henna leaf (Lawsonia inermis) on drug metabolising phase I and phase II enzymes, antioxidant enzymes, lipid peroxidation and chemically induced skin and forestomach papillomagenesis in mice. *Mol. Cell. Biochem.* 245:11–22.
5. Milobedzka, J., Kostanecki, S.V., Lampe, V. 1910. Zur Kenntnis des Curcumins. *Berichte der deutschen Chemischen Gesellschaft* 43(2):2163–2170.
6. Srimal, R.C., Dhawan, B.N. 1973. Pharmacology of diferuloyl methane (curcumin), a non-steroidal anti-inflammatory agent. *J. Pharm. Pharmacol.* 25(6):447–452.
7. Jain, S.K., DeFilipps, R.A. 1991. Medicinal Plants of India. Reference Publishers, Algonac, MI.
8. Ammon, H.P., Wahl, M.A. 1991. Pharmacology of Curcuma longa. *Planta Med.* 57(1):1–7.
9. Vogel, A., Pelletier, J. 1815. Examen chimique de la racine de Curcuma. *J. Pharm.* 1:289–300.
10. Daube, F.V. 1870. Uber curcumin, den farbstoff der Curcumawurzel. *Ber Deutsch Chem Ges.* 3:609–13.
11. Lampe, V., Milobedzka J. 1913. Studien uber Curcumin. *Ber. Deut. Chem. Ges.* 46:2235–2237.
12. Srinivasan, K.R. 1952. The coloring matter in Turmeric. *Curr. Sci.* 21:311–312.
13. Kunchandy, E., Rao, M.N.A. 1990. Oxygen radical scavenging activity of curcumin. *Int. J. Pharm.* 58(3):237–240.
14. Moghadamtousi, S.Z., Kadir, H.A., Hassandarvish, P., Tajik, H., Abubakar, S., Zandi, K. 2014. A review on antibacterial, antiviral, and antifungal activity of curcumin. *Biomed. Res. Int.* 2014:1–12.
15. Parvathy, K.S., Negi, P.S., Srinivas, P. 2009. Antioxidant, antimutagenic and antibacterial activities of curcumin-beta-diglucoside. *Food Chem.* 115(1):265–271.
16. Neelofar, K., Shreaz, S., Rimple, B., Muralidhar, S., Nikhat, M., Khan, L.A. 2011. Curcumin as a promising anticandidal of clinical interest. *Can. J. Microbiol.* 57(3):204–210.
17. Pan, M.H., Lin-Shiau, S.Y., Lin, J.K. 2000. Comparative studies on the suppression of nitric oxide synthase by curcumin and its hydrogenated metabolites through down-regulation of IkB kinase and NFkB activation in macrophages. *Biochem. Pharmacol.* 60(11):1665–1676.
18. Babu, P.S., Srinivasan, K. 1995. Influence of dietary curcumin and cholesterol on the progression of experimentally induced diabetes in albino rat. *Mol. Cell Biochem.* 152(1):13–21.
19. Awasthi, S., Srivatava, S.K., Piper, J.T., Singhal, S.S., Chaubey, M., Awasthi, Y.C. 1996. Curcumin protects against 4-hydroxy-2-trans-nonenal-induced cataract formation in rat lenses. *Am. J. Clin. Nutr.* 64(5):761–766.
20. Lim, G.P., Chu, T., Yang, F., Beech, W., Frautschy, S.A., Cole, G.M. 2001. The curry spice curcumin reduces oxidative damage and amyloid pathology in an Alzheimer transgenic mouse. *J. Neurosci.* 21(21):8370–8377.
21. Deodhar, S.D., Sethi, R. Srimal, R.C. 1980. Preliminary study on antirheumatic activity of curcumin (diferuloyl methane). *Indian J. Med. Res.* 71:632–634.

22. Suzuki, M., Nakamura, T., Iyoki, S., Fujiwara, A., Watanabe, Y., Mohri, K., Isobe, K., Ono, K., Yano, S. 2005. Elucidation of anti-allergic activities of curcumin-related compounds with a special reference to their anti-oxidative activities. *Biol. Pharm. Bull.* 28(8):1438–1443.

23. Chen, H.W., Huang, H.C. 1998. Effect of curcumin on cell cycle progression and apoptosis in vascular smooth muscle cells. *Br. J. Pharmacol.* 124(6):1029–1040.

24. Ghosh, A.K., Kay, N.E., Secreto, C.R., Shanafelt, T.D. 2009. Curcumin inhibits pro-survival pathways in CLL B-cells and has the potential to overcome stromal protection of CLL B-cells in combination with EGCG. *Clin. Cancer Res.* 15(4):1250–1258.

25. Abusnina, A., Keravis, T., Yougbaré, I., Bronner, C., Lugnier, C. 2011. Anti-proliferative effect of curcumin on melanoma cells is mediated by PDE1A inhibition that regulates the epigenetic integrator UHRF1. *Mol. Nutr. Food Res.* 55(11):1677–1689.

26. Lin, Y.C., Chen, H.W., Kuo, Y.C., Chang, Y.F., Lee, Y.J., Hwang, J.J. 2010. Therapeutic efficacy evaluation of curcumin on human oral squamous cell carcinoma xenograft using multimodalities of molecular imaging. *Am. J. Chin. Med.* 38(2):343–358.

27. Chen, H.W., Lee, J.Y., Huang, J.Y., Wang, C.C., Chen, W.J., Su, S.F., Huang, C.W. et al. 2008. Curcumin inhibits lung cancer cell invasion and metastasis through the tumor suppressor HLJ1. *Cancer Res.* 68(18):7428–7438.

28. Swamy, M.V., Citineni, B., Patlolla, J.M., Mohammed, A., Zhang, Y., Rao, C.V. 2008. Prevention and treatment of pancreatic cancer by curcumin in combination with omega-3 fatty acids. *Nutr. Cancer* 60:81–89.

29. Ohtsu, H., Xiao, Z., Ishida, J., Nagai, M., Wang, H.K., Itokawa, H. 2002. Antitumor agents: Curcumin analogues as novel androgen receptor antagonists with potential as antiprostate cancer agents. *J. Med. Chem.* 45:5037–5042.

30. Rajasekaran, S.A. 2011. Therapeutic potential of curcumin in gastrointestinal diseases. *World J. Gastrointest. Pathophysiol.* 2(1):1–14.

31. Sharma, R.A., Euden, S.A., Platton, S.L, Cooke, D.N., Shafayat, A., Hewitt, H.R., Marczylo, T.H. et al. 2004. Phase I clinical trial of oral curcumin: Biomarkers of systemic activity and compliance. *Clin. Cancer Res.* 10:6847–5684.

32. Perkins, S., Verschoyle, R.D., Hill, K., Parveen, I. 2002. Chemopreventive efficacy and pharmacokinetics of curcumin in the min/+ mouse, a model of familial adenomatous-polyposis. *Cancer Epidemiol. Biomarkers Prev.* 11:535–540.

33. Kaul, S., Krishnakantha, T.P. 1997. Influence of retinol deficiency and curcumin/turmeric feeding on tissue microsomal membrane lipid peroxidation and fatty acids in rats. *Mol. Cell Biochem.* 175:43–48.

34. Aggarwal, B.B., Kumar, A., Bharti, A.C. 2003. Anticancer potential of curcumin: Preclinical and clinical studies. *Anticancer Res.* 23:363–398.

35. Bar-Sela, G., Epelbaum, R., Schaffer, M. 2010. Curcumin as an anti-cancer agent: Review of the gap between basic and clinical applications. *Curr. Med. Chem.* 17(3):190–197.

36. Gillett, C., Fantl, V., Smith, R., Fisher, C., Bartek, J., Dickson, C., Barnes, D., Peters, G. 1994. Amplification and overexpression of cyclin D1 in breast cancer detected by immunohistochemical staining. *Cancer Res.* 54:1812–1817.

37. Adelaide, J., Monges, G., Derderian, C., Seitz, J.F., Birnbaum, D. 1995. Oesophageal cancer and amplification of the human cyclin D gene CCND1/PRAD1. *Br. J. Cancer* 71:64–68.

38. Caputi, M., Groeger, A.M., Esposito, V., Dean, C., De Luca, A., Pacilio, C., Muller, M.R. et al. 1999. Prognostic role of cyclin D1 in lung cancer. Relationship to proliferating cell nuclear antigen. *Am. J. Respir. Cell Mol. Biol.* 20:746–50.

39. Arber, N., Hibshoosh, H., Moss, S.F., Sutter, T., Zhang, Y., Begg, M., Wang, S., Weinstein, I.B., Holt, P.R. 1996. Increased expression of cyclin D1 is an early event in multistage colorectal carcinogenesis. *Gastroenterology* 110:669–974.

40. Bartkova, J., Lukas, J., Muller, H., Strauss, M., Gusterson, B., Bartek, J. 1995. Abnormal patterns of D-type cyclin expression and GI regulation in human head and neck cancer. *Cancer Res.* 55:949–956.

41. Singh, A.K., Sidhu, G.S., Deepa, T., Maheshwari, R.K. 1996. Curcumin inhibits the proliferation and cell cycle progression of human umbilical vein endothelial cell. *Cancer Lett.* 107(1):109–115.

42. Mohan, R., Sivak, J., Ashton, P., Russo, L.A., Pham, B.Q., Kasahara, N. 2000. Curcuminoids inhibit the angiogenic response stimulated by fibroblast growth factor-2, including expression of matrix metalloproteinase gelatinase B. *J. Biol. Chem.* 275(14):10405–10412.

43. Han, S., Chung, S.T., Robertson, D.A., Ranjan, D., Bondada, S. 1999. Curcumin causes the growth arrest and apoptosis of Bcell lymphoma by down regulation of egr-1, C myc, Bcl-X(l),NF-κB, and p53. *Clin. Immunol.* 93(2):152–161.

44. Park, M.J., Kim, E.H., Park, I.C. 2002. Curcumin inhibits cell cycle progression of immortalized human umbilical vein endothelial (ECV304) cells by up-regulating cyclin-dependent kinase inhibitor, p21WAF1/CIP1, p27KIP1 and p53. *Int. J. Oncol.* 21(2):379–383.

45. Shankar, S., Srivastava, R.K. 2007. Involvement of Bcl-2 family members, phosphatidylinositol 3-kinase/AKT and mitochondrial p53 in curcumin (diferulolylmethane)-induced apoptosis in prostate cancer. *Int. J. Oncol.* 30(4):905–918.

46. Anand, P., Kunnumakkara, A.B., Newman, R.A., Aggarwal, B.B. 2007. Bioavailability of curcumin: Problems and promises. *Mol. Pharmaceut.* 4(6):807–818.

47. Wahlstrom, B., Blennow, G. 1978. A study on the fate of curcumin in the rat. *Acta Pharmacol. Toxicol. (Copenhagen)* 43(2):86–92.

48. Shoba, G., Joy, D., Joseph, T., Majeed, M., Rajendran, R., Srinivas, P.S. 1998. Influence of piperine on the pharmacokinetics of curcumin in animals and human volunteers. *Planta Med.* 64(4):353–356.

49. Yang, K.Y., Lin, L.C., Tseng, T.Y., Wang, S.C., Tsai, T.H. 2007. Oral bioavailability of curcumin in rat and the herbal analysis from Curcuma longa by LC-MS/MS. *J. Chromatogr. B Anal. Technol. Biomed. Life Sci.* 853(1–2):183–189.

50. Pan, M.H., Huang, T.M., Lin, J.K. 1999. Biotransformation of curcumin through reduction and glucuronidation in mice. *Drug Metab. Dispos.* 27(4):486–494.

51. Garcea, G., Jones, D.J., Singh, R., Dennison, A.R., Farmer, P.B., Sharma, R.A., Steward, W.P., Gescher, A.J., Berry, D.P. 2004. Detection of curcumin and its metabolites in hepatic tissue and portal blood of patients following oral administration. *Br. J. Cancer* 90(5):1011–1015.

52. Garcea, G., Berry, D.P., Jones, D.J., Singh, R., Dennison, A.R., Farmer, P.B., Sharma, R.A., Steward, W.P., Gescher, A.J. 2005. Consumption of the putative chemopreventive agent curcumin by cancer patients: Assessment of curcumin levels in the colorectum and their pharmacodynamic consequences. *Cancer Epidemiol. Biomarkers Prev.* 14(1):120–125.

53. Kasim, N.A., Whitehouse, M., Ramachandran, C. 2004. Molecular properties of WHO essential drugs and provisional biopharmaceutical classification. *Mol. Pharm.* 1(1):85–96.

54. Cruz-Correa, M., Shoskes, D.A., Sanchez, P., Zhao, R., Hylind, L.M., Wexner, S.D., Giardiello, F.M. 2006. Combination treatment with curcumin and quercetin of adenomas in familial adenomatous polyposis. *Clin. Gastroenterol. Hepatol.* 4(8):1035–1038.

55. Li, L., Ahmed, B., Mehta, K., Kurzrock, R. 2007. Liposomal curcumin with and without oxaliplatin: Effects on cell growth, apoptosis, and angiogenesis in colorectal cancer. *Mol. Cancer Ther.* 6:1276–82.

56. Sahu, A., Kasoju, N., Bora, U. 2008. Fluorescence study of the curcumin-casein micelle complexation and its application as a drug nanocarrier to cancer cells. *Biomacromolecules* 9:2905–2912.

57. Verma, S.P., Salamone, E., Goldin, B. 1997. Curcumin and genistein, plant natural products, show synergistic inhibitory effects on the growth of human breast cancer MCF-7 cells induced by estrogenic pesticides. *Biochem. Biophys. Res. Commun.* 233(3):692–696.

58. Fang, J.Y., Hung, C.F., Chiu, H.C., Wang, J.J., Chan, T.F. 2003. Efficacy and irritancy of enhancers on the in-vitro and in-vivo percutaneous absorption of curcumin. *J. Pharm. Pharmacol.* 55(5):593–601.

59. Dhule, S.S., Penfornis, P., Frazier, T., Walker, R., Feldman, J., Tan, G., He, J., Alb, A., John, V., Pochampally, R. 2012. Curcumin-loaded γ-cyclodextrin liposomal nanoparticles as delivery vehicles for osteosarcoma. *Nanomed. Nanotech. Biol. Med.* 8:440–451.

60. Kakkar, V., Singh, S., Singla, D., Kaur, I.P. 2011. Exploring solid lipid nanoparticles to enhance the oral bioavailability of curcumin. *Mol. Nutr. Food Res.* 55(3):495–503.

61. Ma, Z., Shayeganpour, A., Brocks, D.R., Lavasanifar, A., Samuel, J. 2007. High-performance liquid chromatography analysis of curcumin in rat plasma: Application to pharmacokinetics of polymeric micellar formulation of curcumin. *Biomed. Chromatogr.* 21(5):546–552.

62. Song, L., Shen, Y., Hou, J., Lei, L., Guo, S., Qian, C. 2011. Polymeric micelles for parenteral delivery of curcumin: Preparation, characterization and *in vitro* evaluation. *Colloids Surf. A Physicochem. Eng. Aspects* 390:25–32.

63. Liu, A., Lou, H., Zhao, L., Fan, P. 2006. Validated LC/MS/MS assay for curcumin and tetrahydrocurcumin in rat plasma and application to pharmacokinetic study of phospholipid complex of curcumin. *J. Pharm. Biomed. Anal.* 40(3):720–727.

64. Mosley, C.A., Liotta, D.C., Snyder, J.P. 2007. Highly active anticancer curcumin analogues. *Adv. Exp. Med. Biol.* 595:77–103.

65. Kang, H.J., Lee, S.H., Price, J.E, Kim, L.S. 2009. Curcumin suppresses the paclitaxel-induced nuclear factor-kappaB in breast cancer cells and potentiates the growth inhibitory effect of paclitaxel in a breast cancer nude mice model. *Breast J.* 15:223–229.

66. John, V.D., Kuttan, G., Krishnankutty, K. 2002. Anti-tumour studies of metal chelates of synthetic curcuminoids. *J. Exp. Clin. Cancer Res.* 21(2):219–224.

67. Thompson, K.H., Bohmerle, K., Polishchuk, E., Martins, C., Toleikis, P., Tse, J., Yuen, V., McNeill, J.H., Orvig, C.2004. Complementary inhibition of synoviocyte, smooth muscle cell or mouse lymphoma cell proliferation by a vanadyl curcumin complex compared to curcumin alone. *J. Inorg. Biochem.* 98(12):2063–2070.

68. Sui, Z., Salto, R., Li, J., Craik, C., Ortiz de Montellano, P.R. 1993. Inhibition of the HIV-1 and HIV-2 proteases by curcumin and curcumin boron complexes. *Bioorg. Med. Chem.* 1(6):415–422.

69. Vajragupta, O., Boonchoong, P., Watanabe, H., Tohda, M., Kummasud, N., Sumanont, Y. 2003. Manganese complexes of curcumin and its derivatives: Evaluation for the radical scavenging ability and neuroprotective activity. *Free Radic. Biol. Med.* 35(12):1632–1644.

70. Yadav, V.R., Suresh, S., Devi, K., Yadav, S. 2009. Effect of cyclodextrin complexation of curcumin on its solubility and antiangiogenic and anti-inflammatory activity in rat colitis model. *AAPS Pharm. Sci. Tech.* 10(3):752–762.

71. Rahman, S., Cao, S., Steadman, K.J., Wei, M., Parekh, H.S. 2012. Native and β cyclodextrin-enclosed curcumin: Entrapment within liposomes and their *in vitro* cytotoxicity in lung and colon cancer. *Drug Deliv.* 19(7):346–353.

72. Yun, Y., Cho, Y.W., Park, K. 2013. Nanoparticles for oral delivery: Targeted nanoparticles with peptidic ligands for oral protein delivery. *Adv. Drug Deliv. Rev.* 65(6):822–832.

73. Rao, D.P., Srivastav, S.K., Prasad, C., Saxena, R., Asthana, S. 2010. Role of nanoparticles in drug delivery. *Int. J. Nanotech. App.* 4(1):45–49.

74. Jiang, W., Kim, B.Y.S., Rutka, J.T., Chan, W.C.W. 2008. Nanoparticle-mediated cellular response is size-dependent. *Nat. Nanotechnol.* 3:145–150.

75. Chono, S., Tanino, T., Seki, T., Morimoto, K. 2007. Uptake characteristics of liposomes by rat alveolar macrophages: Influence of particle size and surface mannose modification. *J. Pharm. Pharmacol.* 59(1):75–80.

76. Win, K.Y., Feng, S.S. 2005. Effects of particle size and surface coating on cellular uptake of polymeric nanoparticles for oral delivery of anticancer drugs. *Biomaterials* 26(15):2713–2722.

77. Qiu, Y., Liu, Y., Wang, L., Xu, L., Bai, R., Ji, Y., Wu, X., Zhao, Y., Li, Y., Chen, C. 2010. Surface chemistry and aspect ratio mediated cellular uptake of Au nanorods. *Biomaterials* 31(30):7606–7619.

78. Bartneck, M., Keul, H.A., Singh, S., Czaja, K., Bornemann, J., Bockstaller, M., Moeller, M., Zwadlo-Klarwasser, G., Groll, J. 2010. Rapid uptake of gold nanorods by primary human blood phagocytes and immunomodulatory effects of surface chemistry. *ACS Nano* 4(6):3073–3086.

79. Basnet, P., Hussain, H., Tho, I., Skalko-Basnet, N. 2012. Liposomal delivery system enhances anti-inflammatory properties of curcumin. *J. Pharm. Sci.* 101(2):598–609.

80. Chirio, D., Gallarate, M., Peira, E., Battaglia, L., Serpe, L., Trotta, M. 2011. Formulation of curcumin-loaded solid lipid nanoparticles produced by fatty acids coacervation technique. *J. Microencapsul.* 28(6):537–548.

81. Barik, A., Priyadarsini, K.I., Mohan, H. 2003. Photophysical studies on binding of curcumin to bovine serum albumin. *Photochem. Photobiol.* 77(6):597–603.

82. Ganta, S., Amiji, M. 2009. Coadministration of paclitaxel and curcumin in nanoemulsion formulations to overcome multidrug resistance in tumor cells. *Mol. Pharm.* 6(3):928–39.

83. Bisht, S., Feldmann, G., Soni, S., Ravi, R., Karikar, C., Maitra, A., Maitra, A. 2007. Polymeric nanoparticle-encapsulated curcumin ("nanocurcumin"): A novel strategy for human cancer therapy. *J. Nanobiotechnol.* 5(3):1–18.

84. Letchford, K., Liggins, R., Burt, H. 2008. Solubilization of hydrophobic drugs by methoxy poly(ethylene glycol)-block-polycaprolactone diblock copolymer micelles: Theoretical and experimental data and correlations. *J. Pharmaceut. Sci.* 97(3):1179–1190.

85. Ahmad, Z., Pandey, R., Sharma, S., Khuller, G.K. 2006. Alginate nanoparticles as antituberculosis drug carriers: Formulation development, pharmacokinetics and therapeutic potential. *Indian J. Chest Dis. Allied Sci.* 48:171–176.

86. Pandey, R., Khuller, G.K. 2006. Oral nanoparticle based antituberculosis drug delivery to the brain in an experimental model. *J. Antimicrob. Chemother.* 57(6):1146–1152.

87. Jones, M.C., Leroux, J.C. 1999. Polymeric micelles-a new generation of colloidal drug carriers. *Eur. J. Pharm. Biopharm.* 48(2):101–111.

88. Dandekar, P., Jain, R., Kumar, C., Subramanian, S., Samuel, G., Venkatesh, M., Patravale, V. 2009. Curcumin loaded pH-sensitive nanoparticles for the treatment of colon cancer. *J. Biomed. Nanotechnol.* 5(5):445–455.

89. Rejinold, N.S., Muthunarayanan, M., Divyarani, V.V., Sreerekha, P.R., Chennazhi, K.P., Nair, S.V., Tamura, H., Jayakumar, R. 2011. Curcumin-loaded biocompatible thermoresponsive polymeric nanoparticles for cancer drug delivery. *J. Colloid Interface Sci.* 360(1):39–51.

90. Ueda, H., Kreuter, J. 1997. Optimization of the preparation of loperamide-loaded poly (l-lactide) nanoparticles by high pressure emulsification solvent evaporation. *J. Microencapsul.* 14(15):593–605.

91. Tabata, J., Ikada, Y. 1989. Protein pre-coating of polylactide microspheres containing a lipophilic immunopotentiator for enhancement of macrophage phagocytosis and activation. *Pharm. Res.* 6(4):296–301.

92. Lemarchand, C., Gref, R., Passirani, C., Garcion, E., Petri, B., Muller, R. 2006. Influence of polysaccharide coating on the interactions of nanoparticles with biological systems. *Biomaterials* 27(1):108–118.

93. Banik, N., Hussain, A., Ramteke, A., Sharma, H.K., Maji, T.K. 2012. Preparation and evaluation of the effect of particle size on the properties of chitosan-montmorillonite nanoparticles loaded with isoniazid. *RSC Adv.* 2:10519–10528.

94. Lowe, P.J., Temple, C.S. 1994. Calcitonin and insulin in isobutylcyanoacrylate nanocapsules: Protection against proteases and effect on intestinal absorption in rats. *J. Pharm. Pharmacol.* 46(7):547–552.

95. Lescure, F., Zimmer, C., Roy, D., Couvreur, P. 1992. Optimization of polycyanoacrylate nanoparticle preparation: Influence of sulfur dioxide and pH on nanoparticle characteristics. *J. Colloid Interface Sci.* 154(1):77–86.

96. Devi, N., Maji, T.K. 2009. Microencapsulation of isoniazid in genipin-crosslinked gelatin-A-*k*-carrageenan polyelectrolyte complex. *Drug Dev. Ind. Pharm.* 36(1):56–63.

97. Saikia, C., Hussain, A., Ramteke, A., Sharma, H.K., Maji, T.K. 2014. Crosslinked thiolated starch coated Fe_3O_4 magnetic nanoparticles: Effect of montmorillonite and crosslinking density on drug delivery properties. *Starch/Stärke* 66:1–12.

98. Saikia, C., Hussain, A., Ramteke, A., Sharma, H.K., Maji, T.K. 2014. Carboxymethyl starch-chitosan-coated iron oxide magnetic nanoparticles for controlled delivery of isoniazid. *J. Microencapsul.* 4:1–11. doi: 10.3109/02652048.2014.940015.

99. Athanasiou, K.A., Niederauer, G.G., Agrawal, C. 1996. Sterilization, toxicity, biocompatibility and clinical applications of polylactic acid/polyglycolic acid copolymers. *Biomaterials* 17(2):93–102.

100. Mukerjee, A., Vishwanatha, J.K. 2009. Formulation, characterization and evaluation of curcumin-loaded PLGA nanospheres for cancer therapy. *Anticancer Res.* 29(10):3867–3875.

101. Yallapu, M.M., Gupta, B.K., Jaggi, M., Chauhan, S.C. 2010. Fabrication of curcumin encapsulated PLGA nanoparticles for improved therapeutic effects in metastatic cancer cells. *J. Colloid Interface Sci.* 351(1):19–29.

102. Shaikh, J., Ankola, D.D., Beniwal, V., Singh, D., Kumar, M.N.V.R. 2009. Nanoparticle encapsulation improves oral bioavailability of curcumin by at least 9-fold when compared to curcumin administered with piperine as absorption enhancer. *Eur. J. Pharm. Sci.* 37:223–230.

103. Anand, P., Nair, H.B., Sung, B., Kunnumakkara, A.B., Yadav, V.R., Tekmal, R.R., Aggarwal, B.B. 2010. Design of curcumin-loaded PLGA nanoparticles formulation with enhanced cellular uptake, and increased bioactivity *in vitro* and superior bioavailability *in vivo*. *Biochem. Pharmacol.* 79(3):330–338.

104. Shahani, K., Swaminathan, S.K., Freeman, D., Blum, A., Ma, L., Panyam, J. 2010. Injectable sustained release microparticles of curcumin: A new concept for cancer chemoprevention. *Cancer Res.* 70(11):4443–4452.

105. Grabovac, V., Bernkop-Schnurch, A. 2007. Development and *in vitro* evaluation of surface modified poly(lactide-co-glycolide) nanoparticles with chitosan-4-thiobutylamidine. *Drug Dev. Ind. Pharm.* 33:767–774.

106. Thamake, S.I., Raut, S.L., Ranjan, A.P., Gryczynski, Z., Vishwanatha, J.K. 2011. Surface functionalization of PLGA nanoparticles by noncovalent insertion of a homobifunctional spacer for active targeting in cancer therapy. *Nanotechnology* 22:1–10.

107. Punfa, W., Yodkeeree, S., Pitchakarn, P., Ampasavate, C., Limtrakul, P. 2012. Enhancement of cellular uptake and cytotoxicity of curcumin-loaded PLGA nanoparticles by conjugation with anti-P-glycoprotein in drug resistance cancer cells. *Acta Pharmacol. Sin.* 33(6):823–831.

108. Herold, D.A., Keil, K., Bruns, D.E. 1989. Oxidation of polyethylene glycol by alcohol dehydrogenase. *Biochem. Pharmacol.* 38(1):73–76.

109. Richter, A.W., Akerblom, E. 1983. Antibodies against polyethylene glycol produced in animals by immunization with monomethoxy polyethylene glycol-modified proteins. *Int. Arch. Allergy Immunol.* 70(2):124–131.

110. Safavy, A., Raisch, K.P., Mantena, S., Sanford, L.L., Sham, S.W., Krishna, N.R., Bonner, J.A. 2007. Design and development of water soluble curcumin conjugates as potential anticancer agents. *J. Med. Chem.* 50(24):6284–6288.

111. Kim, C.Y., Bordenave, N., Ferruzzi, M.G., Safavy, A., Kim, K.H. 2011. Modification of curcumin with polyethylene glycol enhances the delivery of curcumin in preadipocytes and its antiadipogenic property. *J. Agric. Food Chem.* 59:1012–1019.

112. Vonarbourg, A., Passirani, C., Saulnier, P., Benoit, J.P. 2006. Parameters influencing the stealthiness of colloidal drug delivery systems. *Biomaterials* 27(24):4356–4373.

113. Sahu, A., Bora, U., Kasoju, N., Goswami, P. 2008. Synthesis of novel biodegradable and self-assembling methoxy poly(ethylene glycol)–palmitate nanocarrier for curcumin delivery to cancer cells. *Acta Biomaterialia* 4(6):1752–1761.

114. Shao, J., Zheng, D., Jiang, Z., Xu, H., Hu, Y., Li, X., Lu, X. 2011. Curcumin delivery by methoxy polyethylene glycol–poly(caprolactone) nanoparticles inhibits the growth of C6 glioma cells. *Acta Biochim. Biophys. Sin.* 43(4):1–8.

115. Yin, H.T., Zhang, D.G., Wu, X.L., Huang, X.E., Chen, G. 2013. *In vivo* evaluation of curcumin-loaded nanoparticles in a A549 xenograft mice model. *Asian Pac. J. Cancer Prev.* 14:409–412.

116. Feng, R., Song, Z., Zhai, G. 2012. Preparation and *in vivo* pharmacokinetics of curcumin-loaded PCL-PEG-PCL triblock copolymeric nanoparticles. *Int. J. Nanomed.* 7:4089–4098.

117. Chae, S.Y., Jang, M.K., Nah, J.W. 2005. Influence of molecular weight on oral absorption of water soluble chitosan. *J. Contr. Release* 102(2):383–394.

118. Muzzarelli, R.A.A. 2009. Chitins and chitosans for the repair of wounded skin, nerve, cartilage and bone. *Carbohydr. Polym.* 76(2):167–182.

119. Kumar, M.N.V.R., Muzzarelli, R.A.A., Muzzarelli, C., Sashiwa, H., Domb, A.J. 2004. Chitosan chemistry and pharmaceutical perspectives. *Chem. Rev.* 104(12):6017–6084.

120. Andrews, G.P., Laverty, T.P., Jones, D.S. 2009. Mucoadhesive polymeric plateform for controlled drug delivery. *Eur. J. Pharm. Biopharm.* 71(3):505–518.

121. Mazzarino, L., Travelet, C., Ortega-Murillo, S., Otsuka, I., Pignot-Paintrand, I., Lemos-Senna, E., Borsali, R. 2012. Elaboration of chitosan-coated nanoparticles loaded with curcumin for mucoadhesive applications. *J. Colloid Interface Sci.* 370(1):58–66.

122. Chabib, L., Martien, R., Ismail, H. 2012. Formulation of nanocurcumin using low viscosity chitosan polymer and its cellular uptake study into T47D cells, *Indonesian J. Pharm.* 23(1):27–35.

123. Kar, S.K., Akhtar, F., Ray, G. Pandey, A.K. 2010. Curcumin nanoparticles and methods of producing the same. School of Biotechnology, Jawaharlal Nehru University, New Delhi, India.

124. Anitha, A., Maya, S., Deepa, N., Chennazhi, K.P., Nair, S.V., Tamura, H., Jayakumar, R. 2012. Curcumin-loaded N,O-carboxymethyl chitosan nanoparticles for cancer drug delivery. *J. Biomater. Sci.* 23:1381–1400.

125. Anitha, A., Maya, S., Deepa, N., Chennazhi, K.P., Nair, S.V., Tamura, H., Jayakumar, R. 2011. Efficient water soluble O-carboxymethyl chitosan nanocarrier for the delivery of curcumin to cancer cells. *Carbohydr. Polym.* 83:452–461.

126. Shelma, R., Sharma, C.P. 2013. *In vitro* and *in vivo* evaluation of curcumin loaded lauroyl sulphated chitosan for enhancing oral bioavailability. *Carbohydr. Polym.* 95(1):441–448.

127. Anitha, A., Deepagan, V.G., Divya Rani, V.V., Menon, D., Nair, S.V., Jayakumar, R. 2011. Preparation, characterization, *in vitro* drug release and biological studies of curcumin loaded dextran sulphate-chitosan nanoparticles. *Carbohydr. Poylm.* 84(3):1158–1164.

128. Sarmento, B., Ribeiro, A., Veiga, F., Ferreira, D. 2006. Development and characterization of new insulin containing polysaccharide nanoparticles. *Colloids Surf. B Biointerfaces* 53(2):193–202.

129. Chen, Y., Mohanraj, V.J., Parkin, J.E. 2003. Chitosan-dextran sulfate nanoparticles for delivery of an anti-angiogenesis peptide. *Lett. Pept. Sci.* 10:621–629.

130. Das, R.K., Kasoju, N., Bora, U. 2010. Encapsulation of curcumin in alginate-chitosan-pluronic composite nanoparticles for delivery to cancer cells. *Nanomed. Nanotech. Biol. Med.* 6(1):153–160.

131. Wanka, G., Hoffmann, H., Ulbricht, W. 1990. The aggregation behavior of poly-(oxyethylene)-poly-(oxypropylene)-poly-(oxyethylene)-block-copolymers in aqueous solution. *Colloid Polym. Sci.* 268(2):101–117.

132. Cabana, A., Aït-Kadi, A., Juhász, J. 1997. Study of the gelation process of polyethylene oxide$_a$-polypropylene oxide$_b$-polyethylene oxideacopolymer (poloxamer 407) aqueous solutions. *J. Colloid Interface Sci.* 190(2):307–312.

133. Wenzel, J.G.W, Balaji, K.S.S., Koushik, K., Navarre, C., Duran, S.H., Rahe, C.H., Kompella, U.B. 2002. Pluronic F127 gel formulations of deslorelin and GnRH reduce drug degradation and sustain drug release and effect in cattle. *J. Contr. Release* 85:51–59.

134. Le, T.M.P., Pham, V.P., Dang, T.M.L., La, T.H., Le, T.H., Le, Q.H. 2013. Preparation of curcumin-loaded pluronic F127/chitosan nanoparticles for cancer therapy. *Adv. Nat. Sci. Nanosci. Nanotechnol.* 4:1–4.

135. Martins, A.F., Bueno, P.V.A., Almeida, E.A., Rodrigues, F.H., Rubira, A.F., Muniz, E.C. 2013. Characterization of N-trimethyl chitosan/alginate complexes and curcumin release. *Int. J. Biol. Macromol.* 57:174–184.

136. Liu, J., Xu, L., Liu, C., Zhang, D., Wang, S., Deng, Z., Lou, W., Xu, H., Bai, Q., Ma, J. 2012. Preparation and characterization of cationic curcumin nanoparticles for improvement of cellular uptake. *Carbohydr. Polym.* 90(1):16–22.

137. Zhou, N., Zan, X., Wang, Z., Wu, H., Yin, D., Liao, C., Wan, Y. 2013. Galactosylated chitosan–polycaprolactone nanoparticles for hepatocyte-targeted delivery of curcumin. *Carbohydr. Polym.* 94(1):420–429.

138. Rejinold, N.S., Sreerekha, P.R., Chennazhi, K.P., Nair, S.V., Jayakumar, R. 2011. Biocompatible, biodegradable and thermo-sensitive chitosan-g-poly (N-isopropylacrylamide) nanocarrier for curcumin drug delivery. *Int. J. Biol. Macromol.* 49(2):161–172.

139. Singhal, A.K., Nalwaya, N., Jarald, E., Ahmed, S. 2010. Colon targeted curcumin delivery using guar gum. *Pharmacognosy Res.* 2(2):82–85.

140. Elias, E.J., Anil, S., Ahmad, S., Daud, A. 2010. Colon targeted curcumin delivery using guar gum. *Nat. Prod. Commun.* 5(6):915–918.

141. Chahatray, R., Sahoo, D., Mohanty, D.P., Nayak, P.L. 2013. Guargum-sodium alginate blended with cloisite 30B for controlled release of anticancer drug curcumin. *World J. Nanosci. Technol.* 2(1):26–32.

142. Shinkai, M. 2002. Functional magnetic particles for medical application. *J. Biosci. Bioeng.* 94(6):606–13.

143. McBain, S.C., Yiu, H.H.P., Dobson, J. 2008. Magnetic nanoparticles for gene and drug delivery. *Int. J. Nanomed.* 3(2):169–180.

144. Laurent, S., Forge, D., Port, M., Roch, A., Robic, C., Vander, E.L., Muller, R.N. 2008 Magnetic iron oxide nanoparticles: Synthesis stabilization, vectorization, physico-chemical characterizations, and biological applications. *Chem. Rev.* 108(6):2064–2110.

145. Neuberger, T., Schopf, B., Hofmann, H., Hofmann, M., Rechenberg, B.V. 2005. Superparamagnetic nanoparticles for biomedical applications: Possibilities and limitations of a new drug delivery system. *J. Magn. Magn. Mater.* 293:483–496.

146. Yallapu, M.M., Othman, S.F., Curtis, E.T., Bauer, N.A., Chauhan, N., Kumar, D., Jaggi, M., Chauhan, S.C. 2012. Curcumin-loaded magnetic nanoparticles for breast cancer therapeutics and imaging applications. *Int. J. Nanomed.* 7:1761–1779.

147. Tran, L.M., Hoang, N.M.T., Mai, T.T., Tran, H.V., Nguyen, N.T., Tran, T.D., Do, M.H. et al. 2010. Nanosized magnetofluorescent Fe_3O_4 curcumin conjugate for multimodal monitoring and drug targeting. *Colloids Surf. A* 371(3):104–112.

9 Plastics of the Future
Innovations for Improvement and Sustainability with Special Relevance to Biomedical Applications

Vinod Pravin Sharma

CONTENTS

9.1　INTRODUCTION

Plastics have molded the modern world and transformed the quality of life. There is no human activity where plastics do not play a key role, from clothing to shelter, from transportation to communication, and from entertainment to healthcare. Because of their many attractive properties such as lightweight, high strength, and ease of processing, plastics meet a large share of materials with bewildering array of needs and that too at a comparatively lesser cost and causing lesser environmental implications. From practically zero during the beginning of the twentieth century, humans today consume more than 150 million tons of plastics per year. Plastics possess a unique combination of properties. Plastics can be super tough, rigid as well as flexible, transparent as well as opaque, and can allow permeation or act as a barrier material. Growing population and material consumption have put severe pressure on our natural resources and fragile ecosystems. The materialistic needs of the present generation are growing and modern plastics offer cost-effective alternative sensors and coatings along with polymer reinforcements of varied types and composition, for storage of consumer items or energy-based device applications.

9.2 REGULATORY GUIDELINES/SPECIFICATIONS

Biobased content is the amount of biobased carbon in the material or product as a fraction weight (mass) or percent weight (mass) of the total organic carbon in the material or product. ASTM Method D6866-05 is the U.S. government–approved method for determining the renewable/biobased content of biobased products. Biobased materials are organic materials in which the carbon comes from contemporary (nonfossil) biological sources. Biodegradable plastics are plastics that can decompose into carbon dioxide, methane, water, inorganic compounds, or biomass via microbial assimilation (the enzymatic action of microorganisms). To be considered biodegradable, this decomposition has to be measured by standardized tests and takes place within a specified period, which varies according to the *disposal* method chosen. The American Society of Testing and Materials (ASTM) has created definitions on what constitutes biodegradability in various disposal environments. Plastics that meet ASTM D6400, for instance, can be certified as biodegradable and compostable in commercial composting facilities. In Europe, the equivalent standardized test criterion is EN 13432. In the United States, there is a biodegradability standard for soil (ASTM D5988), a biodegradability test standard for marine and freshwater (ASTM D6692 and D6691), one for wastewater treatment facilities (ASTM D5271), and one for anaerobic digestion (ASTM D 5511). A number of fossil-fuel-based polymers are certified biodegradable and compostable. Biodegradability is directly linked to the chemical structure, not to the origin of raw materials. What is often less understood is that medical equipment used in healthcare settings inside and outside the operating room—such as hemodialysis machines, wall mount drug-delivery systems, and probe docking stations—may require similar cleaning and disinfection validations. It states that these devices may contribute to secondary cross-contamination by the hands of healthcare workers or by contact with medical instruments that will subsequently come into contact with patients.

Cross-contamination is a growing concern in healthcare settings since infections of patients continue to be prevalent. The FDA expects cleaning and disinfection of any equipment surfaces—such as adjustment knobs, handles, carts, cables, touchscreens, monitors, and keyboards—in a patient-care setting that may become contaminated with blood-borne pathogens or other potentially hazardous organic materials. Reusable devices often have intimate patient contact, become grossly soiled during clinical use, and need to be reprocessed before their next use. Doctors/healthcare personnel and manufacturers of reusable medical devices are to be apprised that these types of devices require cleaning and sterilization processes to be validated before the devices. Under the Seventh Framework Programme, ReBioStent (reinforced bioresorbable biomaterials for therapeutic drug eluting stents) are being developed in collaboration for the production of biodegradable and biocompatible resorbable stents using highly innovative, novel, smart, and multifunctional materials to overcome the shortcomings of the currently available stents. Stents are being developed by a few countries through the functionalization the surface of the stent with antibody fragments that will improve the coating of the stent by endothelial cells. Hypothetically, the endothelial cell coating of the stent will prevent restenosis (narrowing of the artery due to the overgrowth of cells), thereby improving the stent performance. The main focus is the development of unique polymers with defined mechanical properties, biocompatibility, and controlled degradation and aims to prevent common complications associated with conventional stents such as inflammation, in stent restenosis, and thrombosis. In addition, Neurograft is a multinational research project focused on functional spinal cord repair and regeneration as well as nanomesh for soft tissue replacement in the case of hernia using natural and ecologically sustainable biopolymers and electrospun meshes suitable for soft tissue repair.

9.3 GRAPHENE-BASED POLYMERS FOR ELECTRONICS AND DRUG DELIVERY

Nowadays, graphene-based polymers are becoming popular as they serve as a semiconductor with a zero bandgap and exceptionally high charge mobility. Electron mobilities in graphene may reach values that are more than an order of magnitude higher than those encountered in an Si transistor, and thus it opens up the possibility that in the future, graphene may replace silicon as the building block of the electronic industry and revolutionize nanoelectronics. Graphene may be produced through micro-mechanical exfoliation, epitaxial growth of graphene films, chemical vapor deposition, unzipping of carbon nanotubes, or reduction of graphene oxides although with a few limitations and toxicity concerns. In a few cases, supercritical carbon dioxide is used besides other green chemistry principles. There is a great potential for recombinant biopolymers as they mimic the structure of natural proteins and are used for the development of novel bioactive biomaterials with desired properties, which help elucidate molecular interactions in biological systems and elaborate strategies for tissue engineering and drug-delivery purposes. The bioinspired recombinant polypeptides represent a highly promising tool in biomedical research as they are intrinsic constituents of both cells and their natural matrices. It may be characterized in terms of morphology, structure, magnetic properties, drug release, and magnetic drivability with promising results for biomedical applications.

9.4 BIOPLASTICS OR BIOPOLYMERS

Bioplastics are plastics in which 100% of the carbon is derived from renewable agricultural and forestry resources such as corn starch, soybean protein, and cellulose. Most of them are starch and cellulose derivatives, PLA, polycaprolactone (PCL), polybutylene succinate (PBS), and polyhydoxy butyrate (PHB). Nanoscale fillers are layered silicate nanoclays such as montmorillite and kaolinite. Bioplastics are not a single class of polymers but a family of products, which can vary significantly from one another. They differ from traditional plastics, which are derived from fossil fuels or nonrenewable carbon. Not all bioplastics are biodegradable, and not all biodegradable plastics are bioplastics. Reflective mulch based on biodegradable plastics enhances ripening and health compounds in apple fruit by improving light utilization and microclimates through hail net (Overbeck, 2013). Microporous-structured biopolymer scaffolds support tissue cells, while in situ delivering drug molecules makes them potentially useful for therapeutic tissue engineering (Dori, 2014). Chitosan has been one of the most popular biopolymers for the development of drug-delivery systems for various applications due to its promising properties, including high biocompatibility, excellent biodegradability, low toxicity, abundant availability, and low production cost. The tailor-made specifications of chitosan-based PEC drug-delivery systems are readily available in different forms, including nanoparticles, microparticles, beads, tablets, gels, films, and membranes.

There are challenges in increasing the compatibility between clays and polymers as well as attaining complete dispersion of nanoparticles. New nanostructures may be useful to provide active and/or smart properties to packaging systems through antimicrobial properties, mechanical and thermal properties, oxygen-enhancing ability, enzyme immobilization or oxygen levels. This innovative field has advanced toward the molecular and nanoscale design of bioactive systems for regenerative medicine, drug delivery, and tissue engineering (Santo et al., 2012). Interestingly, cartilage has a limited regenerative capacity. The clinical challenge of reconstruction of cartilage defects is now being addressed through the application of nanotechnology through biomimetic cartilage regenerative scaffolds (Erh Hsuin Lim et al., 2014).

In fact, the complex nature of cell–biomaterial interaction requires preclinical functionality testing by studying specific cell responses to different biomaterial properties from morphology and mechanisms to surface characteristics at the molecular level. The bioresorbable scaffolds represent a novel approach in coronary stent technology. Although they have potential advantages, these novel devices may face challenges as well in the coming years during routine clinical practices (Costopoulos et al., 2013).

9.5   SUPER PLASTICS FROM NATURAL FIBERS

Green cars could be made from pineapples and bananas as scientists in Brazil have developed a more effective way to use fibers from these and other plants in a new generation of automotive plastics that are stronger, lighter, and more eco-friendly than plastics now in use (*Science News*, 2011). They described the work that could lead to stronger, lighter, and more sustainable materials for automobiles. Substantial interest and progress in 3D printed biopolymers for varied applications in engineering are being observed. Three-dimensional printing is the process of making a 3D object of virtually any shape from a digital model. It may be used for both prototyping and distributed manufacturing with applications in industrial design, automotive industry, aerospace, architecture, medical industries, tissue engineering, and even food. It provides a biomimetic structural environment that facilitates tissue formation and promotes host tissue integration, including soft and hard tissues (Xiaoming et al., 2014).

9.6   SMART PROSTHESES: ELECTRONICS
RESEARCH AIDS AND ROBOTICS

In our society, it is our social and moral responsibility to be involved in welfare activities under corporate social responsibility (CSR), or otherwise, for the physically challenged human beings. This requirement is due to varied type of incidences or accidents in defense day-to-day activities, congenital disorders, burns, etc., leading to stripping of skin revealing the underlying musculature and skeletal structure. Efforts are being taken to prepare artificial human arm or legs using polymeric material, namely, polyether ether ketones (PEEK) and using pneumatic tubes or biocompatible metallic rods. Increased efforts are needed to improve and solve the problems associated with unexploded landmines in some parts of the world, which has focused attention on the field of prosthetics and orthotics. Greater consciousness about the quality of life of amputees has also promoted research efforts to develop a new generation of products. Some of the technologies being explored for use in advanced prosthesis designs are being drawn from disciplines outside of conventional orthotics and prosthetics development.

Flexible electronics have revealed that conventional, silicon-wafer-based fabrication techniques can be modified to apply electronics to the heterogeneous topography of the skin. Conductive polymer nanocomposites may serve as smart plastics due to their high sensitivity to several kinds of external solicitations such as temperature, strain, and solvent vapors or liquids. To assess human exposure to engineered nanomaterials (ENMs) during the different stages of the life cycle of ENM-containing products, there is a need to estimate their quantities when released to the environment together with toxicity-related parameters such as their size, morphology, and chemical composition. The pulmonary toxic effects induced by inhalation of ENMs are best correlated with the surface area rather than the concentration of the particles. Many in vitro and in vivo studies are currently focusing on understanding the toxic effects of ENMs on different species (rats, fishes, algae, daphnia, bacteria, among eco-toxicological test models). Among these studies, rats as animal models are used for obtaining reference doses.

Sporadic toxicity studies are currently available, which provide complete information on experimental conditions, such as nanoparticles characteristics, animal- or cell-line-related information, exposure duration and frequency, and exposure medium and endpoints observed. These challenges arise due to the following data gaps: lack of sufficient empirical data on the composition of biocorona on the surfaces of nanomaterials; lack of in vitro data that can be used to predict in vivo effects of nanomaterials; and the paucity of descriptors that can specifically be used for nanomaterials. Surface characterization of nanomaterials is generally conducted using scanning electron microscopy, transmission electron microscopy, energy dispersive x-ray, Brunauer–Emmett–Teller (BET) surface analysis, thermogravimetric analysis, and Fourier transform infrared, near-infrared, and Raman spectroscopy. These methods are nowadays used as state-of-the-art technologies, but they are usually complicated, time-consuming, and expensive, thereby making them inappropriate for routine monitoring of ENMs in different environmental media.

9.7 PLASTIC-BASED WEARABLE TECHNOLOGICAL ADVANCEMENTS FOR HEALTH AND BEAUTY

A range of innovative and intelligent devices are being planned, which may allow networking and inter-linkages for the development of specialized cloth that is resistant to dirt, oils, or water droplets. Some devices may provide constant health data, have chameleon-like abilities to change colors, and even take photos with a wink. Such devices may be customizable and connected to the Internet and/or to other devices via Wi-Fi, Bluetooth, or near-field communication. Molding medical devices is a high-end business that has proven more resistant to economic swings and to foreign competition than some other plastics markets. Polyetheretherketone (PEEK) implants such as suture anchor can be molded better (and perhaps faster) with pressurized hot water instead of the usual electrical mold heating. Natural gas contains many of the vital raw materials that are used to manufacture plastics and chemicals. Many experts predict an enormous increase in the production of those plastics most often used in consumer packaging and single-use products. The difficulty of dispersing due to hydrophilic property is overcome by replacing the interlayer clay cations with quarternized ammonium or phosphonium cations preferably with long-chain alkyls. Novel polymers are being synthesized using bioreactors fed with renewable resources from plants or crops such as switchgrass (*Panicum virgatum* L.) with environmentally benign and carbon-neutral source of polymers.

9.8   PORTABLE GAS SENSORS AND OTHER APPLICATIONS

Portable gas sensors can allow searching for explosives, diagnosing medical conditions through a patient's breath, and deciding whether it's safe to stay in a mine. These devices do all this by identifying and measuring airborne chemicals, and a new, more sensitive, smart model is under development at the University of Michigan. The smart sensor could detect chemical weapon vapors or indicators of disease better than the current design. It also consumes less power, crucial for stretching battery life down a mineshaft or in isolated clinics (CHEMEUROPE, n.d.). Eco-materials are also being prepared with the concept of nanotechnology for encapsulation, textiles, and other types of medical or surgical treatments for burns, skin replacement, wound healings, grafting, etc.

9.9   CONCLUSION

Bioplastics are becoming significantly important mainly due to the scarcity of oil, increase in the cost of petroleum-based commodities, and environmental concerns with the dumping of nonbiodegradable plastics in landfills with far-reaching implications on climate change. We have to develop biobased economy from the policy concepts of OECD to link renewable biological resources and bioprocesses through industry-scale biotechnologies to produce sustainable products, job opportunities, and income. Nanocomposites are being developed for making lightweight sensors and flexible batteries, making tumors easier to detect through fluorescent and magnetic properties combined together during MRI, speeding up the healing process for broken bones or orthodontic implants, and manufacturing components with higher strength-to-weight ratios. The transitions from microparticles to nanoparticles lead to a change in its physical as well as chemical properties. Compartmented nanotubes are used to protect drugs from destruction in blood stream, to control delivery with well-defined release kinetics, vector targeting properties, or release mechanism by external or internal stimuli. Nanofibers provide a scaffold on which cells may provide favorable conditions with reinforcing agents for the growth of cells, which may attach to the fibers and grow along them systematically. Degradable polymers for use in bioabsorbable stents has great potential in the future with regard to the chemical and biochemical functionalities in spite of a few limitations such as brittle nature caused by the relatively high glass transition temperature, poor mechanical strength, premature reduction in diameter due to degradation, inflammatory reaction, limited efficiency of drug delivery, and limited shelf life. It is anticipated to have continual improvements in promising innovative, alternative, packaging materials or technologies from renewable origin, such as polyethylene terephthalate from plants. Interdisciplinary sciences are expected to improve the health and quality of life for millions of people by restoring, maintaining, or enhancing tissue and organ functions.

Drawing inspiration from the structure of bones and bamboo, a few researchers have found that by gradually changing the internal structure of metals, they can make stronger, tougher materials that can be customized for a wide variety of applications, from body armor to automobile parts. In spite of several attempts, there is a dearth of information with respect to the cellular response and in-depth toxicity analysis of nanoparticles. The researchers are also interested in using the gradient structure approach to make materials more resistant to corrosion, wear, and fatigue. Nanofibers have applications in electrospinning or template methods ranging from tissue engineering to surface modification of implants. Proper handling, treatment, and disposal of nanomaterials and plastic biomedical wastes after use is important in healthcare control programs. Internationally acceptable standards for management and regulation will help protect healthcare workers, patients, and the community. If properly designed and applied, waste management can be a relatively effective and an efficient compliance-related practice. Rules exist for biomedical waste management and handling, but they need to be implemented in true spirits and with holistic approach. International guidelines are being reviewed periodically, but there is an issue of true implementation in different regions of the globe. The rule makes it mandatory for the healthcare establishments to segregate, disinfect, and dispose their waste in an eco-friendly manner. Any biodegradable plastic mulch that may be eventually approved for use must completely biodegrade into carbon dioxide, water, and microbial biomass within a reasonable timeframe as per regulatory requirements, without forming harmful residues or byproducts.

Biobased or renewable polymers are specially designed material with strategic planning and with a view of environmental sustainability from products found in nature, such as natural fibers, coconut, jute, pine, bagasse, wheat straw, rice husk, saw dust, hemp, and sisal fibers. They are environmentally friendly and, as a contribution of economic emergence, free from traditional adverse side effects. All research involving human subjects should be conducted in accordance with three basic ethical principles: respect for persons, beneficence, and justice. Biobased polymers are attracting increased attention due to environmental concerns and the realization that global petroleum resources are finite. Biobased polymers not only replace existing polymeric products in varied applications but also provide new combinations of properties for new applications. We should develop new innovative methods for cost-effective production, enhanced desired properties to meet the intended demands and commercial applications in a convenient manner. Polycaprolactone powders with regulated sizes from 125 to 250 µm are proposed as a reference material for the biodegradation test by regulatory agencies. In a few countries, biodegradable mulch prepared in compliance with ASTM D 6400, ASTM D 5988-03, etc., is used in certified organic production system as it controls weeds, conserves soil moisture, increases soil temperature, and improves crop yield and quality with few limitations and concern by environmentalists. The cradle-to-grave life of a compostable material should meet the intended demand and life cycle as per usage. Although recycling may be energetically more favorable than composting for a few materials, it may not be practical because of excessive sorting and cleaning requirements.

There is increasing interest in developing biobased polymers and innovative process technologies that may reduce the dependence on fossil fuel and divert to sustainable material basis. In packaging, the major emphasis is on the development of high barrier properties against the diffusion of oxygen, carbon dioxide, flavor compounds, and water vapor.

REFERENCES

Al Salem S.M., Lettieri P., and Baeyens J., Recycling and recovery routes of plastic solid waste: A review. *Waste Manage.* 29, 2625–2643, 2009.

Aschberger K., Micheletti C., Sokull-Klüttgen B., and Christensen F.M., Analysis of currently available data for characterizing the risk of engineered nanomaterials to the environment and human health—Lessons learned from four case studies. *Environ Int* 37(6), 1143–1156, 2011.

CHEMEUROPE. n.d. Smart gas sensors for better chemical detection. http://www.chemeurope.com/en/news/topic/university-of-michigan/ (accessed May 7, 2012).

Chen Y.J., Bioplastics and their role in achieving global sustainability. *J Chem Pharm Res* 6(1), 226–231, 2014.

Corbin A.T., Carol A.M., Jeremy C., Douglas G.H., Jennifer M.K., and Debra A.I., Current and future prospects for biodegradable plastic mulch in certified organic production systems. Organic Agriculture, eOrganic Article, Annual-report, March 10, 2014. www.extension.org/.../growing-the-eorganic-community.

Costopoulos C., Naganuma T., Latib A., and Colombo A., Looking into the future with bioresorbable vascular scaffolds. *Expert Rev Cardiovasc Ther* 11(10), 1407–1416, 2013.

Council for International Organizations of Medical Sciences (CIOMS), World Health Organization (WHO), *International Ethical Guidelines for Biomedical Research Involving Human Subjects*, Geneva, Switzerland, 2002.

Dori Y., *3D Printed Models Assist in Congenital Heart Disease Surgery MDT Medical Design Technology*. Children's Hospital of Philadelphia, Philadelphia, PA, 2014.

Falck G.C.M., Lindberg H.K., Suhonen S. et al., Genotoxic effects of nanosized and fine TiO_2. *Hum Exp Toxicol* 28(6–7), 339–352, 2009.

Geiser M., Rothen-Rutishauser B., Kapp N. et al., Ultrafine particles cross cellular membranes by nonphagocytic mechanisms in lungs and in cultured cells. *Environ Health Perspect* 113(11), 1555–1560, 2005.

Gorrasi, G., Progress in barrier packaging materials: Bio-based nanocomposites as barrier materials for food packaging applications. In Jong-Whan R. (ed.), *Progress in Nanomaterial for Food Packaging*, pp. 20–33, 2014.

Gou N., Onnis-Hayden A., and Gu A.Z., Mechanistic toxicity assessment of nanomaterials by whole-cell-array stress genes expression analysis. *Environ Sci Technol* 44(15), 5964–5970, 2010.

Grodzinska Jurczak M., Zakowska H., and Read A., Management of packaging waste in Poland: Development agenda and accession to the EU. *Waste Manage Res* 22(3), 212–223, 2004.

Hopewell J., Dvorak R., and Kosior E., Plastics recycling: Challenges and opportunities. *Philos Trans R Soc Lond B Biol Sci* 364(1526), 2115–2126, 2009.

Kale G., Kijchavengkul T., Auras R., Rubino M., Selke S.E., and Singh S.P., Compostability of bioplastics packaging materials: An overview. *Macromol Bio Sci* 7(3) 255–277, 2007.

Keller A.A., Wang H., Zhou, D. et al., Stability and aggregation of metal oxide nanoparticles in natural aqueous matrices. *Environ Sci Technol* 44(6), 1962–1967, 2010.

Klien T., Developing biodegradable polymers for the next generation vascular stent. European Medical Device Technology (EMDT), London, U.K., 2014. http://www.emdt.co.uk/daily-buzz/developing-biodegradable-polymers-next-generation-vascular-stent.

Kumar P. and Morawska L., Recycling concrete: An undiscovered source of ultrafine particles. *Atmos Environ* 90, 51–58, 2014.

Kumar P., Mulheron M., and Som C., Release of ultrafine particles from three simulated building processes. *J Nanoparticle Res* 14(4), Article 0771, 2012.

Kumar P., Pirjola L., Ketzel M., and Harrison R.M., Nanoparticle emissions from 11 non-vehicle exhaust sources—A review. *Atmos Environ* 67, 252–277, 2013.

Kumar P., Robins A., and Britter R., Fast response measurements of the dispersion of nanoparticles in a vehicle wake and a street canyon. *Atmos Environ* 43(38), 6110–6118, 2009.

Li X., Cui R., Sun L., Aifantis K.E., Fan Y., Feng Q., Cui F., and Watarai F., 3D-printed bio-polymers for tissue engineering application. *Int J Polym Sci*, Article ID 829145 13. http://dx.doi.org/10.1155/2014/829145.

Lim E.H. et al., Nanotechnology biomemetic cartilage regenerative scaffolds. *Arch Plast Surg* 41(3), 231–240, 2014.

Masahiro F., Ninomiya F., and Kunioka M., Biodegradation of polycaprolactone powders proposed as reference test materials for international standard of biodegradation evaluation method. *J Polym Environ* 15, 7–17, 2007.

Murr L.E. and Garza K.M., Natural and anthropogenic environmental nanoparticulates: Their microstructural characterization and respiratory health implications. *Atmos Environ* 43(17) 2683–2692, 2009.

Mooney B.P., The second green revolution? Production of plant based biodegradable plastics. *Biochem J* 418(2), 219–232, 2009.

Nowack B., Mueller N., Krug H., and Wick P., How to consider engineered nanomaterials in major accident regulations? *Environ Sci Eur* 26(1), 2, 2014.

Overbeck V., Schmitz-Eiberger M.A., Blanke M.M. Reflective mulch enhances ripening and health compounds in apple fruit. *J Sci Food Agric* 93(10), 2575–2579, 2013.

Ray S.S, Environmentally Friendly Polymer, Nanocomposites, *Environmentally Friendly Polymer Nanocomposites: Types, Processing and Properties*. Woodhead Publishing Series in Composites Science and Engineering, Oxford, U.K., 2013.

Rhim J.W. and Park Chiang S.K., Bio nanocomposites for food packaging applications. *Prog Polym Sci* 38(10–11), 1629–1652, 2013.

Science News. 2011. Green cars could be made from pineapples and bananas, In *241st National Meeting & Exposition of the American Chemical Society (ACS)*, Anaheim, CA, March 28, 2011.

Santo V.E., Gomwes M.E., Mano J.F., and Reis R.L., From nano- to micro-scale: Nanotechnology approaches for spatially controlled delivery of bioactive factors for bone and cartilage engineering. *Nanomedicine* 7(7), 1045–1066, 2012.

Song J.H., Murphy R.J., Narayan R., and Davies G.B., Biodegradable and compostable alternatives to conventional plastics. *Philos Trans R Soc Lond B Biol Sci* 364(1526), 2127–2139, 2009.

Tang X.Z., Kumar P., Alavi S., and Sandeep K.P., Recent advances in biopolymers and biopolymer based nanocomposites for food packaging materials. *Crit Rev Food Sci Nutr* 52(5), 426–442, 2012.

U.S. Environmental Protection Agency (USEPA), Proposed category for persistent, bioaccumulative and toxic chemicals. *Fed Regist* 63(192), 53417–53423, 1998.

U.S. Environmental Protection Agency (USEPA), Control of nanoscale materials under the Toxic Substances Control Act, U.S. Environmental Protection Agency, Office of Pollution Prevention and Toxics, Washington, DC, 2014.

10 Biomedical Applications of Microbial Cellulose Nanocomposites

Nazire Deniz Yılmaz

CONTENTS

10.1 INTRODUCTION

Microbial cellulose (MC) is a polysaccharide excreted extracellularly by certain bacteria. The species *Gluconacetobacter xylinus* (or *Acetobacter xylinum* as formerly known) is the most extensively studied cellulose-producing bacteria (Czaja et al., 2006). MC exhibits some unique features such as impressive mechanical strength, crystallinity (Blaker et al., 2010), water-holding capacity, purity, and in situ moldability, which are superior to those of plant cellulose (Klemm et al., 2001). MC presents an ultrafine nanofibril network (Wan et al., 2006). These characteristics render MC, which has been traditionally used in food industry and recently in the production of reinforced paper, valuable for biomedical applications (Shah et al., 2013).

Its applications in artificial blood vessels, temporary skin substitutes, wound dressings (Shah et al., 2013), and scaffolds for tissue engineering of cartilage and bone have been reported. In vitro and in vivo studies have showed that MC is biocompatible. It has been studied as replacement in blood vessels in rats (Grande et al., 2009) and pigs (Bäckdahl et al., 2011). MC has the potential to be used in biodegradable nanocomposites. Different composites of MC have been studied. The component other than MC is determined based on the composite application, including vascular graft or bone regeneration and based on the properties required to be imparted to MC, such as biological activity or antimicrobicity (Shah et al., 2013).

This chapter investigates MC as a component of biomedical nanocomposites. Section 10.2 discusses the properties of MC, as well as the production, modification, and storage methods. Section 10.3 covers MC composite production methods and components incorporated in MC nanobiocomposites. Section 10.4 reviews the fields of biomedical applications of MC composites. This chapter concludes with Section 10.5.

10.2   MC: PROPERTIES; PRODUCTION, MODIFICATION, AND STORAGE METHODS

10.2.1   PROPERTIES OF MC

MC is a polysaccharide that is excreted extracellularly by certain bacteria. Of these bacteria, the species *Gluconacetobacter xylinus* (or *Acetobacter xylinum* as formerly known) is the most extensively studied cellulose producing bacteria since its cellulose production rate justifies commercial interest (Czaja et al., 2006). *A. xylinum*, which is a simple Gram-negative bacterium, synthesizes a good amount of high quality cellulose in the form of twisted ribbons of microfibrillar bundles (Czaja et al., 2006).

MC exhibits some unique features that are superior compared to plant cellulose (Klemm et al., 2001), such as impressive mechanical strength, crystallinity (about 90%) (Blaker et al., 2010), water-holding capacity (around 1000%), purity, and moldability in situ. MC possess an ultrafine nanofibril network structure presenting diameters ranging from 35 to 90 nm (Wan et al., 2006) and its Young's modulus, in the order of 114 GPa, is comparable to that of glass and aramid fibers (Blaker et al., 2010). MC also possesses much higher mechanical properties compared to other natural biodegradable polymers, including collagen, chitosan, chitin, and gelatin (Wan et al., 2007). However, MC fibers show certain similarity to collagen fibers; thus, they are suitable for collagen-mimicking scaffold applications (Blaker et al., 2010). Unlike plant cellulose, MC is free from lignin and other impurities. Cost-efficient production is another positive attribute of MC (Svensson et al., 2005). Characterization efforts of MC are listed in Table 10.1.

The water-retention capacity of never-dried MC is in the order of 1000% compared to that of cotton at 60%. After drying, the water-retention capacity of MC decreases drastically to the level of plant cellulose. Thus, freeze drying is a more viable way of MC storage, where the pore structure is maintained (Klemm et al., 2001).

TABLE 10.1
List of Characterization Methods Applied on MC

Characteristic	Testing Method	References
Mechanical properties	Radial strength and elongation in Krebs solution	Backdahl et al. (2006)
	Radial strength and elongation	Klemm et al. (2001)
	Tensile strength and elongation in distilled water	Million et al. (2008)
	Radial and axial strength and elongation	Putra et al. (2008)
	Wet and dry tensile strength	Zhang and Luo (2011)
	Compression strength in wet state	Svensson et al. (2005)
Laminate strength	Peel test (modified ASTM D 903-93)	Charpentier et al. (2006)
Chemical analysis	X-ray photoelectron spectroscopy	Charpentier et al. (2006), Huang et al. (2010), Pertile et al. (2010), Zimmermann et al. (2011)
	Fourier transformed infrared spectroscopy	Hong et al. (2006), Grande et al. (2009), Wan et al. (2006), Wan et al. (2007), Zhang and Luo (2011)
	Inductively coupled plasma atomic emission spectrometry	Wan et al. (2006)
	Electron spectroscopy for chemical analysis	Svensson et al. (2005)
Cell attachment	In vitro: Alamar Blue Assay™ (smooth muscle cells)	Backdahl et al. (2006)
Cell proliferation	In vitro: Alamar Blue Assay™ (smooth muscle cells)	Backdahl et al. (2006)
	Phase-contrast microscopy	Svensson et al. (2005)
Cell adhesion and proliferation	Colorimetric MTS assay (HMEC-1, N1E-115, and 3T3 cells)	Pertile et al. (2010)
Cell migration	In vitro migration chamber and attractant	Backdahl et al. (2006)
Cell morphology	Laser scanning confocal microscopy	Backdahl et al. (2006), (2011), Svensson et al. (2005)
Morphology	Scanning electron microscopy	Backdahl et al. (2006), Grande et al. (2009), Hong et al. (2006), Huang et al. (2010), Pertile et al. (2010), Wan et al. (2006, 2007), Svensson et al. (2005)
	Transmission electron microscopy	Wan et al. (2007), Svensson et al. (2005)
	Energy-dispersive spectroscopy	Hong et al. (2006), Wan et al. (2006), Backdahl et al. (2011), Blaker et al. (2010), Backdahl et al. (2006), Zimmermann et al. (2011)
	Focused ion beam analysis	Backdahl et al. (2011)

(Continued)

TABLE 10.1 (*Continued*)
List of Characterization Methods Applied on MC

Characteristic	Testing Method	References
	Atomic force microscopy	Grande et al. (2009)
	Energy-dispersive x-ray spectroscopy	Wan et al. (2007)
Crystallinity, crystal size	X-ray diffraction	Hong et al. (2006), Grande et al. (2009), Huang et al. (2010), Grande et al. (2009), Wan et al. (2006, 2007), Zimmermann et al. (2011)
Pore size, fiber orientation, fiber diameter	Scanning electron microscopy—image analysis	Grande et al. (2009)
Fibril orientation	Birefringence-polarized light microscopy	Putra et al. (2008)
Surface area determination	Brunauer–Emmet–Teller model	Blaker et al. (2010)
Thermal analysis	Thermogravimetric analysis	Grande et al. (2009), Svensson et al. (2005)
	Differential scanning calorimetry	Huang et al. (2010)
Porosity determination	Mass–volume calculation	Blaker et al. (2010)
Hydrophillicity	Contact angle measurement	Charpentier et al. (2006), Pertile et al. (2010)
	Water-holding capacity	Huang et al. (2010)
	Rehydration ratio	Huang et al. (2010)
Roughness	Image processing	Klemm et al. (2001)
Rheology	Small amplitude oscillatory test	Huang et al. (2010)
Biocompatibility	Animal model (pig)	Backdahl et al. (2011), Wippermann et al. (2009)
	Animal model (rat)	Klemm et al. (2001)
Biocompatibility	Seeding of HEK cells	Grande et al. (2009)
	Seeding of osteoprogenitor cells	Zimmermann et al. (2011)
	Fluorescence microscopy	Zimmermann et al. (2011)
Histochemical analysis	Haematoxylin-Pertex	Backdahl et al. (2011)

The degradation of MC has not been fully investigated for in vitro or in vivo setting. However, other cellulose-based materials present limited degradation in the human body in contrast to that in soil (Wippermann et al., 2009). The idea of a completely degradable material for a tissue engineering scaffold sounds theoretically ideal. However, there are practical problems in the transportation of degradation products to avoid adverse effects on cell proliferation and induction of inflammatory reactions. The optimization and synchronization of the degradation duration and maintenance of necessary mechanical performance are also difficult (Wippermann et al., 2009).

10.2.2 MC PRODUCTION METHODS

During the biosynthesis of MC, the bacteria secrete single, linear β-1,4-glucan chains through a row of pores located on their outer membrane. First, the β-1,4-glucan chains form subfibrils that consist of 10–15 nascent β-1,4-glucan chains, then microfibrils, and finally microfibril bundles comprising a loosely wound ribbon, which consists of around 1000 individual glucan chains (Czaja et al., 2006).

G. *xylinus* prefers an environment with sufficient oxygen and nutrients as well as a place to attach to. O_2 is necessary for MC synthesis, and increase in O_2 supply boosts MC production. Rise in oxygen concentration also enhances mechanical performance of MC (Backdahl et al., 2011).

Glucose, sucrose, fructose, and mannitol have been used as carbon sources for MC production (Shah et al., 2013). One culture medium widely used for G. *xylinus* is the Hestrine–Schramm medium. This medium is composed of 0.5 wt.% bacto-peptone, 0.5 wt.% yeast extract, 0.27 wt.% disodium hydrogen phosphate (Na_2HPO_4), 0.115 wt.% citric acid, and 2 wt.% D(+) glucose (Putra et al., 2008; Pourramezan et al., 2009).

MC can be synthesized in static and agitated cultures (Bäckdahl et al., 2011). In static cultures, MC is produced at the air–culture medium interface as an assembly of nanofibers that form a pellicle. The pellicle grows and increases its thickness until all cells are entrapped in the pellicle and lose contact with the oxygen in the air (Shah et al., 2013). The type of cellulose produced this way is cellulose I, which consists of parallel β-1,4 glucan chains (Huang et al., 2010). The pellicle has a dense surface side formed on the culture medium–air interface and a gelatinous layer on the opposite side (Backdahl et al., 2006). The downside of production in static cultures is its low production rate (Shah et al., 2013).

The second route for MC production is in agitated cultures. The produced MC is in the form of cellulose II, which consists of antiparallel β-1,4 glucan chains. This type of cellulose is similar to that formed by the mercerization of cellulose I (Huang et al., 2010). The degree of polymerization, crystallinity, and mechanical strength is lower during synthesis in agitated cultures compared to static media (Bäckdahl et al., 2011). However, the production rate increases substantially due to increased access to oxygen (Shah et al., 2013). In this method, particles of sizes ranging from 10 μm to 1 mm and shapes such as spherical, ellipsoidal, or fibrous are generated instead of pellicles (Bäckdahl et al., 2011).

MC can be molded into the desired shape during synthesis. For example, Backdahl et al. (2011) produced a tubular MC using a vertical bioreactor. The bioreactor had a silicon tubing inside that acted as a template and membrane for the delivery of oxygen.

Numerous efforts have been made to enhance MC production by using different MC-producing bacteria strains, carbon sources, alternative inexpensive sources, and supplementary materials (Shah et al., 2013). Klemm et al. (2001) compared cellulose production rate of several A. *xylinum* strains. Among the studied strains, the most productive one was AX5 followed by AATCC 53582 after 8 cultivation days. MC production methods are given in Table 10.2.

TABLE 10.2
List of Production Parameters of MC

Bacteria Strain	Media	Temperature/ pH	Duration	MC Pellicle Width	References
Acetobacter xylinum subsp. sucrofermentas BPR2001 (ATCCXXXX)	Corn steep liquid media	30°C	3 days	3 mm	Backdahl et al. (2006)
A. xylinum subsp. sucrofermentas BPR2001, trade number 700178	Corn steep liquid media, Verticular reactor including silicon tubing	30°C	4 days, 6 days, 9 days	N.S.	Backdahl et al. (2011)
N.S.	CHAOKOH® coconut gel in syrup	N.S.	N.S.	N.S.	Blaker et al. (2010)
Acetobacter xylinum X-2	0.3 wt.% green tea powder (analytical grade) and 5 wt.% sucrose (analytical grade)	pH 4.5	7 days	N.S.	Hong et al. (2006)
Gluconacetobacter saccharivorans (LMG 1582) isolated from a Kombucha tea mat	1.0% (w/v) D-glucose, 1.5% (w/v) peptone, 0.8% (w/v) yeast extract, and 0.3% (v/v) glacial acetic acid	30 C, pH 3.5 (HCl)	21 days	N.S.	Grande et al. (2009)
Gluconacetobacter xylinum (BCRC12335),	1. Mannitol broth medium containing 25 g/L mannitol, 5 g/L yeast extract, and 3 g/L peptone 2. Modified coconut juice media, containing 0.2% acetic acid, 10 Brix soluble solid content adjusted with sucrose	1. 30°C 2. 30°C	1.24 h 2.14 day	N.S.	Huang et al. (2010)
A. xylinum AX5	Hestrin–Schramm medium— static, d-glucose (dextrose)	28°C	10–14 days	N.S.	Klemm et al. (2001)

(Continued)

TABLE 10.2 (*Continued*)
List of Production Parameters of MC

Bacteria Strain	Media	Temperature/ pH	Duration	MC Pellicle Width	References
A. xylinum ATCC 53582	Hestrin–Schramm medium—static culture	30°C, pH 5	4 days	N.S.	Pertile et al. (2010)
A. xylinum ATCC 53582	Hestrin–Schramm medium—static culture	28°C, pH 6	7 days	N.S.	Putra et al. (2008)
Acetobacter xylinum X-2	Static culture containing 0.3% (w/w) green tea powder and 5% (w/w) sucrose	pH 4.5	7 days	N.S.	Wan et al., 2006, Wan et al. (2007)
A. xylinum	Hestrin–Schramm medium	N.S.	10 days	0.6–1 mm (thickness), 3.0–3.7 mm internal diameter	Wippermann et al. (2009)
Acetobacter xylinum subsp. sucrofermentas BPR2001, trade number 700178™	Fructose media with an addition of corn steep liquid (CSL)	30°C	2 days	N.S.	Zimmermann et al. (2011)
G. xylinus (ATCC 10245)	10 g/L Bactopeptone, 10 g/L yeast extract, 4 mm KH_2PO_4, 6 mm K_2HPO_4, and 20 g/L d-glucose dissolved in DI water.	30°C, pH 5.1–5.2	7 days	N.S.	Svensson et al. (2005)

10.2.3 MC MODIFICATION METHODS

The usefulness of implants is based on the interactions between the biomaterial and tissues (Pertile et al., 2010). Porosity, pore size, interconnectivity, and topography, especially in the nanoscale, are critical parameters that determine the attachment, proliferation, and migration of cells (Blaker et al., 2010). In case the materials do not have the necessary bioactivity, surface-modification methods are applied to enhance biocompatibility. Using these methods, properties such as wettability, topography, chemistry, surface charge, and the presence and intensity of hydrophobic/hydrophilic functional groups are altered.

Plasma treatment is one of the surface-modification methods. Pertile et al. (2010) reported higher roughness of MC after nitrogen plasma along with better adhesion and growth of HMEC-1 and N1E-115 cells. However, time-specific effectiveness of the surface modification should also be evaluated.

10.2.4 STORAGE OF MC

After the completion of MC synthesis, it is purified: the bacteria are removed from the cellulose generally via alkalization (Bäckdahl et al., 2011). After purification, MC may be kept in distilled or deionized (DI) water (Hong et al., 2006; Putra et al., 2008). In order to lengthen the shelf life of MC, drying can be applied. Nevertheless, drying drastically decreases the water-holding capacity because of high crystallinity (Huang et al., 2010). So, freeze drying may be preferred for MC storage (Klemm et al., 2001). MC purification and storage methods are given in Table 10.3.

10.3 BIOMEDICAL NANOCOMPOSITES OF MC

10.3.1 MC COMPOSITE PRODUCTION METHODS

MC composite production methods may be classified into three groups: in situ, ex situ, and from dissolved MC solution. In the first method, the reinforcing material is added to the culture during MC synthesis. Then it gets trapped inside the MC fibril network and forms a composite. MC composites, including aloe vera and poly-3-hydroxybutyrate, have been produced by this method. The difficulty with this method is that particles remain suspended in the culture only for a limited time. After they move down, they cannot be entrapped by the MC pellicle that forms on the liquid–air interface (Shah et al., 2013). This problem can be solved by increasing the viscosity of the culture medium (Grande et al., 2009) or by using an agitated medium. However, it is not possible to produce MC pellicles or sheets by using agitated cultures. Another drawback of the in situ composite production is that it is not suitable for incorporation of antibacterial agents such as Ag, ZnO, and TiO_2 in an in situ production due to their toxic effects on MC-producing bacteria (Shah et al., 2013).

In ex situ production, the already synthesized MC is impregnated with the reinforcing material. Different materials, including antibacterial agents, can penetrate and get engrossed in the MC network through physical absorbance and H bonds with the OH groups of MC. Using this method, MC composites of chitosan, gelatin, HAp, and Ag nanoparticles were produced. The difficulty reported with this method is that the reinforcing material should be in the sub-micron size to be able to enter into the MC fibril network, and it should be hydrophilic to combine with MC. Additionally, depending on the structural arrangement of the MC network, a homogeneous distribution of the reinforcement materials may not be provided (Shah et al., 2013).

In the last method, powdered MC is dissolved in a solvent and then the reinforcing material is added. The composite solution is then dried and a composite is produced. This method provides better control of the composition and improved homogeneous distribution. The solvents to dissolve MC include N-methyl morpholine N-oxide, ionic liquids, $ZnCl_2(3H_2O)$, NaOH and LiOH/urea/thiourea. This method has not been extensively tried for MC composite production (Shah et al., 2013). One trial is that of Zhang and Luo (2011). They dissolved MC and alginate in separate Li/urea/thiourea solutions and then blended them to produce bicomponent fibers through the wet spinning method. Table 10.4 lists the production methods of MC composites.

TABLE 10.3
List of Some MC Purification and Storage Methods Reported in the Literature

1st Step	2nd Step	3rd Step	Storage	References
0.1 M NaOH at 60°C for 4 h	Boiled in Millipore™ water	Steam sterilized (1 bar, 120°C) for 20 min	Kept refrigerated until use	Backdahl et al. (2006)
Soaked in DI for 24 h and filtered	Stirred in methanol and filtered (three times)	Stirred in dimethylacedamide and filtered (three times)	N.S.	Charpentier et al. (2006)
Soaked in DI at 90°C for 2 h	Boiled in a 0.5 M NaOH solution for 15 min	Washed with DI for several times and soaked in 1 wt.% NaOH for 2 days. Then pellicles were rinsed with DI to pH 7	Stored in DI at room temperature	Hong et al. (2006)
Boiled in 1.0 M NaOH at 70°C for 90 min	Rinsed repetitively in DI	Water was removed by either freeze drying, solvent exchange, or hot pressing	N.S.	Grande et al. (2009)
Boiled in 0.5 N NaOH for 10 min	Immersed in 0.5 N NaOH for 24 h at room temperature	Rinsed with DI to neutral pH	Freeze dried and placed in a desiccator to keep the moisture content below 2%	Huang et al. (2010)
Boiled in 0.1 N NaOH	N.S.	N.S.	N.S.	Klemm et al. (2001)
2% sodium dodecyl sulfate (SDS) for 12 h at 60°C	Washed with distilled water until complete removal of SDS	Immersed in a 4% NaOH solution—gently shaken—for 90 min at 60°C	After neutralization, the pellicles were autoclaved in distilled water and lyophilized	Pertile et al. (2010)
Soaked in a large amount of distilled water for 1 day	Autoclaved in a 1% (w/v) aqueous solution of NaOH at 121°C for 20 min	Washed several times with distilled water followed by (1) soaking in distilled water for a long period of time to reach pH 7	Stored in distilled water at room temperature prior to use.	Putra et al. (2008)
Immersed in deionized water at 90°C for 2 h	Boiled in a 0.5 M aqueous solution of NaOH for 15 min	Washed with DI several times and soaked in 1% NaOH for 2 days. Finally, the BC pellicles were washed free of alkali	MC composites are freeze dried	Wan et al., (2006), Wan et al. (2007)
Boiled in 0.1 M NaOH at 60°C for 4 h	Steam sterilized (1 bar, 120°C) for 20 min	N.S.	Stored in Ringer's solution	Wippermann et al. (2009)
Soaked in 0.1 M NaOH 60°C for 4 h	Repeatedly rinsed in Millipore™ water	Steam sterilized by autoclaving for 20 min (120°C, 1 bar)	Stored in DI water and refrigerated	Zimmermann et al. (2011)
4% SDS (Fisher) in DI at 70°C for 3 h	4% NaOH in DI at 70°C for 90 min	Rinsed with DI to pH = 7	Stored in DI at room temperature	Svensson et al. (2005)

TABLE 10.4
Components and Production Methods of MC Composites Reported in Literature

Component 1	Component 2	Composite Production Method	References
Bacterial cellulose nanowhiskers	Poly(D,L-lactide), Solvent (dimethyle-carbonate or chloroform)	Ice-microsphere templating technique with thermally induced phase separation, ultrasonication	Blaker et al. (2010)
Cellulon TM	PETG 6763 copolyester, PCTG DN004 coplyester	Plasma and UV/ozone treatment of polyester and impregnation	Charpentier et al. (2006)
MC	CaCl$_2$, HAp	CaCl$_2$-treated BC was rinsed with DI and soaked in a 1.5 × SBF solution at 37°C for 7 or14 days	Hong et al. (2006)
MC	Calcium-deficient HAp powder, CMC	Calcium-deficient HAp nanoparticles were prepared by a wet chemical precipitation method using solutions of calcium nitrate and di-ammonium phosphate salts. HAp was added to CMC solution. Precultivated MC was added	Grande et al. (2009)
MC	Tween 80	The second component was added into MC culture medium	Huang et al. (2010)
MC	Urea	The second component was added into MC culture medium	Huang et al. (2010)
MC	CMC	The second component was added into MC culture medium	Huang et al. (2010)
MC	Fluorescent brightener	The second component was added into MC culture medium	Huang et al. (2010)
MC	Hydroxypropylmethyl cellulose	The second component was added into MC culture medium	Huang et al. (2010)
MC	Polyvinyl alcohol (PVA)	PVA was added to the MC suspension. The composite was low-temperature thermal crosslinked under strain to obtain anisotropy	Millon et al. (2008)
MC	HAp	MC pellicle was phosphorylated, then immersed in a CaCl$_2$ solution at 37°C for 3 days. Then the CaCl$_2$-treated and phosphorylated BC samples were immersed in a 1.5 SBF at 37°C for 7 or 14 days	Wan et al. (2006)

(Continued)

TABLE 10.4 (*Continued*)
Components and Production Methods of MC Composites Reported in Literature

Component 1	Component 2	Composite Production Method	References
MC	HAp	Phosphorylated or unphosphorylated MC pellicle was immersed in a $CaCl_2$ solution at 37°C for 3 days. Then the MC samples were immersed in 1.5 SBF at 37°C for 7 or 14 days	Wan et al., (2007)
BC	Alginate	MC and alginate was dissolved in different Li/urea/thiourea solutions. The MC solution was frozen and then let to thaw before mixing of two solutions. The mixture was filtered and degassed	Zhang and Luo (2011)
MC	Calcium-deficient HAp, CMC	CMC was added to a $CaCl_2$ solution. MC samples were placed in this solution for 24 h at room temperature. The MC samples were then placed in a $CaCl_2$ solution for 24 h at room. Finally, the MC samples were rinsed with DI water. The charged MC samples were immersed in SBF at 37°C	Zimmermann et al. (2011)

10.3.2 Components of MC Composites

MC has the potential to be used in biodegradable nanocomposites. Different composites of MC have been studied. The component other than MC is determined based on the composite application and on the properties required to be imparted to MC, such as biological activity or antimicrobicity (Shah et al., 2013). Components that are incorporated in MC composites are given in Table 10.4.

Composites of MC with collagen or chitosan presented valuable properties for wound dressing and other biomedical applications. MC-carboxymethylcellulose (CMC) composites showed increased metal ion adsorption capacity (Grande et al., 2009). Huang et al. (2010) produced composites of MC-hydroxypropylmethyl cellulose and MC-CMC, which have improved water-holding capacity after drying compared to that of neat MC. MC- HAp composites have been investigated for potential use in bone tissue engineering (Grande et al., 2009). Silver nanoparticles have been incorporated in MC to impart antimicrobial property. Some other components studied in MC composites include gelatin, polyethylene glycol, and aloe vera gel (Shah et al., 2013).

The biomedical performance of MC can be enhanced by making its composites with bioactive polymers, nanomaterials, and alike. These materials endow antibacterial, antiviral, antifungal, biocompatible, and wound-healing properties to MC (Shah et al., 2013).

MC composites of chitin have been produced by in situ and ex situ methods to utilize certain properties of chitin, including absorption of wound exudates, wound-healing effects, tissue engineering scaffolds, drug delivery, antimicrobial, antifungal, and antiviral properties. MC composites showed enhanced cell adhesion and proliferation (Shah et al., 2013).

Collagen possesses high biodegradability, low antigenicity, and cell-binding properties, and its weak mechanical strength may be supported by a combination with MC (Shah et al., 2013). MC-gelatin composites have been developed for tissue engineering applications. MC nanocomposites with enhanced mechanical properties were developed ex situ by soaking MC in polyacrilamide and gelatin solutions (Grande et al., 2009). Alginate and aloe vera are other biopolymers combined with MC. MC-Ag nanocomposites show antibacterial properties that are advantageous for wound-dressing applications. MC composites with metallic oxides such as TiO_2 also present antibacterial properties (Shah et al., 2013).

Nonaggregated ferromagnetic materials can be incorporated in MC for targeted drug-delivery applications (Shah et al., 2013). MC-Au nanocomposites have been developed for usage in biosensors and enzyme immobilization processes (Zhang et al., 2010).

Impregnation of MC with clay particles, including montmorrilonite, resulted in immense increase in mechanical strength, enhanced skin protection, cleansing and antibacterial activity, immobilization of cell toxins produced by various bacteria, and excellent wound-healing and blood-clotting capabilities (Shah et al., 2013).

Blaker et al. (2010) produced MC composites with polylactic acid (PLA) where PLA acted as the matrix. The toughness of PLA, which is a brittle polymer, was increased with the addition of MC. MC-polyvinyl alcohol (PVA) composites have been investigated for blood vessel replacement (Grande et al., 2009).

10.4 BIOMEDICAL MC COMPOSITE APPLICATIONS

10.4.1 ARTIFICIAL BLOOD VESSELS

Artificial blood vessels present an alternative solution to reconstructive problems related with vascular diseases by forming small-caliber tissue-engineered vascular grafts. With today's technology, large arteries can be replaced with synthetic polyester or expanded-polytetraflourethylene (ePTFE) grafts. However, these materials are not suitable for replacement of blood vessels with diameters lower than 6 mm because of the risk of thrombosis formation and occlusion due to the lack of compliance between the graft and the adjacent native vessels (Millon et al., 2008). Therefore, it is necessary to develop new materials that are suitable for these small blood vessels (Backdahl et al., 2006).

To reduce the risk of thrombogenicity, Charpentier et al. (2006) impregnated a woven polyester vascular prosthesis in MC to form an impermeable luminal layer to prevent clot formation. They pretreated the polyester with UV/ozone plasma to improve the attachment of MC.

Cardiovascular tissues include an important amount of the structural proteins elastin and collagen. Here, elastin gives the initial elasticity, whereas the collagen fibers, which have a certain amount of slack, contribute to the arterial wall tension as the vessel is further stretched. Thus, the aortic tissue has a nonlinear exponential and viscoelastic mechanical behavior. Besides, the tensile characteristics of cardiovascular tissue, similar to other soft tissues, are anisotropic, with a higher stiffness in the circumferential, compared to that in the axial, direction (Millon et al., 2008).

Backdahl et al. (2006), who studied MC as a potential scaffold for artificial blood vessels, measured the mechanical properties of MC in Krebs solution and compared it with that of porcine carotid arteries and ePTFE grafts. The MC pellicle was reported to have an asymmetric nanofibrillar network structure similar to collagen. The stress–strain behavior of MC was more similar to that of carotid artery compared to that of ePTFE, which might be due to the similar nanofibrillar architecture. However, the strength, elongation, and Young's modulus values of MC were lower than those of porcine carotid artery. Smooth muscle cells attached to and proliferated on the MC pellicle, though slower than the polystyrene reference surface, and no difference in proliferation was reported to be between the compact and porous sides of MC. Cell migration was observed in the porous side but not in the compact side. However, use of platelet-derived growth factor (PDGF-BB) culture enhanced migration in both sides (Backdahl et al, 2006). The luminal side of the engineered vessel tube was suggested to be the compact side in order for enhanced endothelial cell attachment. This mimics the smooth, dense surface of the basal membrane of a vessel. Meanwhile, the outer side of the tube, which is porous, may improve integration with the host tissue (Backdahl et al, 2006).

Millon et al. (2008) developed a PVA-MC nanocomposite material that mimics the anisotropic exponential stress–strain behavior of the cardiovascular tissue. In order to impart anisotropy, they subjected the composites to certain levels of strain. They obtained a close match between the stress–strain relationship of porcine aorta and that of anisotropic PVA-MC nanocomposite hydrogel. The stiffness of the nanocomposite increases with the increase in thermal crosslinking cycles under strain. The stiffness and anisotropy increases until the strain ratio applied during crosslinking increases to 75%. Incorporation of MC into PVA also increases the stiffness and the anisotropy of the polymer.

As can be expected, the tubular shape is advantageous for vascular replacement. Backdahl et al (2011) applied an MC graft synthesized in the shape of a 6 mm diameter tube as an infrarenal aortic bypass for a pig (see Figure 10.1). They reported no problems associated with mechanical performance and thrombosis.

Klemm et al. (2001) used MC for artificial blood vessels for microsurgery of rat carotid artery with an inner diameter of 1 mm. They reported 100% patency with no signs of coagulation. Four weeks after surgery, the inner surface of MC tube was covered with endogene cells. Similarly, Wippermann et al. (2009) developed MC tubes and used them to replace carotid arteries of pigs and obtained 87.5% patency rate.

Putra et al. (2008) produced MC tubes with the desired length, inner diameter, thickness, and fibril orientation parallel to the tube axis by culturing MC in

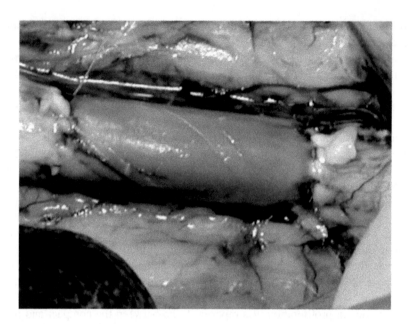

FIGURE 10.1   A 6 mm BC graft as an infrarenal aortic bypass for a pig. (From *Mat. Sci. Eng. C*, 31, Bäckdahl, H., Risberg, B., and Gatenholm, P., Observations on bacterial cellulose tube formation for application as vascular graft, 14–21, Copyright 2011, with permission from Elsevier.)

oxygen-permeable silicone tubes with inner diameters smaller than 8 mm. Fibril orientation increases with the decrease in tube diameter below 8 mm. Above 8 mm, no orientation was obtained. No difference in the orientation was found if the tube was held horizontally or vertically. Strength and modulus are higher in the axial direction, whereas elongation is higher in the radial direction. The MC tube was proposed to be used as a microvessel or soft tissue material.

10.4.2   Wound Healing

Wound-healing systems should provide a suitable environment for epidermal regeneration by forming a barrier against infection and fluid loss (Czaja et al., 2006). The distinctive nanofibrillar structure of never-dried MC makes it a promising matrix for wound healing (Figure 10.2). Thanks to its nanoporous structure, MC not only allows the transfer of antibiotics or other medicines into the wound, but also serves as a barrier against any external infection. The effective hydration and absorption activity of MC provides the necessary moisture balance for the healing period (Czaja et al., 2006).

MC has already found commercial applications under the trade names Biofill, Xcells, Bioprocess (burns and ulcers), and Gengiflex (periodontal diseases) in terms of wound healing. Compared to conventional wound-healing materials, the following advantages have been reported for MC: shorter healing duration, reduced contamination, decreased treatment cost, eliminated pain symptoms,

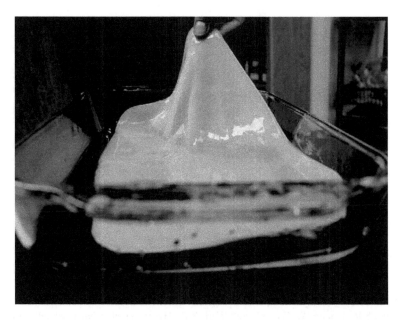

FIGURE 10.2 The never-dried microbial cellulose membrane. (From *Biomaterials*, 27, Czaja, W., Krystynowicza, A., Bielecki, S., and Brown Jr., R.M., Microbial cellulose—The natural power to heal wounds, 145–151, Copyright 2006, with permission from Elsevier.)

enhanced absorption of wound exudates, improved prevention of excessive fluid loss, and easiness of wound inspection due to the transparency of MC (Czaja et al., 2006).

MC-chitin and MC-gelatin composites have been used for wound-healing applications (Shah et al., 2013). MC-collagen and MC-chitosan composites present enhanced properties for wound-dressing applications (Grande et al., 2009).

10.4.3 Bone Tissue Engineering

Bone is a natural composite where HAp mineral crystals reinforce a collagen matrix (Zimmermann et al., 2011). Thus, HAp-collagen nanocomposites have been extensively investigated for bone tissue engineering. Compared to collagen, MC possesses substantially greater strength and modulus and eliminates the risk of cross-infection (Wan et al., 2006).

Among organic polymers, which include silk fibroin and chitosan besides collagen, MC is one of the most recent studied ones for bone applications (Hong et al., 2006). However, MC itself is not feasible for a bone-healing scaffold as the osteoprogenitor cells do not adhere to its surface. This situation can be enhanced by using MC–calcium-deficient HAp composites (Zimmermann et al., 2011). Osteoconductivity and bioactivity of HAp and high strength of MC render MC–HAp composites ideal for bone tissue engineering (Wan et al., 2006).

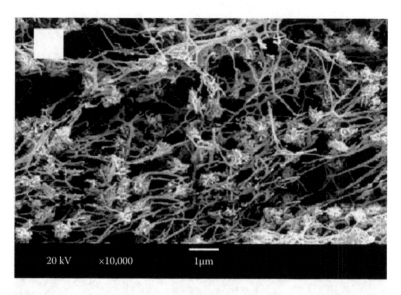

FIGURE 10.3 MC–hydroxyapetite composite. (From *Mater. Lett.*, 60, Hong, L., Wang, Y.L., Jia, S.R., Huang, Y., Gao, C., and Wan, Y.Z., Hydroxyapatite/bacterial cellulose composites synthesized via a biomimetic route, 1710–1713, Copyright 2006, with permission from Elsevier.)

Hong et al. (2006) synthesized MC–HAp, shown in Figure 10.3, in a biomimetic route. First, they immersed MC in CaCl$_2$ solution and then decanted MC in simulated body fluid (SBF) to induce HAp growth.

Wan et al. (2006) used phosphorylation as a means of surface modification of MC to boost calcium phosphate formation. They observed no change in fiber morphology upon phosphorylation. They immersed the phosphorylated and CaCl$_2$-treated MC in SBF to obtain MC–HAp composites. HAp crystals formed on MC fibrils with a crystallite size of 37–43 nm and crystallinity degree of 0.56%–0.79%. The crystallite size and crystallinity rate increased with the increase in the duration of immersion in SBF. After 14 days of immersion in SBF, MC became fully covered by HAp crystals (Figure 10.4). When HAp crystal formation on unphosphorylated MC was investigated by Wan et al. (2007), very little amount of HAp was found to have formed on MC.

Grande et al. (2009) produced MC–calcium-deficient HAp nanocomposites in a static culture in the presence of a mineral phase. CMC was added to suspend HAp by controlling the viscosity of the MC culture. The presence of CMC decreased the average diameter of MC fibers from nearly 120 to 60 nm, whereas the average pore size increased from 0.520 to 0.770 µm. The biocompatibility testing of MC–HAp resulted in 97% viability. The viability of MC increased with the presence of CMC, which was attributed to the change in the fiber diameter and pore size as well as the addition of HAp, as it forms direct chemical bonds with tissues. The crystallinity of HAp and the crystallite size of MC decreased in the composites compared to their pure forms. Grande et al. (2009) stated that further research was necessary to improve the adhesion of cells to MC–HAp nanocomposite scaffolds.

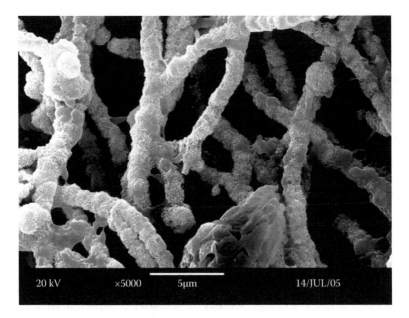

FIGURE 10.4 MC–HAp composite. (From *Compo. Sci. Technol.*, 66, Wan, Y.Z., Hong, L., Jia, S.R., Huang, Y., Zhu, Y., Wang, Y.L., and Jiang, H.J., Synthesis and characterization of hydroxyapatite–bacterial cellulose nanocomposites, 1825–1832, Copyright 2006, with permission from Elsevier.)

10.4.4 CARTILAGE

Articular cartilage consists of a small number of chondrocyte cells in an extracellular matrix, which mainly includes water, collagen type II, and proteoglycans. The main purposes of articular cartilage are to cover the ends of bones in joints to reduce friction during movement and to distribute load (Svensson et al., 2005).

The regenerative capacity of damaged cartilage is limited. Thus, tissue engineering has the potential to provide a scaffold for the repair and regeneration of damaged cartilage. Until today, a variety of natural polymers such as collagen, alginate, hyaluronic acid, fibrin glue, and chitosan as well as synthetic polymers such as PLA, polyglycolic acid, PVA, polyhydroxyethylmethacrylate, and poly(N-isopropylacrylamide) have been studied as scaffold materials for articular cartilages (Svensson et al., 2005).

Among such studies, Svensson et al. (2005) investigated MC as a potential cartilage scaffold. They studied the effect of phosphorylation and sulfonation. They found that phosphorylation and sulfonation increased the compression strength while decreasing tensile strength and elasticity modulus. They found MC to support adherence, growth, and migration of chondrocyte cells.

10.4.5 NERVE

Klemm et al. (2001) used MC tube as a protective layer on sected sciatic nerves of rats. They found better regeneration compared to uncovered sected nerves. Tubular shape has been reported to be advantageous for nerve regeneration (Bäckdahl et al., 2011).

10.4.6 MICROSURGICAL TRAINING

Klemm et al. (2001) have reported that the use of MC tubes during microsurgical training presents a more close-to-reality model compared to rubber membranes and plastic tubes and is advantageous in terms of animal protection by reducing the number of necessary experimental animals.

10.5 CONCLUSION

MC is a polysaccharide excreted extracellularly by certain bacteria, with the species *Gluconacetobacter xylinus* to be the most extensively studied one. MC exhibits some unique features such as impressive mechanical strength, crystallinity, water-holding capacity, purity, and in situ moldability, which are superior to those of plant cellulose. MC presents an ultrafine nanofibril network structure. These characteristics render MC valuable for biomedical applications. Its applications in artificial blood vessels, temporary skin substitutes, wound dressings in deep wounds or burns, scaffolds for tissue engineering of cartilage and bone have been reported. In vitro and in vivo studies showed that MC is biocompatible. It has been studied as replacement in blood vessels in rats and pigs. MC has the potential to be used in biodegradable nanocomposites. Different composites of MC have been studied. Composites of MC with collagen or chitosan presented valuable properties for wound dressing and other biomedical applications. MC-CMC composites showed increased metal ion adsorption capacity. MC–hydroxyapetite composites have been investigated for potential use in bone tissue engineering. Silver nanoparticles have been incorporated in MC to impart antimicrobial property. Some other components studied in MC composites include gelatin, polyethylene glycol, and aloe vera gel.

MC composite production methods may be classified in three groups: in situ, ex situ, and from dissolved MC solution. While the last method provides better control of the composition and improved homogeneous distribution together with a wider spectrum of component materials in terms of chemistry and dimensions, it is the least studied method. Further research pertaining composite production from dissolved MC solutions may provide promise for more sophisticated biomedical composites. In vivo applications of MC composites are also limited to a few studies in contrast to the fact that patency rates higher than 85% were reported. More in vivo studies may provide a better determination of the applicability of MC composites in tissue engineering and other biomedical applications.

REFERENCES

Backdahl, H., G. Helenius, A. Bodin, U. Nannmark, B.R. Johansson, B. Risberg and P. Gatenholm. 2006. Mechanical properties of bacterial cellulose and interactions with smooth muscle cells. *Biomaterials* 27:2141–2149.

Bäckdahl, H., B. Risberg and P. Gatenholm. 2011. Observations on bacterial cellulose tube formation for application as vascular graft. *Materials Science and Engineering* C 31:14–21.

Blaker, J.J., K.-Y. Lee, A. Mantalaris, and A. Bismarck. 2010. Ice-microsphere templating to produce highly porous nanocomposite PLA matrix scaffolds with pores selectively lined by bacterial cellulose nano-whiskers. *Composites Science and Technology* 70:1879–1888.

Charpentier, P.A., A. Maguire, and W.-K. Wan. 2006. Surface modification of polyester to produce a bacterial cellulose-based vascular prosthetic device. *Applied Surface Science* 252:6360–6367.

Czaja, W., A. Krystynowicza, S. Bielecki and R.M. Brown Jr. 2006. Microbial cellulose— The natural power to heal wounds. *Biomaterials* 27:145–151.

Grande, C.J., F.G. Torres, C.M. Gomez, and M.C. Bano. 2009. Nanocomposites of bacterial cellulose/hydroxyapatite for biomedical applications. *Acta Biomaterialia* 5:1605–1615.

Hong, L., Y.L. Wang, S.R. Jia, Y. Huang, C. Gao and Y.Z. Wan. 2006. Hydroxyapatite/ bacterial cellulose composites synthesized via a biomimetic route. *Materials Letters* 60:1710–1713.

Huang, H.-C, L-C. Chen, S.-B. Lin, C.-P. Hsu and H.-H. Chen. 2010. In situ modification of bacterial cellulose network structure by adding interfering substances during fermentation. *Bioresource Technology* 101:6084–6091.

Klemm, D., D. Schumann, U. Udhardt and S. Marsch. 2001. Bacterial synthesized cellulose— Artificial blood vessels for microsurgery. *Progress in Polymer Science* 26:1561–1603.

Millon, L.E., G. Guhados and W. Wan. 2008. Anisotropic polyvinyl alcohol—Bacterial cellulose nanocomposite for biomedical applications. *Journal of Biomedical Materials Research Part B: Applied Biomaterials* 86:444–452.

Pertile, R.A.N., F.K. Andradea, C. Alves Jr. and M. Gama. 2010. Surface modification of bacterial cellulose by nitrogen-containing plasma for improved interaction with cells. *Carbohydrate Polymers* 82:692–698.

Pourramezan, G.Z., A.M. Roayaei and Q.R. Qezelbash. 2009. Optimization of culture conditions for bacterial cellulose production by acetobacter sp. 4B-2. *Biotechnology* 8:150–154.

Putra, A., A. Kakugo, H. Furukawa, J.P. Gong and Y. Osada. 2008. Tubular bacterial cellulose gel with oriented fibrils on the curved surface. *Polymer* 49:1885–1891.

Shah, N., M. Ul-Islam, W.A. Khattak and J.K. Park. 2013. Overview of bacterial cellulose composites: A multipurpose advanced material. *Carbohydrate Polymers* 98:1585–1598.

Svensson, A., E. Nicklasson, T. Harrah, B. Panilaitis, D.L. Kaplan, M. Brittberg and P. Gatenholm. 2005. Bacterial cellulose as a potential scaffold for tissue engineering of cartilage. *Biomaterials* 26:419–431.

Wan, Y.Z., L. Hong, S.R. Jia, Y. Huang, Y. Zhu, Y.L. Wang and H.J. Jiang. 2006. Synthesis and characterization of hydroxyapatite–bacterial cellulose nanocomposites. *Composites Science and Technology* 66:1825–1832.

Wan, Y.Z., Y. Huang, C.D. Yuan, S. Raman, Y. Zhu, H.J. Jiang, F. He and C. Gao. 2007. Biomimetic synthesis of hydroxyapatite/bacterial cellulose nanocomposites for biomedical applications *Materials Science and Engineering* C 27:855–864.

Wippermann, J., D. Schumann, D. Klemm, H. Kosmehl, S. Salehi-Gelani and T. Wahlers. 2009. Preliminary results of small arterial substitute performed with a new cylindrical biomaterial composed of bacterial cellulose. *The European Journal of Vascular and Endovascular Surgery* 37:592–596.

Zhang, S. and J. Luo. 2011. Preparation and properties of bacterial cellulose/alginate blend bio-fibers. *Journal of Engineered Fibers and Fabrics* 6:69–72.

Zhang, T., W. Wang, D. Zhang, X. Zhang, Y. Ma, Y. Zhou and L. Qi. 2010. Biotemplated synthesis of gold nanoparticle–bacteria cellulose nanofiber nanocomposites and their application in biosensing. *Advanced Functional Materials* 20:1152–1160.

Zimmermann, K.A., J.M. LeBlanc, K.T. Sheets, R.W. Fox and P. Gatenholm. 2011. Biomimetic design of a bacterial cellulose/hydroxyapatite nanocomposite for bone healing applications. *Materials Science and Engineering* C 31:43–49.

Index